MORE 4U!

the**clinics.com**

This Clinics series is available online.

Here's what you get:

- Full text of EVERY issue from 2002 to NOW
- Figures, tables, drawings, references and more
- Searchable: find what you need fast

  Search | All Clinics ▼ | for | | GO |

- Linked to MEDLINE and Elsevier journals
- E-alerts

INDIVIDUAL SUBSCRIBERS

LOG ON TODAY. IT'S FAST AND EASY.

Click **Register** and follow instructions

You'll need your account number

Your subscriber account number is on your mailing label

This is your copy of:

THE CLINICS OF NORTH AMERICA

CXXX   **2296532-2**   2   Mar 05

J.H. DOE, MD
531 MAIN STREET
CENTER CITY, NY 10001-001

BOUGHT A SINGLE ISSUE? Sorry, you won't be able to access full text online. Please subscribe today to get complete content by contacting customer service at 800 645 2452 (US and Canada) or 407 345 4000 (outside US and Canada) or via email at elsols@elsevier.com.

NEW!

Now also available for INSTITUTIONS

ELSEVIER

Works/Integrates with MD Co
Available in a variety of pack
14, 31 or 50 Clinics titles
Or Collection upgrade for exi

D1367949

Call today! 877-857-1047 or e-mail: mdc.groupinfo@elsevier.com

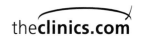

PEDIATRIC CLINICS

OF NORTH AMERICA

Pediatric Hospital Medicine

GUEST EDITORS
Vincent W. Chiang, MD
Lisa B. Zaoutis, MD

August 2005 • Volume 52 • Number 4

SAUNDERS

An Imprint of Elsevier, Inc.
PHILADELPHIA   LONDON   TORONTO   MONTREAL   SYDNEY   TOKYO

W.B. SAUNDERS COMPANY
A Division of Elsevier Inc.

1600 John F. Kennedy Boulevard • Suite 1800 • Philadelphia, Pennsylvania 19103

http://www.theclinics.com

THE PEDIATRIC CLINICS OF NORTH AMERICA   **Volume 52, Number 4**
August 2005   **ISSN 0031-3955**
Editor: Carin Davis   **ISBN 1-4160-2752-1**

The ideas and opinions expressed in *The Pediatric Clinics of North America* do not necessarily reflect those of the Publisher. The Publisher does not assume any responsibility for any injury and/or damage to persons or property arising out of or related to any use of the material contained in this periodical. The reader is advised to check the appropriate medical literature and the product information currently provided by the manufacturer of each drug to be administered to verify the dosage, the method and duration of administration, or contraindications. It is the responsibility of the treating physician or other health care professional, relying on independent experience and knowledge of the patient, to determine drug dosages and the best treatment for the patient. Mention of any product in this issue should not be construed as endorsement by the contributors, editors, or the Publisher of the product or manufacturers' claims.

The Pediatric Clinics of North America (ISSN 0031-3955) is published bi-monthly by W.B. Saunders Company, Corporate and Editorial offices: 1600 JFK Boulevard, Suite 1800, Philadelphia, PA 19103-2822. Accounting and Circulation offices: 6277 Sea Harbor Drive, Orlando, FL 32887-4800. Periodicals postage paid at Orlando, FL 32862, and additional mailing offices. Subscription prices are $135.00 per year (US individuals), $246.00 per year (US institutions), $177.00 per year (Canadian individuals), $320.00 per year (Canadian institutions), $200.00 per year (international individuals), $320.00 per year (international institutions), $68.00 per year (US students), $100.00 per year (Canadian students), and $100.00 per year (foreign students). To receive student/resident rate, orders must be accompanied by name of affiliated institution, date of term, and the signature of program/residency coordinator on institution letterhead. Orders will be billed at individual rate until proof of status is received. Foreign air speed delivery is included in all Clinics subscription prices. All prices are subject to change without notice. POSTMASTER: Send address changes to *The Pediatric Clinics of North America*, W.B. Saunders Company, Periodicals Fulfillment, Orlando, FL 32887-4800. **Customer Service: 1-800-654-2452 (US). From outside of the US, call 1-407-345-4000.** E-mail: hhspcs@harcourt.com.

The Pediatric Clinics of North America is also published in Spanish by McGraw-Hill Inter-americana Editores S.A., Mexico City, Mexico; in Portuguese by Reichmann and Affonso Editores, Rua Comandante Coelho 1085, CEP 21250, Rio de Janeiro, Brazil; and in Greek by Althayia SA, Athens, Greece.

The Pediatric Clinics of North America is covered in *Index Medicus, Excerpta Medica, Current Contents, Current Contents/Clinical Medicine, Science Citation Index, ASCA, ISI/BIOMED,* and *BIOSIS.*

Printed in the United States of America.

GUEST EDITORS

VINCENT W. CHIANG, MD, Assistant Professor of Pediatrics, Harvard Medical School; Chief of Inpatient Services; Pediatric Core Clerkship Director, Division of Emergency Medicine, Children's Hospital Boston, Boston, Massachusetts

LISA B. ZAOUTIS, MD, Assistant Professor of Clinical Pediatrics, University of Pennsylvania School of Medicine; Director of Inpatient Services, Division of General Pediatrics, The Children's Hospital of Philadelphia, Philadelphia, Pennsylvania

CONTRIBUTORS

MICHAEL S.D. AGUS, MD, Instructor in Pediatrics, Harvard Medical School; Director, Intermediate Care Unit, Division of Endocrinology and Critical Care, Children's Hospital Boston, Boston, Massachusetts

CHARLES BERDE, MD, PhD, Department of Anesthesia, Children's Hospital Boston, Boston, Massachusetts

JEAN MARIE CARROLL, RN, BSN, Department of Nursing, The Children's Hospital of Philadelphia, Philadelphia, Pennsylvania

SUSAN E. COFFIN, MD, MPH, Assistant Professor of Pediatrics, Division of Infectious Diseases, University of Pennsylvania School of Medicine; Medical Director, Department of Infection Prevention and Control, Children's Hospital of Philadelphia, Philadelphia, Pennsylvania

CRAIG C. DEWOLFE, MD, Assistant Professor, Department of Pediatrics, George Washington University School of Medicine and Health Sciences; Attending Hospitalist, Children's National Medical Center, Washington, DC

STEPHEN C. EPPES, MD, Clinical Associate Professor, Department of Pediatrics, Thomas Jefferson University, Philadelphia, Pennsylvania; Division of Infectious Diseases, Alfred I. duPont Hospital for Children and Nemours Children's Clinic, Wilmington, Delaware

CHRIS FEUDTNER, MD, PhD, MPH, Department of Pediatrics, The Children's Hospital of Philadelphia, Philadelphia, Pennsylvania

GARY FRANK, MD, MS, Attending Physician, Departments of Pediatrics and Clinical Informatics, Alfred I. duPont Hospital for Children and Nemours Children's Clinic, Wilmington, Delaware

CHRISTINE GRECO, MD, Department of Anesthesia, Children's Hospital Boston, Boston, Massachusetts

MARVIN B. HARPER, MD, Divisions of Infectious Diseases and Emergency Medicine, Children's Hospital Boston, Harvard Medical School, Boston, Massachusetts

MALINDA ANN HILL, MA, Department of Social Work and Family Services, The Children's Hospital of Philadelphia, Philadelphia, Pennsylvania

K. SARAH HOEHN, MD, MBE, Department of Anesthesia and Critical Care Medicine, The Children's Hospital of Philadelphia, Philadelphia, Pennsylvania

TAMMY KANG, MD, Department of Pediatrics, The Children's Hospital of Philadelphia, Philadelphia, Pennsylvania

CHRISTOPHER P. LANDRIGAN, MD, MPH, Research and Fellowship Director, Inpatient Pediatrics Service, Children's Hospital Boston; Director, Sleep and Patient Safety Program, Brigham and Women's Hospital; Assistant Professor, Department of Pediatrics, Harvard Medical School, Boston, Massachusetts

JENNIFER LEMISCH, ATR, BC, LPC, Department of Child Life, Education, and Creative Arts Therapy, The Children's Hospital of Philadelphia, Philadelphia, Pennsylvania

DANIEL J. LICHT, MD, Assistant Professor, Division of Neurology, Department of Pediatrics, The Children's Hospital of Philadelphia, Philadelphia, Pennsylvania

CAROLYN M. LONG, MSW, Department of Social Work and Family Services, The Children's Hospital of Philadelphia, Philadelphia, Pennsylvania

HENRIETTA M. MAHONEY, MD, Senior Resident, Department of Pediatrics, Alfred I. duPont Hospital for Children and Nemours Children's Clinic, Wilmington, Delaware; Department of Pediatrics, Thomas Jefferson University, Philadelphia, Pennsylvania

OSCAR HENRY MAYER, MD, Department of Pediatrics, The Children's Hospital of Philadelphia, Philadelphia, Pennsylvania

NANCY A. MURPHY, MD, Assistant Professor, Department of Pediatrics, University of Utah School of Medicine, Salt Lake City, Utah

JACK M. PERCELAY, MD, MPH, Director, Virtua Inpatient Pediatrics, Ridgewood, New Jersey

DANIEL A. RAUCH, MD, Associate Professor of Clinical Pediatrics, New York University School of Medicine; Director, Pediatric Hospitalist Program, New York, New York

MARY T. ROURKE, PhD, Department of Pediatrics, The Children's Hospital of Philadelphia, Philadelphia, Pennsylvania

THOMAS J. SANDORA, MD, MPH, Division of Infectious Diseases, Children's Hospital Boston, Harvard Medical School, Boston, Massachusetts

GINA SANTUCCI, RN, BSN, Department of Nursing, The Children's Hospital of Philadelphia, Philadelphia, Pennsylvania

SAMIR S. SHAH, MD, Assistant Professor, Department of Pediatrics, Center for Clinical Epidemiology and Biostatistics, University of Pennsylvania School of Medicine; Attending Physician, Divisions of Infectious Diseases and General Pediatrics, The Children's Hospital of Philadelphia, Philadelphia, Pennsylvania

MARY T. SILVIA, MD, Resident, Division of Neurology, The Children's Hospital of Philadelphia, Philadelphia, Pennsylvania

MICHAEL J. SMITH, MD, Fellow, Division of Infectious Diseases, The Children's Hospital of Philadelphia, Philadelphia, Pennsylvania

RAJENDU SRIVASTAVA, MD, FRCP(C), MPH, Assistant Professor, Division of General Pediatrics, Department of Pediatrics, University of Utah School of Medicine; Fellow, Institute for Health Care Delivery Research, Intermountain Health Care, Salt Lake City, Utah

BRYAN L. STONE, MD, Assistant Professor, Division of Pediatric Inpatient Medicine, Department of Pediatrics, University of Utah School of Medicine, Salt Lake City, Utah

JOSEPH I. WOLFSDORF, MB, BCH, Associate Professor, Department of Pediatrics, Harvard Medical School; Director, Diabetes Program and Associate Chief, Division of Endocrinology, Children's Hospital Boston, Boston, Massachusetts

THEOKLIS E. ZAOUTIS, MD, MSCE, Assistant Professor, Department of Pediatrics, Center for Clinical Epidemiology and Biostatistics, University of Pennsylvania School of Medicine; Director, Antimicrobial Stewardship Program; Attending Physician, Division of Infectious Diseases, The Children's Hospital of Philadelphia, Philadelphia, Pennsylvania

DAVID ZIPES, MD, Director, St. Vincent Pediatric Hospitalists, St. Vincent Children's Hospital, Indianapolis, Indiana

CONTENTS

improving pain treatment in pediatric hospitals should be multi-disciplinary and should involve combined use of pharmacologic and nonpharmacologic approaches. Although available information can permit effective treatment of pain for most children in hospitals, there is a need for more research on pediatric analgesic pharmacology, various nonpharmacologic treatments, and different models of delivery of care.

The pediatric hospitalist plays an integral role in providing palliative, end-of-life, and bereavement care for children and families. This article focuses on a multifaceted approach to this domain of care in which the physician is a key member of an interdisciplinary team. We believe that we can improve quality of life and relieve suffering only by paying attention to the medical, emotional, spiritual, and practical needs and goals of dying children and their loved ones.

Bronchiolitis is among the most common and serious lower respiratory tract syndromes that affects young children. In developed countries, the case fatality rate among previously healthy children remains low; in contrast, infants with underlying medical conditions, such as immunodeficiency or chronic lung disease, are at risk of prolonged illness and death. Bronchiolitis is associated with significant morbidity among healthy young children. During the winter season, bronchiolitis is the most common cause of hospitalization among infants. Each year in the United States, approximately 2 per 100,000 infants die as a result of complications associated with bronchiolitis.

Pneumonia is one of the most common infections in the pediatric age group and one of the leading diagnoses that results in overnight hospital admission for children. Various micro-organisms can cause pneumonia, and etiologies differ by age. Clinical manifestations vary, and diagnostic testing is frequently not standardized. Hospital management should emphasize timely diagnosis and prompt initiation of antimicrobial therapy when appropriate. Issues of particular relevance to inpatient management are emphasized in this article.

FORTHCOMING ISSUES

RECENT ISSUES

GOAL STATEMENT

The goal of *Pediatric Clinics of North America* is to keep practicing physicians and residents up to date with current clinical practice in pediatrics by providing timely articles reviewing the state-of-the-art in patient care.

ACCREDITATION

The *Pediatric Clinics of North America* is planned and implemented in accordance with the Essential Areas and Policies of the Accreditation Council for Continuing Medical Education (ACCME) through the joint sponsorship of the University of Virginia School of Medicine and Elsevier. The University of Virginia School of Medicine is accredited by the ACCME to provide continuing medical education for physicians.

The University of Virginia School of Medicine designates this educational activity for a maximum of 90 category 1 credits per year, 15 category 1 credits per issue, toward the AMA Physician's Recognition Award. Each physician should claim only those credits that he/she actually spent in the activity.

The American Medical Association has determined that physicians not licensed in the US who participate in this CME activity are eligible for AMA PRA category 1 credit.

Category 1 credit can be earned by reading the text material, taking the CME examination online at http://www.theclinics.com/home/cme, and completing the evaluation. After taking the test, you will be required to review any and all incorrect answers. Following completion of the test and evaluation, your credit will be awarded and you may print your certificate.

FACULTY DISCLOSURE

Disclosure of faculty financial affiliations: As a provider accredited by the Accreditation Council for Continuing Medical Education (ACCME), the Office of Continuing Medical Education of the University of Virginia School of Medicine must ensure balance, independence, objectivity, and scientific rigor in all its individually sponsored or jointly sponsored educational activities. All authors/editors participating in a sponsored activity are expected to disclose to the readers any significant financial interest or other relationship (1) with the manufacturer(s) of any commercial product(s) and/or provider(s) of commercial services discussed in an educational presentation and (2) with any commercial supporters of the activity (significant financial interest or other relationship can include such things as grants or research support, employee, consultant, stock holder, member of speakers bureau, etc.) The intent of this disclosure is not to prevent authors/editors with a significant financial or other relationship from writing an article, but rather to provide readers with information on which they can make their own judgments. It remains for the readers to determine whether the author's/editor's interest or relationships may influence the article with regard to exposition or conclusion.

The authors/editors listed below have identified no professional or financial affiliations related to their presentation: Michael S. D. Agus, MD; Charles Berde, MD, PhD; Jean Marie Carroll, BSN, RN; Vincent Chiang, MD; Susan E. Coffin, MD, MPH; Carin Davis, Acquisitions Editor; Craig C. DeWolfe, MD; Stephen C. Eppes, MD; Chris Feudtner, MD, PhD, MPH; Gary Frank, MD, MS; Marvin B. Harper, MD; Malinda Ann Hill, MA; K. Sarah Hoehn, MD, MBE; Tammy Kang, MD; Christopher P. Landrigan, MD, MPH; Jennifer Lemisch, ATR, BC, LPC; Daniel J. Licht, MD; Carolyn M. Long, MSW; Oscar Henry Mayer, MD; Henrietta M. Mahoney, MD; Nancy A. Murphy, MD; Jack M. Paecelay, MD, MPH; Daniel A. Rauch, MD; Mary T. Rourke, PhD; Thomas J. Sandora, MD, MPH; Gina Santucci, BSN, RN; Samir S. Shah, MD; Mary T. Silva, MD; Michael J. Smith, MD; Rajendu Srivastava, MD, FRCP, MPH; Bryan L. Stone, MD; Joseph I. Wolfsdorf, MB, BCh; Theoklis E. Zaoutis, MD, MSCE; and, David Zipes, MD.

Disclosure of Discussion of non-FDA approved uses for pharmaceutical products and/or medical devices: The University of Virginia School of Medicine, as an ACCME provider, requires that all authors identify and disclose any "off label" uses for pharmaceutical and medical device products. The University of Virginia School of Medicine recommends that each physician fully review all the available data on new products or procedures prior to instituting them with patients.

All authors who provided disclosures have indicated that they will not be discussing off-label uses except the following:
Michael S. D. Agus, MD will discuss the intravenous use of regular human insulin.
Daniel J. Licht, MD will discuss the use of oxcarbazepine for neuropathic pain, an 'off-label' use both in pediatrics and general medicine, for this medicine that is indicated for complex and simple partial seizures.
Thomas J. Sandora, MD, MPH and Marvin B. Harper, MD will discuss the use of streptokinase, urokinase, and tissue plasminogen activator as intrapleural fibrinolytics when parapneumonic exudates are present.

The following author has not provided disclosure or off-label information.
Christine Greco, MD.

TO ENROLL

To enroll in the *Pediatric Clinics of North America* Continuing Medical Education program, call customer service at **1-800-654-2452** or visit us online at www.theclinics.com/home/cme. The CME program is available to subscribers for an additional fee of $195.00.

PEDIATRIC CLINICS

OF NORTH AMERICA

Pediatr Clin N Am 52 (2005) xiii–xiv

ELSEVIER
SAUNDERS

Preface

Pediatric Hospital Medicine

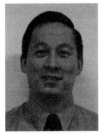 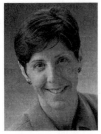

Vincent W. Chiang, MD   Lisa B. Zaoutis, MD
Guest Editors

There were hospitals long before hospitalists. As such, it is remarkable that the field of hospital medicine is growing so quickly. If the field was born when Wachter and Goldman coined the term "hospitalist" in 1996, then pediatric hospital medicine is clearly in the midst of its adolescent growth spurt. With an estimated 1000 pediatric hospitalists to date, this field is already the sixth largest pediatric subspecialty.

As outpatient management of pediatric illness has become increasingly sophisticated and comprehensive, the care of pediatric patients in the hospital setting has had similar shifts. Hospitalization is reserved for patients with a higher severity of illness, patients who require expedited evaluation or more intensive medical support, and patients with complex conditions that may require coordination with multiple specialists at times of acute illness.

In this issue of the *Pediatric Clinics of North America*, the inpatient focus for important topics is provided, including pneumonia, apparent life-threatening events, bone and soft tissue infections, central nervous system infections, diabetes and diabetic ketoacidosis, pain management, infections related to indwelling catheters and devices, and bronchiolitis. Also reviewed are end-of-life issues, medical errors and patient safety, and care of medically complex children. An overview of the growing field of pediatric hospital medicine is included.

doi:10.1016/j.pcl.2005.05.002

We hope that practitioners who care for hospitalized children routinely, occasionally, or infrequently might appreciate this update on medical care in the inpatient setting.

Vincent W. Chiang, MD
Division of Emergency Medicine
Children's Hospital Boston
300 Longwood Avenue
Boston, MA 02115, USA
E-mail address: vincent.chiang@childrens.harvard.edu

Lisa B. Zaoutis, MD
University of Pennsylvania School of Medicine
Division of Emergency Medicine
The Children's Hospital of Philadelphia
Philadelphia, PA 19104-4399, USA
E-mail address: zaoutisl@email.chop.edu

ELSEVIER
SAUNDERS

PEDIATRIC CLINICS
OF NORTH AMERICA

Pediatr Clin N Am 52 (2005) 963–977

Introduction to Pediatric Hospital Medicine

Daniel A. Rauch, MD[a,*], Jack M. Percelay, MD, MPH[b], David Zipes, MD[c]

[a]New York University School of Medicine, NBV-8S4-11, New York, NY 10016, USA
[b]Virtua Inpatient Pediatrics, PO Box 5122, Ridgewood, NJ 07451-5122, USA
[c]St. Vincent Children's Hospital, 2001 West 86th Street, Indianapolis, IN 46260, USA

Since Wachter and Goldman coined the term "hospitalist" in 1996 [1], the field has undergone tremendous growth and change. The National Association of Inpatient Physicians has evolved from 23 founders in 1997 into the Society of Hospital Medicine (SHM), with more than 4000 members by 2005. The American Academy of Pediatrics' (AAP) provisional section on hospital care has become the section on hospital medicine, and the Ambulatory Pediatric Association's (APA) special interest group (SIG) has eschewed its old designation of the hospitalist/inpatient medicine SIG, replacing it with the hospital medicine SIG. The term "hospitalist," the definition of a hospitalist, and the field have been controversial since their beginnings. The National Association of Inpatient Physicians and the AAP's provisional section on hospital care carefully avoided using the term "hospitalist" in their original names. The current use of the term "hospital medicine" reflects the maturation of the field as it begins to define a body of knowledge as opposed to a specific person or job description, a "hospitalist." The field currently boasts an estimated 12,000 hospitalists, with most statistics indicating that approximately 8% t0 10%, or 1000 total, are pediatric hospitalists.

What is a "hospitalist"? The idea and practice of a physician focused on caring for hospitalized patients has existed for some time and, especially in Europe and Canada, is often the predominant model in which physicians care for inpatients. The traditional ward attending physician who has been an omni-

* Corresponding author. New York University, Department of Pediatrics, NBV-8S4-11, New York, NY 10016.

E-mail address: daniel.roach@med.nyu.edu (D.A. Rauch).

doi:10.1016/j.pcl.2005.03.005
pediatric.theclinics.com

present feature of most academic institutions and the oft less-distinguished "house" doctor are well-known examples of this concept in the United States, and they have been in existence for as long as there have been training programs. In 1990, Dr. Vincent Menna stated, "The general pediatrician who specializes in inpatient practice rides the wave of the future [2]." He further suggested that "The continued expansion of clinical knowledge makes it harder and harder for even the most dedicated generalist to stay on top of current diagnostic and therapeutic advances." This notion began to set the stage for the concept that the inpatient service is a unique practice site that requires its own knowledge and skill set. The current definition of a hospitalist is: "Physicians whose primary professional focus is the general medical care of hospitalized patients. Their activities include patient care, teaching, research, and leadership related to Hospital Medicine [3]." This definition reflects the evolution from the original time-based definition of hospitalists as "Physicians who spend at least 25% of their time serving as the physician of record for hospitalized patients who have been referred by primary care physicians and who are referred back to their primary care physicians at the time of discharge" [4].

The early 1990s also saw emerging evidence that hospitalized children were cared for by a small subset of pediatricians [5]. This information was used to argue that residency programs were not providing enough ambulatory experience for trainees. The data also suggested that inpatient medicine was becoming specialized care, however. At the same time, studies demonstrated Dr. Menna's proposition that there was an emerging "knowledge gap" between inpatient and outpatient medicine [6]. There is so much knowledge with which to keep up that physicians must prioritize what they read and what they will use. Primarily outpatient physicians not only care for inpatients less frequently but are also less likely to be current in inpatient knowledge. The average pediatric primary care physician cares for approximately 20 inpatients per year (excluding the newborn nursery) [7], which translates into infrequent care of common inpatient diagnoses and rare familiarity with more complex or less common diagnoses. The Institute of Medicine Report "To Err Is Human: Building a Safer Health System" summarized the deficiencies of care in hospitals and determined that appropriate quality of care was a serious issue [8].

The emergence of hospitalists has coincided with a major overhaul of the graduate medical education system in the United States from one that focused on the educational process to one that demands evidence of educational outcomes as defined in the Accreditation Council for Graduate Medical Education core competencies. Aside from the philosophical alignment with the hospitalist focus on patient outcomes, there is clear synergy of the dedication of experienced clinicians who are constantly available with the attainment of the core competencies. The new limitations on work hours for residents also has led training institutions to seek new ways to care for inpatients and, to date, hospitalists have been the likely surrogates.

A constellation of economic forces also contributed to changes in primary care and inpatient practice. Changing health care finances and the emergence of managed care organizations gave rise to tremendous productivity pressures in the outpatient setting and dictated that only the sickest of the patients "qualified" for hospital care. Decreased rates of admission and decreased lengths of stay worked synergistically to increase patient complexity in outpatient and inpatient settings. Increased pressures on primary care providers to increase volume and complexity of care with decreased levels of reimbursement while meeting ever increasing mandates of quality health maintenance impacted physician quality of life and availability to the inpatient service.

Ample evidence accumulated from the adult literature touted the benefits of hospital medicine, including improvements in length of stay, resource use, and morbidity and mortality. Although fewer in number, pediatric hospitalist studies showed similar results, and pediatric departments increasingly used hospitalist services. In a 1998 survey, fully 50% of academic department chairs claimed to have hospitalist services, and another 27% were planning to implement them in the near future [9].

The growth of hospital medicine over the last 10 years has been astronomical—it is the fastest growing health care specialty in the country. In the mid 1990s there were an estimated 800 hospitalists; currently there are an estimated 12,000 practicing hospitalists, which makes hospital medicine a larger field than gastroenterology, dermatology, pulmonary care, and allergy. As the field of hospital medicine has evolved, specific models of care delivery also have evolved to address shifts in compensation and employer type and optimize communication strategies to limit the loss of information (dubbed "voltage drop") when patients transition from inpatient to outpatient settings and vice versa.

Current status

National data regarding pediatric hospitalist experiences come from a 2002 AAP random survey of 1626 member pediatricians (response rate 59%) [10]. Office-based pediatricians ($n = 654$) reported their experiences with pediatric hospitalists. Forty percent of pediatricians were affiliated with hospitals with full-time pediatric hospitalists, and they referred 45% of their general pediatric ward inpatients to hospitalists. Use of hospitalists by pediatricians varied significantly, with 40% reporting no referrals to pediatric hospitalists and 38% reporting referral of all patients. Nationally, approximately 18% (0.40×0.45) of AAP members who practice in an office setting refer their general ward inpatients to pediatric hospitalists. Of the pediatricians who used pediatric hospitalists ($n=158$), 68% reported that pediatric hospitalists increase quality of patient care. Common reasons for referrals to pediatric hospitalists included better care provided by pediatric hospitalists because of full-time hospital presence (61%) and specialization in inpatient care (53%). Overall, most (87%) pediatricians were satisfied with the care that pediatric hospitalists provided to their patients, and 83% believed that their patients were satisfied with this care.

Individual programs have reported similar—if not higher—satisfaction results. More accurate data to assess the volume of care provided by pediatric hospitalists nationally are not currently available.

Because of the relative infancy of the field, varying definitions of a hospitalist, and the rapid growth in numbers of pediatric hospitalists, it is difficult to quantify the number of pediatricians who are currently practicing as pediatric hospitalists, although best estimates put the current number at approximately 1000. If their growth continues to parallel the growth of internal medicine hospitalists, there will be approximately 3000 by the year 2010. Approximately half of these hospitalists are active members of SHM, AAP, or APA. An SHM survey of hospitalists in 2003–2004 reported data from 206 pediatric hospitalists [11]. They reported their employers as follows: 35% academic institutions, 33% hospitals or hospital corporations, and 13% multispecialty group. Median salaries averaged $130,000/year across all employment types and ranged from $107,000/year in academic settings to $167,000/year in multispecialty group settings. An AAP section on hospital medicine salary survey conducted in 2002 reported data from 120 pediatric hospitalists and revealed median starting salaries of $110,000/year and median salaries with 5 years' experience of $130,000/year [12]. Practice settings included general pediatric inpatient units (97%), emergency department consultations (53%), normal newborn nursery (36%), subspecialty inpatient service (21%), and pediatric intensive care unit (17%) among others, with an average clinical workload of 48 hours/week.

As the surveys indicate, there is a tremendously wide range of practice settings and job descriptions for individuals who are dubbed "pediatric hospitalists." One common model is the pediatric hospitalist who is the attending physician on the general pediatric ward of an academic children's hospital [13,14]. This is an expansion of the role traditionally filled by the teaching attending physician. The hospitalist is on service for 3 to 11 months out of the year compared with the typical 1 to 2 months per year fulfilled by the traditional ward attending physician. The hospitalist is typically available throughout the day to supervise pediatric residents (or nurse practitioners or physician assistants) who provide most of the direct patient care and the nighttime coverage. Hospitalists typically care for a range of 10 to 20 patients, but the optimal workload is a controversial topic and varies by patient acuity, teaching responsibilities, and ancillary resources (eg, housestaff, physician extenders, phlebotomy and intravenous services, computer resources, nurses, case managers). Patients under a hospitalist's care can be expected to range from children with general pediatric problems, such as gastroenteritis, bronchiolitis, and asthma, to children with more complex medical needs who require a hospitalist's expertise at coordinating the input from multiple subspecialists and health care providers. As hospitalists become more entrenched in the daily functioning of the hospital, other roles are being added, such as consulting or co-managing surgical or medical subspecialty patients and providing procedural sedation. Teaching is a major activity of academic hospitalists, and data demonstrate the educational benefit of hospitalists [15,16]. The academic hospitalist is also expected to participate in research and, like all hospitalists, logistics and systems issues related to inpatient care.

In contrast to the academic hospitalist, the pediatric hospitalist in a community hospital may have a different job description. In a community-based teaching program, the hospitalist may supervise family practice, transitional interns, medical students (generally as an elective rotation), nurse practitioners, physician assistants, or pediatric residents on a smaller, general ward with limited subspecialty availability. A common model for hospitalist programs is a "spoke and hub" model, in which the academic or larger children's hospital functions as the "hub" and the smaller, satellite hospitals function as the "spokes." The satellite programs are in the surrounding communities where pediatric hospitalists work, with or without residents, caring for general pediatric inpatients. Children who require subspecialty or critical care are generally transferred to the "hub" institution, although less acute needs may be fulfilled by phone consultation or a traveling subspecialist. These affiliations can be advantageous to all persons involved, including patients. High-quality local pediatric care is provided so families can stay close to home, residents have a supervised experience in a community setting, tertiary care bed availability is preserved for the high-acuity patients, and the referral base necessary to support a complete set of pediatric subspecialists is preserved.

Responsibilities beyond managing patients on the general ward vary from program to program and may include attending deliveries, caring for infants in the well-baby and special care nurseries, covering an urgent care area, consulting in the emergency room, and managing patients in a smaller pediatric intensive care unit. Staffing models vary from 24/7 in-house presence (absolutely necessary, in the authors' opinion, for an institution with a large delivery service staffed by hospitalists), to a hospitalist on call from home, to residents taking call in-house with attending back-up coverage. The breadth of pediatric practice opportunities in a community hospital setting seems to be a large part of the attraction for hospitalists. The pediatric hospitalist can be equally comfortable managing a premature infant or a teenager on an insulin drip in the pediatric intensive care unit, consulting on complex cases in the emergency room, and providing inpatient care on the pediatric ward. In this setting, the hospitalist must be cognizant of individual and institutional limitations and standards of care in the community. He or she must know when consults, referrals, or transfers must take place. Like the academic hospitalist, the community hospitalist must be expert clinically and must be equally skilled in addressing the logistics and systems issues of hospital care. Other responsibilities, such as teaching, research, committee membership, and outreach, vary from program to program.

A growing trend involves hospitalists who function primarily in the subspecialty venue. For example, pediatric hospitalists may provide after-hours coverage in a neonatal or pediatric intensive care unit. This is particularly valuable in a smaller community intensive care unit in which, unlike a neonatal nurse practitioner, a hospitalist is able to multi-task and assist in the emergency room and pediatric ward when not occupied in the neonatal intensive care unit.

Pediatric hospitalists also have been used successfully in pediatric intensive care unit settings, with one report suggesting that pediatric hospitalists led to improved outcomes when compared with traditional resident coverage [17]. In all of these instances, the hospitalist must have appropriate back-up and support from the appropriate subspecialist or must be able to transfer a patient readily to an institution that can provide the appropriate care. Based on the authors' experience, on-site response time for neonatal or pediatric intensive care unit coverage should not exceed 30 minutes with immediate phone availability 24/7. Hospitalists can be a valuable adjunct but are not meant to substitute for intensivists, neonatologists, or any other subspecialists.

The internal medicine hospitalist world has seen the development of "subspecialty" hospitalists who specialize in cardiology, hematology, neurosurgery, and various other subspecialties. The major rate-limiting step is the number of inpatients for any given specialty, which is more of an issue with pediatrics than internal medicine. There have been some preliminary forays in pediatric subspecialty hospitalists. In these models, a hospitalist works specifically in one field under the direction of the subspecialists to provide hospital care to the subspecialty patients. This model can help alleviate manpower issues related to resident limitations and subspecialist shortages. It remains to be seen whether this is a viable long-term career option. Interested practitioners would seem more inclined to pursue the full subspecialty training rather than continue to practice in the more subsidiary role. A more appealing structure may be rotating a group of hospitalists through various subspecialty fields, which would appeal to the diverse interests of hospitalists and ultimately would create a cadre of highly skilled inpatient physicians with significant depth and breadth of postgraduate training.

Economically, pediatric hospitalist programs based on the general pediatric ward rarely, if ever, generate enough income from professional billing to support themselves. Independent of the concerns that pediatric care is undervalued compared with adult care (Medicaid rates of reimbursement are generally significantly lower than MediCare rates), much of the work and value of pediatric hospitalists is unbillable, including systems improvements (eg, developing pathways, providing education, serving on committees, sleeping in house to be available for emergencies), decreased length of stay, decreased use of resources, and, likely, better outcomes. Many programs have begun to multi-task to find alternative sources of revenue. Examples include normal newborn services, sedation services, and emergency room or urgent care services.

Most hospitalist programs (adult and pediatric) require financial support for the less financially tangible services they provide to the hospital system as a whole, however. Depending on the particular program, the support may come from the hospital, the department of pediatrics, insurance companies, or some larger physician group. Time will tell whether other methods, such as revising the value assigned to inpatient codes or creating a diagnosis-related group-like system for the professional component of hospital care to make hospital medicine more financially viable, will be developed.

In contrast to internal medicine hospitalists, few commercial, national, pediatric hospitalist entities are in existence. Most programs are developed locally to meet to the specific needs and culture of the community. Individuals interested in establishing a pediatric hospitalist program in their own institution are encouraged to contact SHM, the AAP, and the APA because each organization provides unique but equally valuable information and each has a different perspective. Likewise, these organizations are excellent starting points for physicians interested in pursuing careers as pediatric hospitalists.

Looking ahead

The future for pediatric hospital medicine has never been brighter. The rapid growth of the field has positioned it as the fastest growing field in pediatrics, and the current number of practitioners—approximately 1000—places it as the sixth largest pediatric subspecialty [18]. In the near future, pediatric hospital medicine will continue to take on further trappings of a well-defined subspecialty. There are already active pediatric hospital medicine activities within the AAP, APA, and SHM, and each organization devotes specific time to pediatric hospital medicine during their annual meetings. The success of the Pediatric Hospitalists in Academic Settings meeting in San Antonio, Texas in 2003 spurred a tri-sponsored meeting by the AAP, APA, and SHM in Denver in the summer of 2005 that will be the first—and hopefully largest—of a regularly scheduled pediatric hospital medicine meeting. A textbook already exists, "Pediatric Hospital Medicine: Textbook of Inpatient Management," and a second, "Comprehensive Pediatric Hospital Medicine," is in the finishing stages. The journal *Pediatric Emergency Care* has added a hospital medicine section and pertinent articles have been published in journals such as *Pediatrics*, *Archives of Pediatrics and Adolescent Medicine*, and *Ambulatory Pediatrics*.

Fellowships such as those at Children's Hospital Boston, DC Children's National Medical Center, and University of California, San Diego, will continue to develop and generate a corps of academically trained practitioners with research experience who are needed to help take the next steps that are necessary to bring the field to maturity. A rapidly growing number of experienced pediatric hospitalists whose commitment to the field already has done much to catalyze the growth of hospital medicine. SHM has established an adult and pediatric core curriculum task force whose goal is to define the core base of knowledge that defines hospital medicine, and fellowships will help to delineate a specific set of skills and knowledge base for the practice of pediatric hospital medicine.

Research topics include further evaluation of the impact of hospital medicine on the care of hospitalized children in terms of cost, resource use, safety, and patient outcomes and the impact of hospitalists on the patient/family experience, medical teaching, and hospital activities. A pediatric hospital medicine collaborative research network (Pediatric Research in the Inpatient Setting) has been developed designed to mimic the success of Pediatric Research in Office Settings in addressing outpatient topics. Hospitalists also are uniquely situated for bench to bedside research and applications of new technologies. Most modern hospitalists are in the infancy of their careers, and the future likely will bring them into the ranks of senior faculty, division heads, and other thought leaders with the ability to impact child health further.

Of equal importance to the academic and clinical growth of hospital medicine is the financial viability of the field. Studies consistently show a 12% to 15% cost savings, largely through reduced length of stay, when hospitalist programs are initiated [13,14]. These savings clearly plateau, however, after 2 years from implementation of a hospitalist program, at which point institutions must balance the relative value of hospitalists in terms of patient care and the myriad other benefits to the hospital system versus a typical shortfall in direct patient revenue compared with the costs of a hospitalist program. The most recent SHM compensation and productivity survey demonstrated a cost of approximately $60,000 per hospitalist (salary minus patient revenue) [11]. How hospitalist services should be supported and by whom—whether by the hospital, insurance industry, changes in inpatient reimbursement, referring physicians, or a combination of these or some as-yet to be determined mechanism—are significant questions for the future and viability of hospital medicine.

A long-term question for the field is whether it will become or should become a board-certified subspecialty—a specialty with an added qualification similar to geriatrics or sports medicine—or maintain the status quo. Traditional subspecialties involved organ-based systems. The American Board of Pediatrics recognizes several subspecialties that are based on specific patient populations or location of care, however, such as adolescent medicine, emergency pediatrics, and critical care. The obstacles to achieving official subspecialty status are significant, and the potential attainment of board certification is many years ahead. The similarities between the current state of affairs and the early years of emergency medicine and the critical care fields cannot be ignored, however. It is a source of active debate in the pediatric hospitalist movement whether a 3-year fellowship is necessary to function as a pediatric hospitalist. The research component could be clinical research or quality improvement-, patient safety-, or management-type activities. The requirement to complete a 3-year fellowship would be a significant deterrent for graduating residents to pursue a career as pediatric hospitalist, as it has been in other subspecialties. Alternatives to hospitalist fellowship include hospital medicine–based residency tracks, a single additional clinical year, and working within the structure of current general academic pediatric fellowships by focusing the clinical component on inpatient work. Most likely, the pediatric hospitalist movement will follow the lead of the adult hospitalists in this arena. If the adult hospitalists decide a fellowship is unnecessary, it is unlikely that the pediatric hospitalists would impose this additional training requirement. Similarly, if the adult hospitalists create a standard such as a formal sub-board or competency program, pediatrics is likely to follow suit.

Society of Hospital Medicine

SHM, originally named the National Association of Inpatient Physicians, was founded in 1997 shortly after the term "hospitalist" was first coined by Wachter and Goldman. In 2003, the name was changed from National Association of Inpatient Physicians to the Society of Hospital Medicine to reflect the field's popularity and acceptance of hospital medicine within the medical field. SHM is affiliated with the American College of Physicians and, as of 2004, has more than 4000 dues-paying members. Its headquarters are located in Philadelphia, Pennsylvania. SHM is the fastest growing medical society in the country, and hospital medicine is the fastest growing medical specialty. SHM estimates that there are approximately 12,000 practicing hospitalists and predicts that the number will reach approximately 30,000 by the end of the decade. Most surveys conclude that 8% to 10% of hospitalists are pediatric hospitalists, with most being internists.

SHM was developed specifically to assist hospitalists in all aspects of their practice and enhance the delivery of health care to their patients. SHM's stated goals are to (1) promote high quality care for all hospitalized patients, (2) promote education and research in hospital medicine, (3) promote teamwork to achieve the best possible care for hospitalized patients, (4) advocate a career path that will attract and retain the highest quality hospitalists, (5) define the competencies, activities, and needs of the hospital medicine community, and (6) support, propose, and promote changes to the health care system that lead to higher quality and more efficient care for all hospitalized patients. SHM holds an annual meeting that lasts 2 days with a 1 day pre-course. The annual meeting has a dedicated pediatric track and most nonclinical topics are relevant to internists and pediatricians. SHM has begun a national leadership conference with the goal of teaching the necessary survival skills for leading hospitalist groups and promoting positive change within hospital systems. Most of SHM's members are internists, but family practice, medical subspecialties, and pediatrics comprise a sum total of approximately 15%. Affiliate membership is open to health care administrators, allied health professionals, health care analysts, medical librarians, and others interested in hospital medicine.

Despite the fact that pediatric hospitalists make up only 10% of SHM members, SHM has demonstrated a tremendous commitment to pediatric hospitalists. There has been a pediatric hospitalist on the board since the beginning of the organization, and there is a pediatric hospitalist on most of SHM's 20 committees and task forces. A pediatric committee oversees and coordinates pediatric hospital medicine activities within SHM. SHM has several resources available to the pediatric hospitalist, including a members-only LISTSERV, a Website, and a bimonthly publication, *The Hospitalist*, all with devoted pediatric content. Topics on the LISTSERV range from billing to patient care, and the bimonthly newsletter is full of clinically relevant information and job advertisements and practice profiles. Each issue features a pediatric section with review of recent literature and pediatric-specific articles. In association with the adult core curriculum task force, a pediatric core curriculum task force has been developed. The goal of the task forces is to define the core competencies of pediatric hospital medicine and divide the competencies into three main areas: clinical, procedural, and systems issues. Upon completion, a book comprising SHM's definition of core competencies will be published that may be used as a reference guide or may be a step toward an added qualification certificate or potential board certification for pediatric hospitalists.

SHM has fostered and maintained working relations with the two other main organizations that represent pediatric hospital medicine: (1) the AAP's section on hospital medicine and (2) the APA's pediatric hospital medicine SIG. As the field of hospital medicine continues to grow, the importance of the three leading organizations that represent pediatric hospitalists increases. They all support different facets of pediatric hospital medicine, and the leaders of each organization have developed a close and mutually beneficial working relationship. Of the three organizations, SHM tends to play the largest advocacy role for hospital medicine locally and nationally and gets much more involved in the business aspects of hospital medicine. SHM develops policy and position statements that address the concerns and issues of hospitalists, advocates on behalf of hospitalists before other medical societies, government, and regulatory agencies, and works with the media to represent the interests of hospitalized patients and the field of hospital medicine. SHM's biannual survey is the largest and most comprehensive survey of hospitalists and provides the most accurate productivity and compensation data. There is discussion between the APA section on hospital medicine and SHM about publishing an annual pediatric hospitalist literature review that could be a compilation of the ongoing literature review in *The Hospitalist*. SHM has been cultivating relations with the National Association of Children's Hospitals and Related Institutions. SHM also is part of the pediatric research in the inpatient setting network. Along with the section on hospital medicine, SHM has a jointly sponsored pediatric hospital medicine LISTSERV. SHM is a part of the national advisory board, which consists of most of the national medical organizations, including the AAP.

Membership can be achieved by filling out the application on the SHM Website (www.hospitalmedicine.org) or by calling 800-843-3360 or 215-351-2742. Membership benefits are described on the Website and include all the activities mentioned previously, including access to the productivity and compensation survey.

American Academy of Pediatrics

The AAP was founded in 1930. It is committed to the attainment of optimal physical, mental, and social health and well-being for all infants, children, adolescents, and young adults. Organizationally, the AAP is composed of three major entities: chapters, sections, and committees. Traditionally, chapters represent the grassroots of the organization, whereas sections represent subspecialties and special interests, and committees review and write policies. Sections may be based on a discipline (eg, hematology), a specific interest (eg, adoption), or a subpopulation of pediatricians (eg, residents). Typically, sections provide educational activities in their particular field for section members and AAP members at large. Sections also may sponsor and review policy statements and technical reports.

Focused hospitalist activity within the AAP began in 1998 when approximately 75 interested pediatricians initiated the process to form a new section, originally named "the proposed Provisional Section on Hospitalists." Hospitalists were a controversial and relatively new concept in 1998, and there was concern that hospitalists would "steal" patients from primary care pediatricians. People also were concerned as to the long-term impact that hospitalists would have on the practice of pediatrics. It was uncertain what impact surrendering one's inpatient activities would have on the pride and professionalism of the primary care pediatrician. Ultimately, the proposed section was approved with the cautious and less controversial title of "provisional section on hospital care," which was viewed as the sister section to the already existing committee on hospital care.

Shortly after the formation of the provisional section on hospital care, as part of the AAP's effort to improve collaboration between sister sections and committees, a section liaison member was appointed to the committee on hospital care. This was the first formal and titled input that hospitalists had on the decision-making organs of the AAP, although realistically many of the former members of the committee on hospital care were practicing hospitalists in disguise ("inpatient attendings"). Using the gradual and kind approach familiar to most pediatricians, the provisional section on hospital care membership grew. Educational programs sponsored by the provisional section on hospital care at the annual meeting were well received, and many of the initial concerns regarding hospital medicine receded as adult and pediatric hospitalist programs became more popular nationally and the value that hospitalists could provide to the system became more apparent. In 2002, the provisional section on hospital care was approved as the section on hospital care, and in 2004, the section changed its name to the section on hospital medicine, which reflected the rise and general acceptance of hospital medicine as a unique discipline. Currently, membership is open to all who are interested in hospital medicine, and there are no set criteria in terms of patient volumes, time spent as a hospitalist, or additional training that is required to be a member of the section.

By January 2005, membership in the section had more than quadrupled from its original 75 members and currently boasts 320 pediatricians. The section has become the focal point for hospitalist activity within the AAP, and it regularly reviews policy statements that impact the care of hospitalized children. In addition to education activities at the national conference and exhibition, the section produces a well-received biannual newsletter and sponsors a pediatric hospital medicine LISTSERV with more than 300 participants that covers everything from clinical and administrative questions to job postings and continuing medical education opportunities and publishes (free of charge) job ads in the newsletter. LISTSERV membership is currently open to all but the section Web page, with its associated hospitalist resources of sample pathways, salary surveys, presentations, practice management and quality improvement tools, and is a members-only benefit. Communication with chapters, an important part of any hospitalist's activities, is maintained through section liaisons with each individual chapter.

Research is an important endeavor for the section on hospital medicine, and the section is a co-sponsor, along with the APA and SHM, of the pediatric research in the inpatient setting network, the periodic survey of fellows previously discussed. As noted earlier, the section on hospital medicine has been involved with policies that may affect hospitalized patients and, accordingly, has authored a set of guiding principles for pediatric hospitalist programs that include the following six recommendations:

1. All pediatric hospitalist programs should be based on voluntary referrals.
2. Each pediatric hospitalist program should be designed to meet the unique needs of the patients, families, and physicians in the community it serves.
3. Physicians who serve as hospitalists should be board certified in pediatrics or have equivalent qualifications.
4. Pediatric hospitalist programs should include in their design provision for appropriate outpatient follow-up of patients on discharge.
5. Pediatric hospitalist programs should provide for timely and complete communication between the hospitalist and the physicians responsible for a patient's outpatient management, including the primary care physician and all involved subspecialists.
6. Pediatric hospitalist programs should include data collection and outcome assessment capabilities to monitor their performance and are encouraged to contribute to research studies that involve the care of hospitalized children.

Future activities, goals, and directions of the section on hospital medicine will be determined by its membership and developments in the field of hospital medicine. Targeted projects currently include continued membership growth and educational programming at the national conference and exhibition, growth of pediatric research in the inpatient setting, further development of the Website, LISTSERV, and newsletter, development of inpatient coding resources and reassessment of the relative values assigned to inpatient codes, pursuit of an equip module for pediatric hospitalists to use for the QI activities necessary for renewal of Pediatric Boards, repetition of the tripartite pediatric hospitalist conference (first one to take place July 2005 in Denver), and continued successful collaboration with the AAP committee on hospital care and the pediatric hospitalist entities of SHM and the APA.

The strong cooperation among the three organizations that represent pediatric hospitalists, the APA, SHM and AAP has been a hallmark of the success of the section on hospital medicine and the pediatric hospital medicine movement as a whole. Within the structure of this three-legged stool, the section on hospital medicine aims to serve as the umbrella organization that represents pediatric hospitalists above all as pediatricians first and hospitalists, researchers, or educators second. Hospitalists take pride in the care they provide to hospitalized children, and they advocate strongly for hospital care that allows each child to reach his or her optimal physical and mental health. To join the AAP section on hospital medicine, contact the AAP on their Website (www.aap.org) or by calling 800-433-9016.

Ambulatory Pediatric Association

The APA was founded in 1961 and has the mission statement "to improve the teaching of general pediatrics, to improve services in general pediatrics and to affect public and government opinion regarding issues vital to teaching, research, and patient care in general pediatrics." Although the name may imply otherwise, the APA is the academic home for all pediatric generalists, regardless of their site of practice. Scientific presentations at the first meeting in 1961 included presentations on hospital services for children. Over the years, the APA has spun off several organizations, including the Association of Pediatric Program Directors, the Societies for Adolescent Medicine, Developmental Pediatrics, and Behavioral Pediatrics, and the Council on Medical Student Education in Pediatrics. It is actively engaged in teaching, patient care, and research in general pediatrics and has more than 2000 members, including physicians, nurses, nurse practitioners, epidemiologists, educators, and other health care professionals. The organization has standing committees, ten geographic regions, and many SIGs. The hospitalist/inpatient medicine SIG was started in 2001 and changed to the hospital medicine SIG in 2004 to conform to the names of the SHM and AAP section of hospital medicine. The hospital medicine SIG provides a home for hospitalists and others interested in inpatient medicine, particularly regarding teaching and research. The SIG spurred the APA sponsored conference, "Pediatric Hospitalists in Academic Settings," in November 2003. By providing a flexible structure for its annual meeting, the SIG allows for an agenda that can be changed up to the meeting date. The pediatric research in the inpatient setting network, although sponsored by SHM, AAP section on hospital medicine, and the APA, finds its home within the hospital medicine SIG. The Pediatric Academic Societies annual meeting, which includes the APA, American Pediatric Society, and Society for Pediatric Research, has a hospitalist plenary session for the presentation of scientific abstracts. The APA also publishes a journal, *Ambulatory Pediatrics*, which provides a forum for interesting and cutting-edge work in academic general pediatrics.

Membership can be achieved by filling out the application on the APA Website (www.ambpeds.org). Membership benefits include all the activities of any SIG and region and participation in the APANET LISTSERV, a forum for academic discussions in general pediatrics, and announcements relevant to APA members.

Summary

This article provides a brief summary of the past, present, and future of pediatric hospital medicine. In its short history, it already has made an impact on the way pediatrics is practiced and taught. There is no denying Dr. Menna's prescience when he wrote his opinion in 1990. As the field continues to emerge and mature, the current leadership is cognizant of the obstacles ahead and the need to maintain the goal of the well-being of all children. Maintaining that goal means redoubling efforts to maintain contact with primary care providers for continuity of care in and out of the hospital. Only by promoting patient- and family-centered care, inclusive of all providers, can children's health best be served.

References

[1] Wachter RM, Goldman L. The emerging role of "hospitalists" in the American health care system. N Engl J Med 1996;335:514–7.

[2] Menna VJ. Inpatient care: the general pediatrician's future. Pediatr Rev 1990;12(6):165–6.

[3] Society of Hospital Medicine. Available at: http://www.naiponline.org/presentation/apps/indlist/intro.asp?flag=6. Accessed January 15, 2005.

[4] Wachter RM. Hospitalists: their role in the American health care system. J Med Pract Manage 1997;13:123–6.

[5] Meltzer SM, Grossman DC, Rivara FP. Physician experience with pediatric inpatient care in Washington State. Pediatrics 1996;97:65–70.

[6] Wofford JL, et al. Improved reading efficiency for general internists dividing medical literature between hospitalist and ambulatory practices. J Gen Intern Med 1998;13(Suppl 1):76.

[7] Zipes D. What is a hospitalist? In: Perkin RM, Swift JD, Newton DA, editors. Pediatric hospital medicine: textbook of inpatient management. Philadelphia: Lippincott Williams & Wilkins; 2003. p. 3.

[8] Kohn LT, Corrigan JM, Donaldson MS, editors. To err is human: building a safer health system. Washington, DC: National Academy Press; 2000.

[9] Srivastava R, Landrigan C, Gidwani P, et al. Pediatric hospitalists in Canada and the United States: a survey of pediatric academic department chairs. Ambul Pediatr 2001;1(6):338–9.

[10] Percelay J, O'Connor K, Neff J. Pediatricians' attitudes toward and experiences with pediatric hospitalists: a national survey [abstract 1304]. Presented at the annual meeting of the Pediatric Academic Societies, Seattle, WA. May 6, 2003.

[11] Society of Hospital Medicine. Survey of hospitalist productivity and compensation. Philadelphia: Society of Hospital Medicine; 2003.

[12] American Academy of Pediatrics. AAP periodic survey. Elk Grove Village, IL: AAP; 2002.

[13] Bellet PS, Whitaker RC. Evaluation of a pediatric hospitalist service: impact on length of stay and hospital charges. Pediatrics 2000;105(3 Pt 1):478–84.

[14] Landrigan CP, Srivastava R, Muret-Wagstaff S, et al. Impact of a health maintenance organization hospitalist system in academic pediatrics. Pediatrics 2002;110(4):720–8.

[15] Landrigan CP, Muret-Wagstaff S, Chiang VW, et al. Senior resident autonomy in a pediatric hospitalist system. Arch Pediatr Adolesc Med 2003;157(2):206–7.

[16] Homme JH. How pediatric hospitalist programs can affect graduate medical education. Pediatr Ann 2003;32(12):822–4.

[17] Tenner PA, Dibrell H, Taylor RP. Improved survival with hospitalists in a pediatric intensive care unit. Crit Care Med 2003;31(3):847–52.

[18] American Board of Pediatrics. Workforce/statistics. Number of diplomats certified. Available at: http://www.abp.org/stats/numdips.htm. Accessed January 15, 2005.

ELSEVIER
SAUNDERS

PEDIATRIC CLINICS
OF NORTH AMERICA

Pediatr Clin N Am 52 (2005) 979–993

The Safety of Inpatient Pediatrics: Preventing Medical Errors and Injuries Among Hospitalized Children

Christopher P. Landrigan, MD, MPH[a,b,c],*

[a]*Inpatient Pediatrics Service, Children's Hospital Boston, 300 Longwood Avenue, Boston, MA 02115, USA*
[b]*Sleep and Patient Safety Program, Brigham and Women's Hospital, 221 Longwood Avenue, Boston, MA 02115, USA*
[c]*Department of Pediatrics, Harvard Medical School, 260 Longwood Avenue, Boston, MA 02115, USA*

In 1999, the Institute of Medicine released a landmark report, "To Err is Human," which brought unprecedented public attention to bear on the safety of American health care. It estimated that medical errors cause between 44,000 and 98,000 deaths each year in the United States [1], making medical error the sixth to ninth leading cause of death [2]. Although the precision of this estimate has been a source of some controversy [3–5], injuries caused by medical errors are unquestionably common.

"To Err is Human" found that errors most often result from complex system failures rather than aberrant actions of individual providers. Fundamental re-design of the health care system must occur if patient safety is to improve substantively. The United States President and Congress publicly accepted the recommendations of the Institute of Medicine and issued directives to study patient safety further and implement systematic improvements. Unfortunately, despite considerable investment, patients seem to be no safer currently than when the Institute of Medicine report was released 6 years ago, in large part because of difficulties implementing proven patient safety solutions [6].

Dr. Landrigan has conducted research on the incidence of adverse events and complications in patients with bronchiolitis that was supported by grants from Medimmune, Inc.

* 221 Longwood Avenue, Boston, MA 02115.

E-mail address: christopher.landrigan@childrens.harvard.edu

This article explores the current state of knowledge about the safety of hospitalized patients in general and patients in pediatric settings in particular. It discusses approaches to evaluating patient safety and reviews the current literature on adverse events and errors in hospitals. The article also discusses strategies proven effective in reducing medical errors and some of the barriers to implementing these strategies that must be overcome.

Cognition and complexity in the genesis of errors

Over the past several decades, understanding of the nature of errors in complex systems has changed dramatically. Historically, errors in medicine have been viewed principally as individual failings. Consequently, serious errors leading to patient harm often were blamed on individual providers at the front line of care, with little attention paid to deeper flaws in the design of health care systems that potentiated error. As the focus of health care providers on the problem of patient safety has sharpened, however, awareness of the inherent limitations of human thought processes and the complexity of hospital systems has grown. Individual errors by front-line providers do not occur in a vacuum; rather, they are the product of an individual's working conditions and environment, which are predominantly determined by systemic designs and processes beyond the individual's immediate control [7].

The dual roles of human cognitive processes and complexity in error are the foundations of human factors engineering, a discipline that has emerged from roots in cognitive psychology and engineering. Human factors engineering evaluates the cognitive and physical parameters of human functioning and the interface between humans and the complex environment in which they work. Human cognitive processes can be divided schematically into "active" and "automatic" modes of processing [7–9]. When confronted with a novel problem that requires intensive thought to solve, we use the active mode of thinking. This mode is slow, labor intensive, and prone to certain types of well-characterized, experimentally reproducible mistakes. If, for example, a hospitalist recently admitted a child with respiratory distress who unexpectedly turned out to have a bacterial pneumonia as the cause of respiratory distress, there is an increased probability of jumping to the conclusion that the next child who comes in with respiratory distress has a bacterial pneumonia, rather than broadly considering all possibilities on the differential diagnosis. This is referred to as the "availability heuristic." Similar errors in probabilistic thinking are common and well described elsewhere [7–9].

Errors also occur in the "automated mode" of processing. When possible, we preferentially use an automated mode to complete routine, highly over-learned tasks so that we can focus our active attention on other problems. Driving is an example of such a task. Experienced drivers do not need to focus actively on the road the entire time they are behind the wheel; most of the time, they can operate a vehicle with little conscious attention paid to how much they are depressing the accelerator or turning the wheel or even their speed and route of travel. During an emergency, or when a novel situation arises, however, it is necessary to move into an active mode of thinking. A common error that occurs as a consequence of operating in an automated mode is accidentally driving past one's intended highway exit. This is a failure to re-engage the active mode of thinking, known as a "capture slip," one of many well-defined types of "slips" and "lapses" [7–9]. Slips and lapses are particularly likely to occur when an individual is distracted, overworked, or sleep deprived.

Complexity in systems also leads to error. As an illustrative example in the hospital setting, it is useful to consider the medication delivery system, which typically consists of many discrete steps (eg, a physician writes an order for a drug, a nurse transcribes the order into a medication administration record, a unit clerk faxes the order to the pharmacy, a pharmacist receives the fax, the pharmacist selects a drug from the stocks, the pharmacist mixes the drug, and so forth). If there are 25 steps in total and each of these steps is performed correctly 99% of the time, the net probability of a medication order making it through the 25 steps without any error occurring is only 78% ($0.99^{25} = 0.78$). An error would occur in 22% of all orders written. Most studies have found the error rate to be somewhat lower than this (as described later), because many steps in the medication delivery process occur with more than 99% success rates and because feedback loops potentially can decrease error rates. Despite this, however, some risk as the result of complexity remains.

James Reason, a leader in the field of human factors engineering, has suggested the following model to explain the occurrence of errors and adverse events in complex systems (Fig. 1) [10]. When an erroneous action, or "trigger," occurs, there are typically multiple safety nets in place that can potentially prevent harm. These safety nets are themselves flawed, however, and periodically, an error slips through every safety net and causes harm.

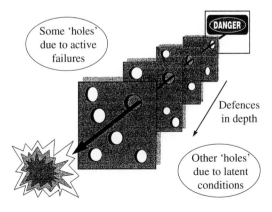

Fig. 1. Reason's Swiss cheese model. (*From* Reason J. Managing the risks of organizational accidents. Burlington (VT): Ashgate Publishing Company; 2000; with permission.)

In sum, the cognitive processes of even the best-intentioned, most motivated physicians are fallible, and errors in problem solving and task execution are common. The complexity of medical care delivery greatly compounds the possibility of errors occurring. How often, then, do significant errors actually occur in clinical practice? How often do they lead to harm? Most importantly, what can be done to prevent them?

Definitions

Before discussing the epidemiology of medical errors and adverse events in detail, it is necessary to clarify some terminology:

"Adverse event" is defined as any injury that is the result of medical management, whether it was ("preventable adverse event") or was not ("nonpreventable adverse event") caused by an error. Injuries caused by an underlying disease process rather than medical management are not adverse events.

"Medical error" is any error in the delivery of medical care, whether it has the potential to cause harm or not.

"Near miss" (sometimes also called a potential adverse event) is a medical error that has significant potential to cause harm but does not, either because it is intercepted before reaching the patient ("intercepted near miss") or because the patient had sufficient physiologic reserve to avoid detectable harm despite it having reached the patient ("nonintercepted near miss"). A "near miss" is a serious error that nearly causes harm.

"Serious medical errors" are all errors that do harm or have significant potential to do harm (ie, preventable adverse events + near misses). Errors with little or no potential for harm are not serious medical errors, nor are nonpreventable adverse events.

To clarify these terms, Fig. 2 depicts their relationships graphically.

Approaches to evaluating patient safety

Several approaches to evaluating patient safety have been used in research and clinical settings. To evaluate safety epidemiologically, it is possible either to look primarily for injuries that occur as a consequence of therapy and then determine what fraction of these were caused by errors (the "adverse events approach") or to look primarily for medical errors and then determine what fraction of these cause harm (the "medical errors approach"). The adverse events approach was used in the Harvard Medical Practice and Utah-Colorado studies

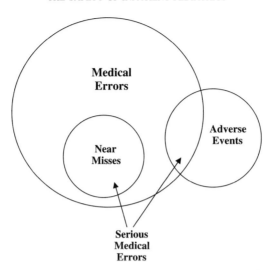

Fig. 2. Relationship between adverse events and medical errors. Not all medical errors result in adverse events, and not all adverse events are the result of errors. Near misses are errors with significant potential to cause harm that are either intercepted before reaching the patient or absorbed by the patient without apparent harm. Serious medical errors include near misses and the subset of adverse events that are preventable (ie, the result of error). (*Adapted from* Bates DW, Makary MA, Teich J, et al. Asking residents about adverse events in a computer dialogue: how accurate are they? Joint Commission Journal on Quality Improvement 1998;24:197–202; with permission.)

(described later) that informed the Institute of Medicine's report. The principal advantage of this approach is that ultimately, it is harm to the patient that matters; an emphasis on "harm" helps focus efforts on errors that are most immediately concerning. A major disadvantage of this approach, however, is that the infrequency of preventable adverse events within a single institution often precludes their measurement as sensitive indicators of the safety of specific care processes or of the success of patient safety interventions within a single center. Consequently, many studies of medication errors and interventions within a single institution have used the "medical errors approach." The basis of this approach is that whereas most potentially harmful errors are intercepted before reaching the patient or are absorbed by the patient without causing clinically apparent harm, injurious and noninjurious errors have common roots within the system. Errors that do not cause harm offer free lessons into how to improve systems of care. Some literature supports this supposition and describes the quantitative relationship between adverse events and errors (see the later section on adverse drug events and medication errors in hospitals). This article addresses data derived from the adverse events and medical errors approaches.

Although not the focus of this article, it should be noted that in addition to epidemiologic methods, it is also possible to seek to improve safety by taking an intensive investigative approach to individual serious errors or processes of care within a hospital. Root cause analysis is a method of identifying retrospectively all of the steps leading up to a serious error and determining what active and "latent" errors (ie, underlying fundamental system flaws) might have contributed to it [11–13]. Failure mode and effects analysis is a method of prospectively charting out all steps in a care process and determining where errors might be introduced [14,15]. Both analyses seek to redesign care processes to minimize the occurrence of errors by addressing systemic flaws identified. The primary strength of failure mode and effects analysis and root cause analysis is that they structure careful analyses of individual problems that address active errors committed by providers at the "sharp" end of care (ie, at the point of care) and errors at the "blunt" end (ie, working conditions and systemic determinants that caused a provider to make a mistake). Because they can address only one error or process at a time, however, they cannot be used as epidemiologic tools, and any conclusions drawn are likely to be influenced by the subjective concerns of the investigators at the time of the analysis and by prevailing institutional priorities. Despite these limitations, however, both approaches have been used to great effect in individual hospitals and in industrial settings to make improvements.

Adverse events in hospitalized patients

The practice of medicine suffers from a high incidence of serious errors and adverse events. The Harvard Medical Practice Study found in a chart review of 30,000 admissions that 3.7% of patients hospitalized in New York State in 1984 experienced an adverse event during medical treatment [16]. Medications, wound infections, operative complications, and diagnostic mistakes were the most common causes of adverse events. Seventy-one percent of adverse events caused short-term disability, 3% caused permanently disability, and 14% led to death; 69% of the injuries detected were judged to be preventable (ie, caused by an error in care) [7,17].

Subsequent studies have found adverse event rates similar to or even more than those identified in this study. In a review of 15,000 randomly selected hospital charts in Utah and Colorado in 1992, Thomas and colleagues [18] found that 2.9% of patients suffered an adverse event. This study used the same medical review abstraction methodology as the Harvard Medical Practice Study. Using a more inclusive chart review methodology, the Quality in Australia Health Care Study found that a much higher proportion of all patients (13%) suffered an adverse event, half of which were caused by human errors [19].

It is important to point out that the number of events identified in all of these studies was much higher than the number reported through typical hospital mechanisms. Many institutions identify adverse events primarily through the filing of incident reports by staff [20–22]. Incident reporting has been found to identify only 6% of all adverse events identified using more active surveillance methodologies [23–28]. Medical errors in pediatric patients in particular have been found to be underreported [29].

Financial impact of adverse events

Adverse events are not only harmful but also expensive. The Harvard Medical Practice Study estimated that the annual cost of adverse events to New York State was $878 million. Bates and colleagues [30] concluded that for a 700-bed hospital, the annual costs of adverse drug events (ADEs)—the subset of adverse events caused by medications—and preventable ADEs were $5.6 million and $2.8 million, respectively. At a national level, hospital-based ADEs have been estimated to cost $2 billion per year [30,31]. Other work has estimated the annual cost of drug-related morbidity and mortality to be as high as $76.6 billion, with most of this cost ($47 billion) attributable to hospital admissions [32]. For comparison, $45 billion is spent on diabetes care each year in the United States [32].

Pediatric inpatient adverse events

More limited data exist to measure the incidence of adverse events among pediatric inpatients. The Harvard Medical Practice Study included pediatric patients and found that 12.91 adverse events occurred per 1000 discharges for all patients aged 0 to 15 years [33]. More recently, several studies have used the Agency for Health Care Research and Quality's "Patient Safety Indicators," a series of markers of possible adverse events that are coded in administrative and billing databases (eg, foreign body left in after procedure, failure to rescue, iatrogenic pneumothorax, infection as a result of medical care, birth trauma), to evaluate the incidence of specific adverse events across multiple pediatric hospitals [34–36]. Patient safety indicator events were associated with significant (and often substantial) increases in charges, length of stay, and in-hospital deaths. Miller and Zhan [35] estimated that in the year 2000, patient safety indicator events led to more than $1 billion in charges in pediatric hospitals.

The major advantage of using administrative data to identify patient safety hazards is that such data are collected routinely in many pediatric inpatient settings, and as such, data from many hospitals can be examined efficiently. Some exploration of variation between hospitals also can be attempted, although with caution given the variability between institutions in administrative coding practices. Because only adverse events that are coded are captured, however, and because it is often not possible in such studies to validate possible adverse events detected, this method is neither sensitive nor highly specific. For example, "failure to rescue" (death because of a complication rather than a primary diagnosis) occurred 703 times per 10,000 discharges in one study [35]. Although this rate is concerning, it is unclear whether all "failures to rescue" were coded, and it is unclear whether "failure to rescue" truly indicates a preventable adverse event, a problem pointed out by Sedman and colleagues [36]. Nevertheless, the patient safety indicators represent an important method of identifying certain patient safety hazards and tracking the effects of high-level changes over time.

Of relevance to pediatric hospitalists, some work also has been conducted to measure rigorously the incidence of complications and adverse events in inpatients with bronchiolitis, one of the most common diseases treated by pediatric hospitalists. Willson and colleagues [37] conducted an analysis of clinical data from inpatients with bronchiolitis at ten children's hospitals. The study found that 79% of all patients suffered a complication in care; 24% suffered a serious complication. Complications were associated with prolonged length of stay and increased hospital costs. The database used in this study did not allow differentiation of adverse events from complications caused by natural progression of disease, but a prospective study by McBride and colleagues [38] of 143 consecutive patients admitted with bronchiolitis found that nine preventable adverse events (ie, adverse events caused by errors in care) occurred per 100 admissions; among critically ill patients, 68 preventable adverse events occurred per 100 admissions. Patients in the intensive care unit who suffered adverse events had an increased length of stay. Studies to evaluate the incidence and nature of adverse events in other common pediatric conditions are needed.

Adverse drug events and medication errors in hospitals

ADEs are some of the most common types of adverse events and perhaps the best studied. Patients frequently suffer injuries secondary to medication use [39,40], a substantial fraction of which are caused by errors in medication ordering or administration [39,41]. The ADE Prevention Study found that 6.5% of hospitalized adults suffered an ADE, of which 28% were preventable [39,42]. Preventable ADEs are common, but medication errors that do not lead to harm are more common still. Only a small fraction of all medication errors cause ADEs. Study of noninjurious errors can be useful, however, because even apparently trivial data can provide insights into latent systemic flaws that lead to injury.

Some of the earliest work that systematically evaluated the incidence of medication errors in hospitals was conducted by pharmacist researchers. Lesar and colleagues [43] found that an average of 3.1 errors occurred per 1000 orders; 58% of these were classified as potentially harmful. Folli and colleagues [44] and a study by the Institute of Medicine [45] documented a slightly higher rate of 4.7 errors per 1000 orders. Both studies included only medication errors that were detected and prevented in the pharmacy, however, which represent only a fraction of all medication errors.

A study that used trained data collectors to observe nurses administering medications found a higher rate of errors: one medication administration error per patient per day [46]. Although this high rate of errors is concerning, it represents only a fraction of all medication errors, because only errors that occurred at the administration stage of the medication delivery process were captured. It did not look for errors in physician ordering, transcribing, or pharmacist dispensation of drugs.

To capture more comprehensively all errors in the medication delivery process, Bates and colleagues [47] prospectively studied errors in an adult hospital by reviewing all medication order sheets, charts, and medication administration records for a cohort of inpatients and soliciting reports from clinical staff. This intensive surveillance methodology identified 5.3 errors per 100 orders, a rate ten times higher than that detected in the pharmacist studies. Twenty-five ADEs were identified, of which 5 were preventable.

Medication errors in inpatient pediatric settings

Hospitalized children may be especially prone to medication errors for several reasons. First, whereas many adult medications have standard doses, virtually all pediatric medications are weight based, which introduces the potential for serious errors caused by miscalculations or misplaced decimal points. Second, many pediatric medications must be mixed by pharmacists or nurses in the hospital at the time of use, which provides a second opportunity for miscalculation. Third, many pediatric medications come in multiple formulations (eg, acetaminophen infant drops and children's elixir), which creates the possibility of over- or underdosing because of confusion regarding the medication's concentration. Finally, children often have less ability than adult inpatients to recognize and communicate an error or adverse event themselves.

Using the methodology pioneered by Bates and colleagues, Kaushal and colleagues [48] performed a study of medication errors in two academic pediatric institutions. The rates of medication errors and ADEs were similar, but a threefold higher rate of potential ADEs (near misses) was found. During the course of the study, 10,778 orders were reviewed and 616 medication errors were identified (5.7%). Of these errors, roughly 1 in 5 (115) were near misses, and a total of 5 erroneous orders caused harm (1% of errors). Although a rate of 5 injuries per 10,000 orders (or 1 per 200 admissions) initially may sound reassuring, one should recognize that these data were collected on select wards over the space of only a handful of weeks. Were such rates to be extrapolated up to a national level, at which there were 36,610,535 admissions in 2003 to 5764 registered hospitals [49], the absolute incidence of preventable ADEs would be of a similar magnitude to the rate of preventable drug-related injuries estimated by "To Err is Human."

Of importance for hospitalists, 74% of all errors in the medication delivery process and 91% of near misses in that study were committed by physicians writing orders. A comparison of rates of errors across various inpatient settings is presented in Table 1. Although the rates of all errors per 100 orders were similar across settings, serious errors were much more common in intensive care environments. Elevated rates in these settings are most likely a product of the greater fragility of patients in neonatal and pediatric intensive care units and the intensity of medical therapies used in their care.

Additional comprehensive studies of pediatric medication errors and ADEs largely have supported these findings [50]. A study of 3312 orders that used a

Table 1
Comparison of rates of errors and serious errors (near misses plus preventable adverse events) in
various inpatient pediatric settings

	Error rate per 100 orders $(P=.31)$	Serious error rate per 100 orders $(P<.001)$
Medical ward	6.0	0.8
Surgical ward	4.7	0.4
PICU	5.7	1.3
NICU	5.5	2.8

Abbreviations: NICU, neonatal intensive care unit; PICU, pediatric intensive care unit.
Data from Kaushal R, Bates DW, Landrigan C. Medication errors and adverse drug events in pediatric inpatients. JAMA 2001.

similar methodology but somewhat more inclusive definitions of errors found 784 errors (24%) [51]. Most of these errors were intercepted. In this study, 83% percent of the errors identified occurred at the prescribing stage. A study of 1197 admissions that was restricted to chart review without medication order review or staff reports identified 7.5 ADEs and 9.3 potential ADEs per 1000 patient days [52]. In all of these studies, decimal point misplacements and miscalculations of doses have been found to be important sources of serious errors in the care of pediatric patients.

Preventing medical errors and injuries

Three primary strategies exist to decrease the number of injuries caused by medical errors. The first is to prevent errors from occurring, the second is to intercept errors before they reach the patient, and the third is to mitigate the harm of errors that do reach the patient. Over the past decade, numerous studies have demonstrated the effectiveness of interventions to improve safety. In 2001, the Agency for Health Care Research and Quality sponsored an evidence-based assessment of 79 published patient safety interventions [53]. A full review of the report is well beyond the scope of this article, but selected key practices and studies relevant to inpatient pediatric work environments are highlighted here.

Medication safety

Computerized physician order entry consistently has been found to prevent and intercept serious medical errors in adult and pediatric inpatient settings. Bates and colleagues [54,55] demonstrated that computer order entry with decision support (eg, automated allergy checking and drug-drug interaction checking) decreased rates of serious medication errors by 55% initially; rates decreased by 81% after full implementation of iterative improvements in decision support. Rates of all medication errors fell 83%. Evans and colleagues [56] found that ADEs caused by antibiotics decreased 70% after implementation of a computerized physician order entry system. In a pediatric hospital, King and colleagues [57] found that introduction of a computerized physician order entry system was associated with a 40% reduction in medication errors. Potts and colleagues [58] found that near misses decreased 41% and medication prescribing errors decreased 99% after introduction of a computerized physician order entry system in a pediatric intensive care unit.

Other technologic tools have been less well studied, but many seem to hold promise to improve safety further. The use of an enhanced, structured computer sign-out was found in one study to reduce the risk of adverse events associated with cross-coverage of patients by house staff less familiar with them [59]. Studies also have suggested possible roles for computerized adverse event detection systems, bar coding, and smart intravenous pumps [53].

Using clinical pharmacists to monitor ordering also has proved effective in decreasing serious errors. Leape and colleagues [60] found that clinical pharmacists who participated in intensive care rounds decreased preventable ADE rates by 66%. A study by Kaushal and colleagues [50,61] found that introduction of ward-based clinical pharmacists in pediatric hospitals led to a fivefold reduction in serious medical errors in intensive care unit settings but no significant improvement in ward settings.

Reducing nosocomial infections

The use of maximal sterile barriers (ie, mask, cap, sterile gloves, gown, and large drape) and antiseptic-impregnated catheters has been found to reduce significantly the risk of nosocomial infections. Nosocomial bloodstream infections differ from noninfectious adverse events because the precise timing of their origin (and the nature of a break in sterile technique or other error that may have caused them) usually cannot be determined. Therefore, it is not clear what percentage of nosocomial infections may be preventable, because some may occur despite perfect sterile technique and catheter maintenance. Despite this uncertainty regarding the precise proportion of preventable infections, however, interventions to reduce sterile breaks and decrease the risk of subsequent infection have been proved to enhance patient safety. A study by Raad and colleagues [62] found that use of maximal sterile barriers decreased the number of catheter-related infections from 0.5 to 0.08 per 1000 catheter days. A meta-analysis of the effectiveness of antiseptic-coated catheters found that their use was associated with an almost twofold decrease in the odds of developing a catheter-related bloodstream infection [63].

Improving working conditions

Recent studies have evaluated the effect of interventions in the working conditions of health care personnel as a means of preventing errors. The Harvard Work Hours, Health, and Safety Group recently found that reducing interns' sleep deprivation substantially improved patient safety in a medical and cardiac intensive care unit. Compared with interns whose consecutive work was limited to 16 hours, interns who worked traditional schedules with recurrent 30-hour shifts slept less, had twice as many attentional failures at night, and made 36% more serious medical errors, including more than five times as many serious diagnostic errors [64,65]. Studies of nurses' work hours and workload likewise have suggested that as working conditions become more difficult, error rates increase [53,66].

Future work

Altogether, a convincing literature has emerged to demonstrate that serious medical errors and preventable adverse events are common in health care. Computerized order entry, clinical pharmacists, improved infection control, and amelioration of sleep deprivation and adverse working conditions have proved effective in decreasing serious errors.

Three immediate challenges in improving pediatric inpatient safety are (1) validating interventions tested in nonpediatric hospital settings, (2) identifying additional strategies to make ongoing improvements, and, most importantly, (3) effectively disseminating those interventions that have proved successful. Adoption of many interventions that have proved effective in the reduction of medical error has been slow. Computerized order entry, for example, one of the most widely studied and proven interventions in health care, was in use in only 5% of hospitals in 2003 [6]. Clinical pharmacists are underused. Techniques to reduce nosocomial infections are not used frequently. Housestaff continue to work recurrent shifts of 30-hours in a row.

As a consequence, the public has yet to experience convincingly the effects of the extensive patient safety research conducted over the past decade [6]. Most Americans report feeling dissatisfied with the quality of American health care, and roughly half believe that it is unsafe [67]. To improve substantially the safety of pediatric inpatient care, we must find efficient and effective ways of translating improvements into practice. Patient safety must grow from an interest of a few to a core responsibility of all health care providers. Only at that time will the potential for safety interventions to improve significantly the health of hospitalized children be realized.

References

[1] Institute of Medicine. To err is human: building a safer health system. Washington, DC: National Academy Press; 1999.
[2] Kochanek KD, Murphy SL, Anderson RN, et al. Deaths: final data for 2002. Natl Vital Stat Rep 2004;53(5):1–115.
[3] Brennan TA. The Institute of Medicine report on medical errors: could it do harm? N Engl J Med 2000;342:1123–5.

[4] Leape LL. Institute of Medicine medical error figures are not exaggerated. JAMA 2001; 284:95–7.

[5] McDonald CJ, Weiner M, Hui SL. Death due to medical errors are exaggerated in Institute of Medicine report. JAMA 2000;284(93):95.

[6] Altman DE, Clancy C, Blendon RJ. Improving patient safety: five years after the IOM report. N Engl J Med 2004;351(20):2041–3.

[7] Leape LL. Error in medicine. JAMA 1994;272:1851–7.

[8] Reason J. Human error. Cambridge (MA): Cambridge University Press; 1990.

[9] Rasmussen J, Jensen A. Mental procedures in real-life tasks: a case study of electronic trouble shooting. Ergonomics 1974;17(3):293–307.

[10] Reason J. Managing the risks of organizational accidents. Burlington (VT): Ashgate Publishing Company; 2000.

[11] Rex JH, Turnbull JE, Allen SJ, et al. Systematic root cause analysis of adverse drug events in a tertiary referral hospital. Jt Comm J Qual Improv 2000;26(10):563–75.

[12] Bagian JP, Gosbee J, Lee CZ, et al. The Veterans Affairs root cause analysis system in action. Jt Comm J Qual Improv 2002;28(10):531–45.

[13] Shojania KG, Wald H, Gross R. Understanding medical error and improving patient safety in the inpatient setting. Med Clin North Am 2002;86(4):847–67.

[14] McDermott RE, Mikulak RJ, Beauregard MR. The basics of FMEA. Portland (OR): Resources Engineering, Inc.; 1996.

[15] DeRosier J, Stalhandske E, Bagian JP, et al. Using health care failure mode and effect analysis: the VA National Center for Patient Safety's prospective risk analysis system. Jt Comm J Qual Improv 2002;28(5):248–67.

[16] Brennan TA, Leape LL, Laird N, et al. Incidence of adverse events and negligence in hospitalized patients: results from the Harvard medical practice study I. N Engl J Med 1991; 324:370–6.

[17] Leape LL, Lawthers AG, Brennan TA, et al. Preventing medical injury. QRB Qual Rev Bull 1993;19(5):144–9.

[18] Thomas EJ, Studdert DM, Burstin HR, et al. Incidence and types of adverse events and negligent care in Utah and Colorado. Med Care 2000;38(261):271.

[19] Wilson RM, Harrison BT, Gibberd RW, et al. An analysis of the causes of adverse events from the quality in Australian health care study. Med J Aust 1999;170(9):411–5.

[20] Berry LL, Segal R, Sherrin TP, et al. Sensitivity and specificity of three methods of detecting adverse drug reactions. Am J Hosp Pharm 1988;45:1534–9.

[21] Faich GA. National adverse drug reaction reporting, 1984–1989. Arch Intern Med 1991; 151:1645–7.

[22] Rogers AS, Israel E, Smith CR, et al. Physician knowledge, attitudes, and behavior related to reporting adverse drug events. Arch Intern Med 1988;148(1596):1600.

[23] Cullen DJ, Bates DW, Small SD, et al. The incident reporting system does not detect adverse drug events: a problem for quality improvement. Jt Comm J Qual Improv 1995;21:541–8.

[24] Scott HD, Thacher-Renshaw A, Rosenbaum SE, et al. Physician reporting of adverse drug reactions: results of the Rhode Island adverse drug reaction reporting project. JAMA 1990; 263(13):1785–8.

[25] Classen DC, Pestotnik SL, Evans RS, et al. Computerized surveillance of adverse drug events in hospital patients. JAMA 1991;266:2847–51.

[26] Bates DW, Makary MA, Teich JM, et al. Asking residents about averse events in a computer dialogue: how accurate are they? Jt Comm J Qual Improv 1998;24:197–202.

[27] Bates DW, O'Neil AC, Boyle D, et al. Potential identifiability and preventability of adverse events using information systems. J Am Med Inform Assoc 1994;1:404–11.

[28] Bates DW, O'Neil AC, Petersen LA, et al. Evaluation of screening criteria for adverse events in medical patients. Med Care 1995;33:452–62.

[29] Taylor JA, Brownstein D, Christakis DA, et al. Use of incident reports by physicians and nurses to document medical errors in pediatric patients. Pediatrics 2004;114(3):729–35.

[30] Bates DW, Spell N, Cullen DJ, et al. The costs of adverse drug events in hospitalized patients: Adverse Drug Events Prevention Study Group. JAMA 1997;227:307–11.

[31] Classen DC, Pestotnik SL, Evans RS, et al. Adverse drug events in hospitalized patients: excess length of stay, extra costs, and attributable mortality. JAMA 1997;277:301–6.

[32] Johnson JA, Bootman JL. Drug-related morbidity and mortality: a cost-of-illness model. Arch Intern Med 1995;155:1949–56.

[33] Leape LL, Brennan TA, Laird N, et al. The nature of adverse events in hospitalized patients: results of the Harvard Medical Practice Study II. N Engl J Med 1991;324:377–84.

[34] Miller MR, Elixhauser A, Zhan C. Patient safety events during pediatric hospitalizations. Pediatrics 2003;111(6 Pt 1):1358–66.

[35] Miller MR, Zhan C. Pediatric patient safety in hospitals: a national picture in 2000. Pediatrics 2004;113(6):1741–6.

[36] Sedman A, Harris JM, Schulz K, et al. Relevance of the Agency for Healthcare Research and Quality patient safety indicators for children's hospitals. Pediatrics 2005;115(1):135–45.

[37] Willson DF, Landrigan CP, Horn SD, et al. Complications in infants hospitalized for bronchiolitis or respiratory syncytial virus pneumonia. J Pediatr 2003;143(5 Suppl):S142–9.

[38] McBride SC, Chiang VW, Goldmann DA, et al. Preventable adverse events in infants hospitalized with bronchiolitis. Pediatrics, in press.

[39] Bates DW, Cullen D, Laird N, et al. Incidence of adverse drug events and potential adverse drug events: implications for prevention. JAMA 1995;274:29–34.

[40] Lazarou J, Pomeranz BH, Corey PN. Incidence of adverse drug reactions in hospitalized patients: a meta-analysis of prospective studies. JAMA 1998;279:1200–5.

[41] Bates DW, Leape LL, Petrycki S. Incidence and preventability of adverse drug events in hospitalized adults. J Gen Intern Med 1993;8:289–94.

[42] Leape LL, Bates DW, Cullen DJ, et al. Systems analysis of adverse drug events. JAMA 1995;274:35–43.

[43] Lesar TS, Briceland LL, Delcoure K, et al. Medication prescribing errors in a teaching hospital. JAMA 1990;263(2329):2334.

[44] Folli HL, Poole RL, Benitz WE, et al. Medication error prevention by clinical pharmacists in two children's hospitals. Pediatrics 1987;79:718–22.

[45] Institute of Medicine. Crossing the quality chasm: a new health system for the 21st century. Washington, DC: National Academic Press; 2001.

[46] Allan EL, Barker KN. Fundamentals of medication error research. Am J Hosp Pharm 1990; 47(555):571.

[47] Bates DW, Boyle DL, Vander Vliet MB, et al. Relationship between medication errors and adverse drug events. J Gen Intern Med 1995;10(199):205.

[48] Kaushal R, Bates DW, Landrigan C. Medication errors and adverse drug events in pediatric inpatients. JAMA 2001;285:2114–20.

[49] American Hospital Association. Fast facts on US hospitals from AHA hospital statistics. Available at: http://www.aha.org/aha/resource_center/fastfacts/fast_facts_US_hospitals.html. Accessed March 3, 2005.

[50] Kaushal R, Jaggi T, Walsh K, et al. Pediatric medication errors: what do we know? What gaps remain? Ambul Pediatr 2004;4(1):73–81.

[51] Marino BL, Reinhardt K, Eichelberger WJ, et al. Prevalence of errors in a pediatric hospital medication system: implications for error proofing. Outcomes Manag Nurs Pract 2000;4(3): 129–35.

[52] Holdsworth MT, Fichtl RE, Behta M, et al. Incidence and impact of adverse drug events in pediatric inpatients. Arch Pediatr Adolesc Med 2003;157(1):60–5.

[53] Agency for Healthcare Research and Quality. Making health care safer: a critical analysis of patient safety practices. AHRQ Publication No. 01–E058. Washington, DC: Agency for Healthcare Research and Quality; 2001.

[54] Bates DW, Teich J, Lee J, et al. The impact of computerized physician order entry on medication error prevention. J Am Med Inform Assoc 1999;6(313):321.

[55] Bates DW, Leape LL, Cullen DJ, et al. Effect of computerized physician order entry and a team intervention on prevention of serious medication errors. JAMA 1998;280(15):1311–6.
[56] Evans RS, Pestotnik SL, Classen DC, et al. A computer-assisted management program for antibiotics and other antiinfective agents. N Engl J Med 1998;338(4):232–8.
[57] King WJ, Paice N, Rangrej J, et al. The effect of computerized physician order entry on medication errors and adverse drug events in pediatric inpatients. Pediatrics 2003;112(3 Pt 1):506–9.
[58] Potts AL, Barr FE, Gregory DF, et al. Computerized physician order entry and medication errors in a pediatric critical care unit. Pediatrics 2004;113(1 Pt 1):59–63.
[59] Petersen LA, Orav EJ, Teich JM, et al. Using a computerized sign-out program to improve continuity of inpatient care and prevent adverse events. Jt Comm J Qual Improv 1998;24(2): 77–87.
[60] Leape LL, Cullen DJ, Clapp MD, et al. Pharmacist participation on physician rounds and adverse drug events in the intensive care unit. JAMA 1999;282:267–70.
[61] Kaushal R, Bates D, McKenna KJ, et al. Ward-based clinical pharmacists and serious medication errors in pediatric inpatients. In: Proceedings of the Annual Meeting of the National Academy of Health. 2003.
[62] Raad II, Hohn DC, Gilbreath BJ, et al. Prevention of central venous catheter-related infections by using maximal sterile barrier precautions during insertion. Infect Control Hosp Epidemiol 1994;15(4 Pt 1):231–8.
[63] Veenstra DL, Saint S, Saha S, et al. Efficacy of antiseptic-impregnated central venous catheters in preventing catheter-related bloodstream infection: a meta-analysis. JAMA 1999;281(3):261–7.
[64] Lockley SW, Cronin JW, Evans EE, et al. Effect of reducing interns' weekly work hours on sleep and attentional failures. N Engl J Med 2004;351(18):1829–37.
[65] Landrigan CP, Rothschild JM, Cronin JW, et al. Effect of reducing interns' work hours on serious medical errors in intensive care units. N Engl J Med 2004;351(18):1838–48.
[66] Rogers AE, Hwang WT, Scott LD, et al. The working hours of hospital staff nurses and patient safety. Health Aff (Millwood) 2004;23(4):202–12.
[67] Agency for Healthcare Research and Quality, and Harvard School of Public Health. National survey on consumers' experiences with patient safety and quality information. Menlo Park, CA: Kaiser Family Foundation; 2005.

ELSEVIER
SAUNDERS

PEDIATRIC CLINICS
OF NORTH AMERICA

Pediatr Clin N Am 52 (2005) 995–1027

Pain Management for the Hospitalized Pediatric Patient

Christine Greco, MD, Charles Berde, MD, PhD*

Department of Anesthesia, Children's Hospital Boston, 300 Longwood Avenue, Room 555, Boston, MA 02115, USA

Assessment and management of pain and other symptoms is a central aspect of pediatric hospital medicine. Although hospitals may differ in the division of responsibilities and chain of command for pain management, pediatric hospitalists should become involved in the establishment of protocols and in ensuring a safe and effective standard of care for infants and children in their hospitals. In general hospitals in which adults and children are cared for together, it is essential to have a set of protocols for pain and symptom management specifically for infants and children.

A report of a patient experiencing pain requires assessment of causes, mechanisms, and factors that influence pain experience and pain-related behaviors. In some situations, primary attention is directed to relieving the underlying cause (eg, pain caused by an excessively tight cast may be relieved by bivalving or replacing the cast). In other situations, an underlying cause is established (eg, pain caused by extensive surgery, a major fracture, or advanced cancer with compression of multiple tissues), and primary attention is directed to analgesic administration for symptomatic relief. In other circumstances, efforts at diagnostic evaluation and analgesic intervention may proceed in parallel.

Pediatric hospitals should make uniform assessment of pain part of their standard of care. Validated self-report measures are available for use with most children aged 4 and older and involve photos or drawings of faces [1–3] or a slide rule with increasing color intensity that signifies increasing pain intensity [4] (Figs. 1 and 2). For children who are unable to use self-report, several behavioral scales are available for infants and nonverbal children [5] and even

---

* Corresponding author.

E-mail address: Charles.Berde@childrens.harvard.edu (C. Berde).

0031-3955/05/$ – see front matter © 2005 Elsevier Inc. All rights reserved.
doi:10.1016/j.pcl.2005.04.005
pediatric.theclinics.com

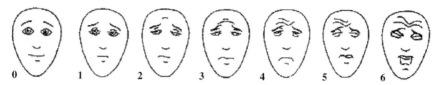

Fig. 1. Faces pain scale.

for preterm neonates [6]. Although behavioral measures are useful, they can be overly sensitive to fear or anxiety in the acute setting and can underrate persistent pain relative to self-report [7].

Recently the Joint Commission on Accreditation of Health Care Organizations has mandated that health care facilities should implement uniform pain assessment and systematic efforts at improving pain treatment interventions. Some pediatric hospitals have reported on their programs to minimize pain whenever possible [8]. The spirit of these initiatives is entirely laudable. We caution, however, that too literal interpretation of use of a specific pain score (eg, Visual Analog Score pain score >4) as a trigger for intervention in every case is not evidence based and not realistic. Whereas every effort should be made to relieve pain whenever feasible and safe to do so, all persons who manage pain on a daily basis must acknowledge that for a minority of patients with some severely painful conditions (eg, mucositis after bone marrow transplantation, scoliosis surgery, severe sickle cell vaso-occlusive episodes), there are situations in which attempts to relieve pain, even with optimally titrated administration of systemic opioids and adjuvant medications, result in either pain scores >6 or oversedation and hypoventilation with attempts to achieve lower pain scores. For occasional patients who have extensive surgery, especially neonates, postoperative ventilation for a day may be the safest way to provide adequate analgesia. For other patients, this option is not feasible. Even with physicians and nurses practicing in a state-of-the art manner, good pain relief is occasionally not achievable. To promise otherwise is disingenuous.

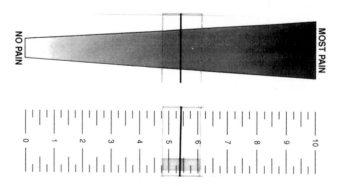

Fig. 2. Colored analogue scale.

Principles of analgesic pharmacology in infants and children

Several factors produce age-related differences in responses to analgesics [9].

- Neonates and young infants have delayed maturation of hepatic enzyme systems involved in drug metabolic inactivation. Analgesics metabolized in the liver, such as opioids and amino-amide local anesthetics, have a prolonged elimination half-life in newborns. Rates of maturation of individual enzyme functions vary, but for most analgesics, metabolism has matured by approximately age 6 months.
- Glomerular filtration and renal tubular secretion are reduced in the first several weeks of life, which results in slower elimination of opioids and their active metabolites.
- Neonates and young infants have reduced levels of α_1-acid glycoprotein and albumin. This factor leads to decreased plasma protein binding for many drugs and results in greater concentrations of pharmacologically active unbound drug.
- Infants have immature ventilatory reflexes in response to hypoxia and hypercarbia and have increased risk of hypoventilation in response to opioids.

Nonopioid analgesics

Mechanisms of action

The term "nonopioid analgesic" refers to acetaminophen, aspirin, nonsteroidal anti-inflammatory drugs (NSAIDs), and selective cyclo-oxygenase 2 (COX-2) inhibitors. COX enzymes convert arachidonic acid to various prostanoid products that have diverse physiologic roles, including increasing pain and hypersensitivity, fostering inflammation and fever, regulating regional blood flow, and protecting gastric mucosal integrity. Several subtypes or iso-enzymes of the COX enzymes have been identified, and these subtypes differ in their distribution and function in various peripheral tissues and in the central nervous system. Aspirin and the NSAIDs act on a broad spectrum of COX enzymes. Aspirin's irreversible inhibition of COX-1 in platelets contrasts with the reversible action of the NSAIDs, which accounts for the much longer duration of aspirin's antihemostatic actions. The COX-2 inhibitors were developed specifically to inhibit the COX isoenzyme subtype 2, which is expressed preferentially in leukocytes and other cell types involved in inflammation and in neurons and glial cells in the peripheral and central nervous systems [10,11]. Although these drugs commonly are regarded as "peripheral" analgesics, analgesia from all of these drugs involves a combination of peripheral and central actions. In particular, acetaminophen's analgesic actions seem to occur largely via sites within the central nervous system, although there is controversy regarding importance of central COX-3 inhibition in acetaminophen's analgesic effects [12–14].

Acetaminophen

Acetaminophen is the most widely used analgesic and antipyretic agent in infants and children. Unlike aspirin, NSAIDs, and COX-2 inhibitors, it exerts minimal peripheral anti-inflammatory effects. Acetaminophen is effective for mild to moderate pain with good safety margin, and it is often combined with opioids to provide additive analgesic effects [15]. Acetaminophen is available in various formulations, including capsules, tablets, suspensions, and suppositories. Caution should be used to avoid dosing errors with suspensions because the infant drops are more concentrated than the commonly used liquid formulation. Excessive dosing, especially in infants and children with febrile illnesses, hypovolemia, or other risk factors, can precipitate hepatic failure [16]. Typical oral dosing is 10 to 15 mg/kg, although single dosing of 20 mg/kg is sometimes used. Daily maximum dosing has been recommended at 100 mg/kg for children, 75 mg/kg for term infants, and 40 mg/kg for premature infants [17].

Rectal dosing of acetaminophen is sometimes used, especially among children who are unwilling or unable to take oral mediations. The rectal route has slow and somewhat variable absorption [18]. Peak rectal absorption occurs at 70 minutes. Recommended rectal dosing for children is 30 to 45 mg/kg followed by 20 mg/kg every 6 hours. Dosage guidelines for acetaminophen and commonly used NSAIDs are listed in Table 1.

Nonsteroidal anti-inflammatory drugs

Unlike acetaminophen, NSAIDs have prominent anti-inflammatory and analgesic effects. The principle mechanism of action is inhibition of prostaglandin synthesis by reversible blockade of the COX enzyme. The weight-scaled clearances of several NSAIDs are diminished in newborns [19] and younger infants. Conversely, the weight-scaled clearances of several NSAIDs are greater in children ages aged 3 to 8 compared to adults [20]. Beyond age 10, the pharmacokinetic parameters of most NSAIDs resemble those in younger adults.

Table 1
Dosing guidelines for nonsteroidal anti-inflammatory drugs

	Dose <60 kg	Dose >60 kg
Acetaminophen	10–15 mg/kg q 4 h PO	650–1000 mg q 4 h PO
Naproxen	5 mg/kg q 12 h PO	250–500 mg q 12 h PO
Ibuprofen	6–10 mg/kg q 6–8 h PO	400–600 q 6 h PO
Celecoxib	2–4 mg/kg q 12 h PO	100–200 mg q 12hrs PO
Ketorolac	0.5 mg/kg q6–8 h IV, not for >5 d	30 mg q 6–8 h IV, not for >5 d

Dosing guidelines listed herein refer to children >1 year of age.
Further modifications in dosing are required for use of these agents in term and preterm neonates and in infants. Modifications are detailed in the text.
Abbreviations: PO, orally; q; every.

NSAIDs are commonly used for mild to moderate pain and are often used as adjuvants to opioid therapy. Despite marketing claims to the contrary, NSAIDs are fairly similar to each other in peak analgesic effect when administered at equitoxic doses [21]. No evidence exists that any NSAID or selective COX-2 inhibitor is "stronger" than older agents, such as ibuprofen or naproxen. There is also no "magic" associated with parenteral routes; ketorolac is not uniquely stronger than any of the oral NSAIDs as an analgesic [21]. NSAIDs do produce good analgesia for patients with a various types of pain. In paradigms in which postsurgical patients are randomly assigned to receive NSAID or placebo, with parenteral opioids as rescue analgesics, the NSAID groups typically show lower pain scores and a 30% to 40% reduction in opioid use [22]. Contrary to common belief, a standard dose of many NSAIDs produces more effective analgesia than 30 to 60 mg of codeine in adults after surgery. (Other reasons to disparage codeine are presented later.) Unlike opioids, NSAIDs are not associated with respiratory depression, sedation, or tolerance, and they can be especially helpful in reducing excessive sedation and urinary retention caused by opioids.

Despite these benefits, NSAIDs can produce significant risks and side effects, including nephropathy, gastropathy, and bleeding caused by platelet dysfunction. In general, short-term use of NSAIDs is well tolerated by children, with low incidence of side effects [23,24]. The risks of renal and hepatic toxicity are increased by hypovolemia or cardiac failure. Prolonged use of NSAIDs incurs a significant risk of gastrointestinal bleeding, although with still a lower risk overall compared to adults [25,26]. Information regarding safety and efficacy of NSAIDs for analgesia in neonates and young infants is limited [27]. Most of the available information regarding pharmacokinetics and safety of NSAIDs in neonates has been derived from studies of their use for closure of a patent ductus arteriosus. In that setting, ibuprofen may be somewhat safer than indomethacin [28].

A common use of NSAIDs has been for analgesia after tonsillectomy [29]. In theory, an analgesic that produces less risk of nausea and vomiting, sedation, or respiratory depression would be attractive in this patient group, and a large number of studies have shown good analgesia and a reduction in opioid use with several different NSAIDs. A primary risk associated with this operation is immediate and delayed bleeding from the tonsillar bed, however, which at times can be life threatening. Although several individual clinical trials did not report increased risk of bleeding complications, most lacked sufficient statistical power to show a change in the frequency of clinically important bleeding. Two meta-analyses have reached different conclusions regarding these risks; one found a threefold increase in the risk of requiring a second operative procedure to obtain hemostasis and the other reported no significant increase in risk [30,31]. Our view, and the view of otolaryngology colleagues at our institution, is that the potential risks from NSAIDs outweigh the benefits for children undergoing tonsillectomy. Those who dispute this view point out that giving more doses of opioids can increase the risk of hypoventilation in children with degrees of obstructive sleep apnea, and the true frequency of life-threatening airway obstruction and hypoventilation in different subgroups of children after tonsillectomy remains to be determined.

Another important area of dispute concerns the effects of NSAIDs on bone healing in children with fractures or children who have undergone types of surgery that require active bone formation, such as posterior fusion and instrumentation for scoliosis [32–34]. Prostanoids play essential roles in osteoblast activation and new bone formation. Studies in vitro and in animals have raised theoretical concerns, and a small number of case-controlled series in adults have suggested a higher frequency of non-union with NSAID use. Critics of these studies have suggested that NSAID use may be more common among patients with more severe pain, with ongoing inflammatory disorders, or with other risk factors for non-union. Other researchers have suggested that a few doses or a few days of NSAID use are unlikely to influence dramatically the overall course of bone healing, which occurs over months, rather than days. Children also are overall much less prone to difficulty with fracture healing or non-union than adults who undergo similar operations. Our recommendation is to adopt a middle course pending more specific data on clinical outcomes and risks. For children at high risk for non-union or impaired bony fusion, NSAIDs probably should be avoided. Conversely, for children who are at comparatively low risk of non-union, who have had severe and difficult to control side effects from opioids, or who have significantly increased risks from opioids, an NSAID or COX-2 inhibitor is administered for 1 to 2 days postoperatively. Some studies suggest that selective COX-2 inhibitors are less likely to inhibit bone formation than traditional NSAIDs [32,33].

Ketorolac is the most commonly used parenteral NSAID in the United States. It is often used in postoperative patients either alone or as an adjuvant to opioids [22]. It is not uniquely stronger than other NSAIDs but may be convenient for administration during or at the end of surgery. Recommended dosing of ketorolac is 0.25 to 0.5 mg/kg every 6 hours. Safety and efficacy data are limited for younger infants [35].

Selective COX-2 inhibitors have been shown to provide analgesia and anti-inflammatory effects similar to traditional NSAIDs, with a lower short-term incidence of gastropathy [36,37] and with milder effects on in vitro measures of platelet function [38]. The incidence of renal toxicity associated with selective COX-2 inhibitors, however, seems to be similar to other NSAIDs. Recent reports of cardiovascular complications in adults with some of the COX-2 inhibitors [39] have prompted withdrawal of two of these drugs, rofecoxib and valdecoxib, from the market. Although these complications were originally seen in trials with prolonged use, subsequent studies have reported complications even with perioperative use in adults undergoing cardiac surgery [40]. Whether these agents pose any significant cardiovascular or thrombotic risk in infants and children remains unknown. These adverse events may reflect alteration of the balance among prostaglandins, thromboxanes, and prostacyclins. For certain subgroups of patients, such as children with hemarthroses caused by hemophilia, the benefits COX-2 inhibitors for providing analgesia with a reduced risk of bleeding seem clear. For other groups of children, including children with hypercoagu-lability disorders, Moya-Moya disease, or Kawasaki's disease, COX-2 inhibitors probably should be avoided, pending further study. Postoperative analgesic trials with COX inhibitors in children have yielded mixed results [41,42]. For chronic administration for children and adolescents with arthritis who have experienced significant gastrointestinal bleeding, clinicians may consider prescribing either a COX-2 inhibitor, some the modified salicylates with relatively mild gastric effects, including salsalate, diflunisal, or choline-magnesium salicylate [43], or some of the NSAIDs with milder gastric effects, such as etodolac or nambutone, along with gastric protective interventions, including acid blockers, misoprostol, and sucralfate.

Opioids

Opioids are commonly used for the treatment of moderate to severe pain in adults and children. Historically, children received inadequate doses of opioids [44], partly because of a limited understanding of drug metabolism and limitations in the ability to assess pain in children. Pharmacokinetic studies of opioids and advancements in developmental neuroanatomy have led to more appropriate dosing and the widespread use of opioids for pain management in children.

Neonates and preterm infants have unique differences in opioid pharmaco-kinetics compared with older infants and children [45–47]. Premature and term neonates have immature hepatic enzyme systems, which lead to decreases in conjugation of opioids [48]. Glomerular filtration is reduced in the first week of life, which results in slower elimination of opioid metabolites. These factors lead to a longer duration of clinical effects of opioids in young infants. For example, the terminal elimination half-life of parenteral morphine in adults and older children is approximately 2 hours, compared to 6 to 8 hours in neonates and roughly 10 hours in premature infants [49].

Infants younger than 2 or 3 months of age—and especially premature infants—may have an increased risk of hypoventilation and respiratory depres-sion in response to opioids [50]. Some studies in animal models suggested that increased passage of opioids across the blood-brain barrier in infants may account for age-related increases in respiratory depression. Other studies have argued that the respiratory depressant effects of opioids are more likely, however, because of intrinsic age-related pharmacodynamic differences in opioid actions on their receptors and not because of greater blood-brain barrier permeability [51]. Young infants, particularly those with underlying chronic lung disease, have a diminished ventilatory response to hypoxia and hypercarbia. Based on pharmacokinetic and pharmacodynamic considerations, infants younger than 3 months of age who are receiving opioids should have reduced weight-scaled doses and infusion rates compared to older children. They also should have additional nursing observation and cardiorespiratory monitoring for signs of respiratory depression.

The specific choice of opioids depends in part on desired route of administration and adverse effects. Various routes of administration of opioids are available, including oral, intravenous (IV), intramuscular, subcutaneous, and transdermal. Oral administration is commonly used for mild to moderate pain and should provide effective analgesia provided that gastrointestinal absorption is intact. IV administration is useful for rapidly escalating pain or when patients are unable to tolerate oral intake. Additional routes are discussed later.

Codeine is a commonly used oral analgesic and is available in pill form and elixir. It is also used as an antitussive. Codeine is extensively metabolized in the liver, with a portion of it demethylated to morphine. Codeine is considered a weak opioid and is usually combined with acetaminophen, which enhances its analgesic effect. Textbooks often state that codeine has a ceiling effect, which is controversial. In practice, however, dose escalation beyond 2 mg/kg is not recommended because of a high frequency of side effects. Typical doses for children are 0.5 to 1 mg/kg orally every 4 hours. Overall, codeine is a weaker analgesic than commonly believed [52]. A large percentage of children (estimated as 36% in a recent pediatric study [53]) show remarkably inefficient hepatic conversion of codeine to morphine. In these subjects, codeine is essentially inert as an analgesic. For this reason, we discourage use of codeine for most patients with moderate or severe pain. One specific convenient feature of codeine is that combination formulations with acetaminophen can be prescribed over the telephone (with a mailed script to follow) more readily than most opioids.

Oxycodone may be administered alone or in combination with acetaminophen. Although previously recommended for mild to moderate pain, subsequent studies showed that oxycodone dosing can be escalated for moderate to severe pain much like morphine or other strong opioids. Oxycodone is also available as an elixir for patients who are unable to swallow pills and as a sustained-release preparation for the treatment of chronic pain. It undergoes hepatic metabolism to oxymorphone. Immediate-release tablets are prescribed commonly for moderate to severe pain in doses of 0.1 to 0.2 mg/kg every 4 hours.

Morphine is widely used and is typically a first choice for parenteral use in children. Oral elixirs, tablets, and sustained-release tablets are commonly used for children with pain or air hunger caused by cancer. Morphine undergoes hepatic conversion to metabolites, including morphine 6- and 3-glucuronides, which contribute to analgesia and side effects. These metabolites are excreted renally. Accumulation of these metabolites accounts for much of the exaggerated and prolonged response to morphine seen among patients with renal failure. Morphine and most other opioids release histamine locally and systemically. Erythema and hives along the course of a vein proximal to an IV site do not imply allergy to morphine. Hypotension can occur because of several physiologic processes, including (1) histamine-mediated vasodilation, (2) direct inhibition of sympathetic nerve activity, which leads to reductions in arterial and venous tone and reduced sympathetic stimulation of cardiac inotropy and chronotropy, and (3) reduction in baroreceptor-mediated reflex responses. Hypotension caused by morphine and other opioids is more problematic in patients who have hypovolemia or in other patients who depend on basal sympathetic tone to maintain blood pressure. The duration of analgesic action of morphine is generally 3 to 4 hours. Because of wide individual variation in opioid requirements and metabolism, opioids should be dosed according to age, weight, and side effects and should be titrated to effect [45,46]. Dosing guidelines for parenteral and oral morphine can be found in Table 2.

Hydromorphone is similar to morphine in many respects. It is approximately five to six times as potent as morphine in steady state when given intravenously in children [54]. It is often used in patients with renal insufficiency because of decreased accumulation of active metabolites when compared to morphine. Despite common teaching and despite apparent differences in individual patients, available data do not suggest any general population differences between morphine and hydromorphone in their frequency of producing either central or peripheral opioid side effects [55].

Meperidine has excitatory cardiac and central nervous system effects, particularly with repeated dosing. Accumulation of normeperidine, an active metabolite, can cause hyperreflexia, agitation, dysphoria, and seizures. Life-threatening reactions are associated with the use of meperidine in patients taking monoamineoxidase inhibitors and may include hyperpyrexia, metabolic and hemodynamic derangements, excitability, seizures, and coma. Because of these adverse effects and lack of specific advantages as an analgesic, meperidine in our practice is generally restricted to use in small doses of 0.25 mg/kg intravenously in the treatment of rigors associated with administration of blood products or treatment of postanesthetic shivering. The plasma elimination half-life is 3 to 4 hours.

Fentanyl is approximately 70 to 100 times more potent than morphine in single-dose administration and approximately 30 to 50 times as potent via prolonged infusions. Fentanyl provides less histamine release and somewhat less vasodilation in critically ill subjects. Because of its rapid onset and comparatively brief duration of action with initial bolus dosing, it is useful for the treatment of pain associated with brief procedures, such as lumbar punctures, dressing changes, and bone marrow aspirations, either by itself or in combination with benzodiazepines or short-acting general anesthesia [56]. Repeated dosing or continuous infusions result in prolonged duration of action [57]. (For a discussion of the concept of "context-sensitive half-times" for opioids, see references [58–60].) Rapid administration, particularly with high doses, may produce glottic and chest wall rigidity [61] and sometimes can be treated with naloxone, although in other cases, neuromuscular blockade and assisted ventilation are required. Typical doses used for brief, painful procedures in nonintubated patients should be administered in increments of 0.5 μg/kg every 1 to 2 minutes to a full dose of approximately 1 to 3 μg/kg. Careful observation, cardiorespiratory monitoring, and immediate availability of airway equipment and clinicians with advanced airway skills are recommended.

Transdermal fentanyl is an alternative route of administration for the treatment of cancer pain in selected children who have either a better side-

Table 2
Initial dosing guidelines for opioids

Drug	Equianalgesic doses		Usual starting intravenous or subcutaneous doses and intervals		Parenteral oral dose ratio	Usual starting oral doses and intervals	
	Parenteral	Oral	Child <50 kg	Child >50 kg		Child <50 kg	Child >50 kg
Codeine	120 mg	200 mg	NR	NR	1:2	0.5–1.0 mg/kg every 3–4 h	30–60 mg every 3–4 h
Morphine	10 mg	30 mg (long-term); 60 mg (single dose)	Bolus: 0.1 mg/kg every 2–4 h; Infusion: 0.03 mg/kg/h	Bolus: 5–8 mg every 2–4 h; Infusion: 1.5 mg/hr	1:3 (long-term); 1:6 (single dose)	Immediate release: 0.3 mg/kg every 3–4 h; Sustained release: 20–35 kg; 10–15 mg every 8–12 h; 35–50 kg; 15–30 mg every 8–12 h	Immediate release: 15–20 mg every 3–4 h; Sustained release 30–45 mg every 8–12 h
Oxycodone	NA	15–20 mg	NA	NA	NA	0.1–0.2 mg/kg every 3–4 h	5–10 mg every 3–4 h
Methadone[a]	10 mg	10–20 mg	0.1 mg/kg every 4–8 h	5–8 mg every 4–8 h	1:2	0.1–0.2 mg/kg every 4–8 h	5–10 mg every 4–8 h
Fentanyl	100 µg (0.1 mg)	NA	Bolus: 0.5–1.0 µg/kg every 1–2 h; Infusion: 0.5–2.0 µg/kg/h	Bolus: 25–50 µg every 1–2 h; Infusion: 25–100 µg/h	NA	NA	NA
Hydromorphone	1.5–2 mg	6–8 mg	Bolus: 0.02 mg every 2–4 h; Infusion: 0.006 mg/kg/h	Bolus: 1 mg every 2–4 h; Infusion: 0.3 mg/h	1:4	0.04–0.08 mg/kg every 3–4 h	2–4 mg every 3–4 h
Meperidine (pethidine)[b]	75–100 mg	300 mg	Bolus: 0.5–1.0 mg/kg every 2–3 h	Bolus: 50–75 mg every 2–3 h	1:4	2–3 mg/kg every 3–4 h	100–150 mg every 3–4 h

Doses are for patients over 6 months of age. In infants under 6 months, initial per-kilogram doses should begin at roughly 25% of the per-kilogram doses recommended here. Higher doses are often required for patients receiving mechanical ventilation. All doses are approximate and should be adjusted according to clinical circumstances. Recommendations are adapted from previous summary tables, including those of a consensus statement from the World Health Organization and the International Association for the Study of Pain.

Abbreviations: NA, not applicable; NR, not recommended.

[a] Methadone requires additional vigilance because it can accumulate and produce delayed sedation. If sedation occurs, doses should be withheld until sedation resolves. Thereafter, doses should be substantially reduced, the interval between doses should be extended to 3 to 12 hours, or both.

[b] The use of meperidine should generally be avoided if other opioids are available, especially with long term use, because its metabolite can cause seizures.

Adapted from Berde CB, Sethna NF. Analgesics for the treatment of pain in children. N Engl J Med 2002;347:1094–103.

effect profile with fentanyl compared with several other opioids or difficulty with oral opioids but do not require parenteral access for other purposes [62]. After initial application, there is relatively constant release of fentanyl that then diffuses across skin layers. Approximately 12 to 24 hours are necessary to achieve steady state; therefore, transdermal fentanyl is primarily indicated for opioid-tolerant patients with relatively constant pain. It should not be used to treat acute pain, particularly among opioid-naïve patients; adverse events have occurred with use in opioid-naïve patients after surgery or major trauma. Because transdermal fentanyl cannot be titrated rapidly upward or downward in dose, most patients need an additional opioid by a different route for breakthrough pain. Oral transmucosal fentanyl has been used for rapid onset for brief painful procedures in children [63] and for cancer breakthrough pain in adults [64–66].

Several analogues of fentanyl have been developed with shorter durations of action, including sufentanil, alfentanyl, and remifentanil [67]. Their indications are predominantly for use in the operating room or for selected patients in the intensive care units who require short-term analgesia with rapid cessation of effect before planned extubation. Although they have been used for brief painful procedures, their use generally should be restricted to clinicians with considerable experience and advanced airway skills.

Methadone is a long-acting opioid with a widely variable elimination half-life, ranging from approximately 6 to 30 hours. Methadone's prolonged duration of action makes it a convenient drug to provide steady plasma concentrations with less frequent IV boluses compared to morphine, hydromorphone, or fentanyl [68]. The bioavailability of methadone ranges from 60% to 90% and is available in elixir preparation, which makes it useful in providing prolonged duration analgesia (similar to sustained-release formulations of other opioids) for children with cancer or other forms of severe chronic pain who are unable to swallow pills. Methadone is uniquely useful and uniquely challenging to titrate because it is really a combination drug. Methadone is prepared commercially as a racemic mixture of d and l isomers. The l-isomer acts largely as a mu opioid. The d-isomer of methadone acts as an antagonist at the N-methyl-aspartate subgroup of excitatory amino acid receptors in the brain, spinal cord, and in peripheral nerves [69]. Blockade of N-methyl-aspartate receptors reduces pain and hyperalgesia in many forms of inflammatory and neuropathic pain and partially prevents or reverses tolerance to mu opioids.

The result of these multiple actions is that the potency ratio of methadone to morphine and other opioids differs, depending on the type of pain involved and a patient's degree of opioid tolerance [70–72]. Stated another way, methadone seems to be more potent among opioid-tolerant patients when compared to opioid-naïve patients. In single-dose IV administration, morphine and methadone are roughly equipotent at peak effect, but methadone is longer acting. For opioid-naïve subjects after surgery, the average daily requirement of IV methadone tends to be approximately one third that of IV morphine. Conversely, in some patients who have cancer and have high opioid tolerance, the equipotent daily dose of IV methadone may be as little as 10% to 15% of the previous daily IV morphine dose. Careful titration and monitoring of respiratory depression is necessary when dosing with methadone because of incomplete cross-tolerance and slow but variable clearance. If a patient shows oversedation or even mild hypoventilation with methadone, it may be necessary to hold a next dose for a considerable time period or dramatically reduce subsequent doses rather than just make small incremental adjustments in the dose or the dosing interval.

Butorphanol, nalbuphine, and buprenorphine show variable degrees of partial agonist activity at the kappa and sigma receptors and antagonist activity at the mu receptor. They have moderate analgesic potency but cannot be titrated effectively to relieve severe pain in opioid-tolerant patients, and they show a relatively flat dose-response curve with respect to analgesia and respiratory depression compared to pure mu receptor agonists, although respiratory depression can occur with higher doses of buprenorphine when used as an analgesic in opioid-naïve infants and children [73]. All of these agents can precipitate withdrawal symptoms when used in opioid-tolerant patients. Buprenorphine is also being used increasingly as maintenance therapy for treatment of opioid addiction. The most common side effects are nausea, sedation, and dysphoria. Nalbuphine is used in some centers to treat patients who experience moderate pain associated with sickle cell vaso-occlusive episodes; efficacy is somewhat controversial [74,75]. We make extensive use of nalbuphine in the treatment of itching and nausea from epidural opioids [76,77]. Table 2 provides dosing guidelines for commonly used opioids.

Intermittent opioid boluses

Intermittent parenteral boluses of opioids result in wide variations in plasma opioid concentration. During the dosing period, patients can experience an increase in pain just before their next scheduled opioid dose, when their plasma opioid concentration is relatively low [78]. Shortly after receiving the next scheduled opioid dose, patients then can experience relatively good analgesia but with associated opioid side effects caused by high plasma opioid concentrations. To avoid the wide fluctuations in opioid plasma concentrations, analgesia, and side effects, continuous infusions and patient- or nurse-controlled analgesia are often used.

Continuous opioid infusions

Continuous infusions of opioids have been shown to provide effective postoperative pain relief in children [79–83]. Continuous opioid infusions result in near-constant state plasma opioid concentrations; however, this may be suboptimal in circumstances in which there are wide fluctuations in pain intensity. In these circumstances, additional opioid boluses are often necessary to provide additional analgesia, particularly when patients are undergoing potentially painful procedures. For example, a continuous infusion may provide good analgesia to a patient who recently underwent a thoracotomy and is lying still in bed. Additional boluses would be necessary, however, if the patient required chest physiotherapy or had frequent coughing. Morphine, hydromorphone, and fentanyl are the most commonly used opioids for continuous infusions. Initial morphine starting dose for continuous infusion is typically 0.025 mg/kg/h for children, although individual patients vary considerably in their effective infusion rates [79,80]. Neonates and young infants require lower starting infusion rates, ranging from as low as 0.005 mg/kg/h in preterm neonates to 0.015 mg/kg/h in infants aged 2 to 6 months [80–83].

Patient- and nurse-controlled analgesia

Patient-controlled analgesia (PCA) involves a delivery system that administers comparatively small preset doses of opioid, usually intravenously, whenever a patient depresses an attached button. A lockout period between doses, typically 5 to 10 minutes, prevents administration of repeated doses in a short time period. PCA devices also may administer a basal or continuous infusion along with these boluses and may have additional lockout features that set maximum doses over a longer time period, typically either 1 hour or 4 hours. PCA has been shown to be safe and effective in children aged 7 and older [84]. Although selected children aged 4 to 6 years may use PCA effectively, there is a higher frequency of failed analgesia in this age group, commonly because of lack of understanding of the causal connection between pushing a button and getting pain relief. PCA is widely used for various acute painful conditions, such as postoperative pain, cancer pain [85], and pain from sickle cell vaso-occlusive episodes. Some studies that compared PCA to continuous infusions suggested that PCA tends to produce either similar or lower pain scores, but with lower overall opioid dosing and lower opioid-related side effects compared to continuous infusions [86], although other studies have not supported this conclusion [87]. PCA is commonly used for cancer pain and palliative care in home and hospital settings.

The original concept behind PCA in adults was that having patients push their own buttons helped to ensure safety. If a patient is too sleepy to push the button, dosing ceases, the plasma concentrations fall, and the dosing is regulated in a safe range. Administration by surrogates has generated more controversy. Nurse-controlled analgesia is commonly used for infants and children who are cognitively or physically unable to push the button. Available evidence suggests that this is an efficient and safe way to titrate opioids in these patient groups, and a growing consensus favors use of nurse-controlled analgesia at pediatric centers worldwide [88,89]. Parent-controlled analgesia seems well established for children with advanced cancer or in palliative care for various illnesses. The use of parent-controlled analgesia outside of palliative care is more controversial. Advocates point out that parents know their children best and are good judges of when their child is in pain. This argument is especially compelling for children with developmental disabilities or children who have previously undergone multiple operative procedures.

Advocates of parent-controlled analgesia also note that in some hospitals with higher patient-to-nurse ratios, waiting for a child's nurse to push the button may result in delays in providing analgesia. Critics point out that nurses, unlike most parents, have extensive expertise in weighing the risks and benefits of opioids and are in a position to make better assessments of factors that may increase risk in opioid dose titration. They note that parents are not trained in these assessments and that their lack of objectivity may predispose to over-medication in some cases. We are aware of several critical incidents, including respiratory arrests and deaths, around the United States and in other countries associated with parent-controlled analgesia. Our view is that if parent-controlled analgesia in opioid-naïve subjects is to be considered, it should be approached with considerable caution, with a program for education of parents, protocols for frequent nursing observations, and potentially with use of electronic monitoring [89].

Currently, parent-controlled analgesia in our hospital is predominantly restricted to patients with cancer or in palliative care. PCA is administered as bolus dosing with or without a background continuous infusion. NSAIDs and acetaminophen are often used along with PCA to reduce total opioid use. Patients with mild to moderate pain typically experience good analgesia with on-demand PCA use. Patients with severe pain often require continuous infusion with their PCA to control their pain adequately. A relatively larger ratio of basal rate to bolus dosing is often used for patients with pain caused by cancer, sickle cell disease, or other chronic disease to provide effective analgesia without the need for frequent on-demand boluses. Studies in postoperative patients have shown that patients sleep better with nighttime background infusions, but in some of these studies they also have more frequent but self-limited brief desaturation episodes [90]. Morphine and hydromorphone are the most commonly used opioids for PCA. Fentanyl is also used in PCA. Typical starting opioid doses for PCA (and nurse-controlled analgesia) are listed in Table 3.

Opioid side effects and management

All opioids produce a range of side effects, including constipation, nausea and vomiting, pruritus, sedation, respiratory depression, and urinary retention

Table 3
Typical starting doses for patient-controlled analgesia

Drug	Bolus dose (μg/kg)	Continuous rate (μg/kg/h)	4-hour limit (μg/kg)
Morphine	20	4–15	300
Hydromorphone	5	1–3	60
Fentanyl	0.25	0.15	4

The usual lockout interval is 7 minutes.

[79]. Although individual patients may tolerate one opioid better than another, few data suggest that population prevalences of these side effects differ greatly among the commonly used opioids. Left untreated, in some cases the side effects of opioids can be as distressing as the pain for which they are being prescribed. Side effects should be anticipated and treated aggressively.

Constipation is nearly universal among patients who receive opioids. Unless there is diarrhea or other specific contraindication, stimulant laxatives should be prescribed per routine whenever patients are anticipated to require more than one to two doses of opioids [91]. Some evidence exists that oral naloxone can be effective in treating opioid-induced constipation. Novel enterally constrained [92–94] or peripherally constrained [95–97] opioid antagonists show outstanding promise in adult clinical trials in preventing opioid-induced bowel dysfunction in acute and chronic use.

Nausea and vomiting are caused by agonist activity at opioid receptors in the chemoreceptor trigger zone. Ondansetron is a selective $5-HT_3$ receptor antagonist and often is used in the treatment of nausea and vomiting. Phenothiazines, butyrophenones, and a related drug, metoclopramide, have been used for many years for treatment of nausea and vomiting. These drugs occasionally can produce extrapyramidal reactions, which can be treated with either centrally acting antihistamines, such as diphenhydramine, or central anticholinergics, such as benztropine. Droperidol is no longer recommended because of the risk of QT prolongation. Recent evidence supports the use of ultra–low-dose naloxone infusions (0.25 μg/kg/h) to reduce the frequency and severity of nausea while not antagonizing analgesia in adults [98] and children [99] who receive opioids. At these naloxone infusion rates, compared to placebo, there was no change in either opioid use or pain scores. These naloxone infusion rates are more than 20-fold below the infusion rates that typically produce measurable reversal of analgesia or respiratory depression. The mechanisms underlying this differential action involve different affinities and dose-response relationships for actions of opioids and antagonists on coupling of opioid receptors to either stimulatory or inhibitory G-proteins [100,101]. For patients who are opioid tolerant, it remains to be determined whether even lower starting naloxone infusion rates should be used to avoid precipitating withdrawal symptoms.

Opioid-induced pruritus can be distressing. It is often treated with antihistamines, such as diphenhydramine, although evidence is stronger for treatment with mu receptor antagonists, such as nalbuphine or ultra–low-dose infusions of naloxone, at the same rate of 0.25 μg/kg/h recommended for prevention of nausea and vomiting [99]. Antihistamines also can exacerbate sedation, constipation, and urinary retention.

Among children with advanced cancer, fatigue and somnolence are common [102–104]. Opioids are one among many factors that exacerbate these symptoms. In adults with cancer, HIV, and other serious illnesses, a robust amount of literature supports the use of stimulant drugs, such as methylphenidate, to antagonize somnolence and fatigue [105,106]. Methylphenidate provides additional analgesia and a rapid onset of antidepressant action [107]. It is typically dosed in the morning and midday or in a sustained-release formulation in the morning. Common opioid side effects and management are listed in Table 4.

Monitoring of patients receiving opioids

Opioids can be administered safely to infants and children provided safety protocols are in place [108]. Close nursing observation with standardized sedation scales and vital sign assessments is essential for all patients. Cardiorespiratory monitoring with alarms that sound in a centralized nursing station should be considered for certain patients. Infants who are younger than 6 months or older infants who have a history of apnea or prematurity should have cardiorespiratory monitoring when receiving opioids. Other types of patients in whom cardiorespiratory monitoring should be considered include opioid-naïve patients who are receiving continuous opioid infusions or patients with conditions that might place them at especially high risk for opioid-induced respiratory depression, such as a history of obstructive sleep apnea or certain craniofacial anomalies.

Table 4
Management of common opioid side effects

Side effect	Comments	Drug dosage
Nausea	Exclude other processes (eg, bowel obstruction) Consider switching to different opioid Use antiemetics	Metoclopramide 0.1–0.2 mg/kg PO/IV q 6 h Ondansetron 10–30 kg: 1–2 mg IV q 8 h >30 kg: 2–4 mg IV q 8 h Naloxone infusion 0.1–0.25 μg/kg/h Prochlorperazine 10–40 mg: 2.5 mg PR 1–3 times per day Adult: 2.5–10 mg IV/IM q 12 h 25 mg PR q 12 h
Pruritus	Exclude other causes (eg, drug allergy) Consider switching to different opioid Use antipruritics	Diphenhydramine 0.5 mg/kg PO/IV q 6 h Nalbuphine 10–20 μg/kg/dose IV q 6 h Naloxone infusion 0.1–0.25 μg/kg/h Hydroxyzine Child: 0.5–1 mg/kg PO q 6 h Adult: 25–75 mg/dose PO/IM q 6 h
Sedation	Add nonsedating analgesic (eg, ketorolac) and reduce opioid dose Consider switching to different opioid	Methylphenidate 0.05–0.2 mg/kg PO bid (morning and midday dosing) Dextroamphetamine 5–10 mg every day
Constipation	Regular use of stimulant and stool softener laxatives	Ducosate Child: 10–40 mg PO daily Adults: 50–200 mg PO daily Dulcolax Child: 5 mg PO/PR daily Adult: 10 mg PO/PR daily

Abbreviations: bid, twice a day; PO, orally; PR, rectally; q, every.

Local anesthesia

Uses of local anesthesia [109] in children include topical anesthesia for needle procedures or suture of lacerations, infiltration anesthesia for various procedures, including postoperative wound infiltration by surgeons, and various types of regional anesthesia primarily performed by anesthesiologists, including blockade of major nerves or plexuses, epidural anesthesia, and spinal anesthesia (see later section on postoperative pain). Pediatric hospitalists should have a familiarity with local anesthetic pharmacology and safety issues and with several forms of topical anesthesia and infiltration anesthesia [109,110]. Although they do not perform more specialized forms of regional anesthesia themselves, it is helpful for pediatric hospitalists to develop a basic familiarity with the uses, indications, and potential complications of these approaches, because they are being used widely for children postoperatively.

A predominant mechanism of local anesthetic action is via blockade of voltage-gated sodium channels. Blockade of sodium channels inhibits initiation and propagation of action potentials. If administered in excessive doses or if there is inadvertent intravascular injection, local anesthetic agents can generate serious reactions, including seizures, ectopy, arrhythmias, and severe myocardial depression. Dosing guidelines are detailed in Table 5. These dosing limits are particularly an issue for neonates and infants, both for single-dose administration and infusions. Inability to aspirate blood from a syringe does not exclude the possibility of needle placement in a vein, because veins may collapse upon aspiration. With infiltration anesthesia, continuous advancing or withdrawal of the needle during injection (so that the needle tip cannot remain in a vein for a significant fraction of the entire injection) is more effective in preventing intravascular injection and allows the infiltration to be accomplished more quickly than fixing the needle in one place and repeatedly aspirating. Buffering of lidocaine can reduce the pain of infiltration. Local anesthetic-induced seizures and myocardial depression are intensified greatly by hypoxemia, hypercarbia, or acidosis. If a patient develops twitching or other premonitory signs of toxicity, clinicians should administer supplemental oxygen immediately. If any doubt exists about adequacy of ventilation, the clinician should initiate assisted ventilation. Benzodiazepines, including lorazepam, midazolam, and diazepam, are first-line agents to stop local anesthetic-induced seizures.

Table 5
Local anesthetic dosing guidelines for infiltration anesthesia

Drug	<6 mo of age	>6 mo of age
Lidocaine	4 mg/kg	5 mg/kg
Bupivacaine	1.5 mg/kg	2 mg/kg

Suggested doses are intentionally more conservative than those listed in some textbooks and refer to non–epinephrine-containing solutions. Epinephrine 5 μg/mL (1:200,000) may increase the maximum safe doses by approximately 30% in children >6 months of age.

Nonpharmacologic approaches to pain management

In patients of all ages, the experience of pain and distress is modified by fear, anxiety, expectation, meaning of the pain, and various biologic/temperamental variables. Despite the extent of detail and emphasis in the preceding section, it must be emphasized that pain is best treated by individualized combination of drug therapies, various physical interventions, and use of a range of psychological approaches, including relaxation training, hypnosis and self-hypnosis, and several other cognitive-behavioral pain management interventions. Evidence supports various cognitive-behavioral approaches for brief painful procedures [111], pain caused by surgery [112], and various chronic pain conditions, including headaches, abdominal pain, and complex regional pain syndromes [113–118]. In our view, cognitive-behavioral intervention skills should be taught as a basic part of pediatric residency education [119,120]. Pediatric hospitalists should take a lead role in efforts to provide resources for pediatric inpatient care, including ready availability of clinicians with specific expertise in these areas, including child psychologists and child-life specialists [121]. Various complementary and alternative therapies are commonly used in pediatric hospitals [122]. Further research is needed to establish the risks, benefits, and costs of many of these interventions [123].

Specific painful conditions in infants and children

Acute postoperative pain

Depending on the type of surgery and patient-specific factors, postoperative pain may be treated with varying combinations of oral or IV opioids, acetaminophen, NSAIDs or COX-2 inhibitors, and regional anesthesia. For mild pain in patients who are able to tolerate oral intake postoperatively, oral dosing of opioids is preferred. Often, acetaminophen or NSAIDs or both are used with opioids to provide additional analgesia without additional opioid side effects. For more severe pain or for patients who cannot tolerate oral intake, IV opioids are usually necessary. For example, some patients who undergo a tonsillectomy typically have mild to moderate pain, but others require IV opioids for the first night until able to take oral opioids. Use of NSAIDs is controversial for these patients. Patients who have undergone spinal fusion usually have severe pain and require PCA therapy for several days postoperatively. Often, patients are placed on a basal rate and a cardiorespiratory monitor for the first several days and then receive plain PCA therapy. Patients are advised to dose their PCA just before getting out of bed or before starting physical therapy. Sometimes small doses of benzodiazepines are helpful for muscle spasms after spinal fusions. After several days of IV opioids, most patients who experience postoperative pain use less total daily opioids and are able to transition to oral opioids. Often, bolus doses of opioids are necessary for breakthrough pain while patients transition to oral opioids.

In adults, epidural analgesia and other forms of regional anesthesia are key components of efforts to improve and accelerate postoperative recovery [124]. Epidural infusions [125] are useful for infants and children who undergo major thoracic, abdominal, and pelvic operations. Continuous peripheral [126,127] or plexus [128,129] infusions are also useful for children who undergo major extremity orthopedic operations. Epidural infusions commonly involve combinations of local anesthetics with either opioids [125] or clonidine [130]. Opioids and clonidine act on receptors involved in pain transmission in the spinal dorsal horn. They provide markedly synergistic analgesia when combined with dilute local anesthetic infusions. An extensive body of literature confirms that these approaches can be applied with excellent safety and efficacy for infants and children and can improve the course of postoperative recovery for many types of surgery [125,131–133]. Detailed discussion of these issues is presented elsewhere [134]. Pediatric hospitalists often collaborate in the care of children who are receiving epidural, plexus, or peripheral nerve infusions and should be aware of potential physiologic effects and side effects (eg, vasodilation or motor blockade from local anesthetics, itching, sedation or hypoventilation from epidural opioids) and the impact of these infusions on postoperative assessments (eg, assessment of a tight cast or compartment syndrome in patients after orthopedic surgery).

Painful procedures

Brief diagnostic and therapeutic procedures are a major aspect of pediatric hospital practice [135–138]. Every hospital that cares for children should develop a regular multi-tiered program for management of these procedures. Topical analgesics such as EMLA [139], which is a eutectic mixture of local anesthetics lidocaine and prilocaine, lidocaine cream or tetracaine gel [140], lidocaine iontophoresis [141], and several others under current investigation [142] should be used for various minor needle procedures. Cognitive-behavioral interventions, such as guided imagery and hypnosis, also have been shown to be effective for procedural pain [143,144]. These techniques are limited in young children or persons with cognitive limitations. Analgesia for more invasive needle procedures, such as lumbar punctures, bone marrow biopsies and aspirates, and central venous line insertions or removals, generally should involve the use of either conscious sedation or general anesthesia. Procedural sedation often is performed safely by oncologists and pediatricians with the use of specific sedation protocols according to the American Academy of Pediatrics guidelines, although considerable controversy remains over several specific aspects of these guidelines [145–148]. Involvement by pediatric anesthesiologists is recommended for children who are at increased risk or require general anesthesia. Our view is that most pediatric centers should have a two-tiered system in which pediatric subspecialists (eg, oncologists, gastroenterologists) perform some sedation procedures and pediatric anesthesiologists are available on a regular basis for more involved procedures or higher risk patients.

Cancer pain

Children with cancer frequently experience pain as a result of tumor at the time of initial diagnosis [149], cancer treatment, or tumor spread with progressive disease [150]. Treatment of cancer often results in painful mucositis and peripheral neuropathies [151,152] and the need for repeated painful needle procedures, such as bone marrow aspirates and lumbar punctures. Treatment of painful procedures is discussed in a previous section.

Mucositis involves painful mucosal inflammation caused by chemotherapy or radiation therapy. Evidence for various preventive or topical therapies has been mixed [153,154]. For cases in which pain persists despite topical therapies, opioids should be used. PCA or nurse-controlled analgesia often is used for patients who undergo bone marrow transplantation; they often have severe pain with swallowing for up to 2 weeks [55]. Tumors can produce pain by infiltrating bone, stretching capsules such as the spleen, or infiltrating viscera and nerves. Leukemias and lymphomas commonly cause pain by infiltration of solid viscera, distention of spleen and liver, or bone marrow infiltration. Exquisite neuropathic pain can be a result of tumor invasion of nerves and plexuses.

For most adults with advanced cancer, a stepwise program of analgesic therapy, as codified by the World Health Organization, can provide good or adequate pain relief with a tolerable side-effect profile [155,156]. The initial formulations of this program involved a three-step "ladder" with nonopioid analgesics, including acetaminophen and NSAIDs, for mild pain, so-called weak opioids, including codeine and low-dose oxycodone, for moderate pain, and so-called strong opioids, especially morphine, for severe pain. Oral dosing of opioids was recommended whenever feasible. Experience with children suggested that this approach also could be effective for most children [157], although a retrospective report on parents' recollections of symptom management before the end of life found that pain and other symptoms, especially fatigue, were common, produced considerable suffering, and at times were not addressed adequately by clinicians [158].

A detailed discussion of analgesic therapy for cancer pain in children is presented elsewhere [150]. For patients with severe pain, oral sustained-release preparations of morphine are convenient for providing near-constant basal analgesic effect with dosing three times daily [159]. Sustained-release formulations of oxycodone and hydromorphone are also available, although they have received less pediatric study. For most of these formulations, if the tablets are crushed, then the sustained-release properties are lost. For young patients and persons who are unable to swallow pills, methadone elixir can provide a prolonged duration of action. Often a prolonged-duration opioid is prescribed along with an immediate-acting opioid, with the former on a schedule and the latter on an as-needed basis. Oral dosing may fail for some patients with rapidly escalating pain and for children who are unable to tolerate oral opioids because of mucositis, vomiting, or ileus, although in some cases, oral-mucosal absorption of morphine elixir may be effective. IV infusions and IV boluses or PCA can permit rapid titration for escalating pain. If limiting side effects are present with one opioid, there may be a role for switching or rotation among different opioids. Key aspects of opioid analgesia for children with cancer include individualized dosing, titration to clinical effect, and proactive treatment of opioid side effects, as detailed previously in the section on opioid side effects.

There remains a small subgroup of children with cancer who require truly massive opioid dose escalation (ie, more than 100-fold above starting infusion rates) [157], who have intolerable side effects with standard dose escalation and side effect management, or who alternate between excessive sedation and inadequate analgesia. In selected cases, regional anesthetic approaches may be considered, although several technical, pharmacologic, logistic, and quality-of-life considerations are involved in a choice of this type of therapy [160]. In our practice, this most commonly involves an implanted intrathecal port for combined infusions of local anesthestic agents, opioids, and clonidine. In many cases, they can provide effective analgesia for patients with unremitting neuropathic pain, pain from tumor involvement of the spine, or refractory abdominal, pelvic, or limb pain. In other situations, in which there is no feasible option to provide adequate analgesia without some degree of sedation, there may be a limited role for infusions of sedatives [161,162]. In our view, sedative infusions should not be a routine aspect of pediatric end-of-life care [163] but should be considered only on an individual basis and only in conjunction with active efforts to relieve pain and suffering by use of opioids and other approaches [164].

Sickle cell vaso-occlusive episodes

Patients with sickle hemoglobinopathies are commonly admitted to hospital with pain, which is most commonly associated with vaso-occlusive episodes, although in each case, clinicians must use the interval history, physical examination, and focused laboratory investigations to evaluate the probability of various other acute processes that may require more specific treatments (eg, osteomyelitis, pneumonia, stroke, priapism, acute cholecystitis or cholelithiasis, splenic sequestration, or various other abdominal emergencies). NSAIDs and opioids should be prescribed for moderate to severe pain, and opioids should be titrated as needed to relieve pain, as limited by severe sedation or hypoventilation. PCA is widely used for these episodes. It should be noted that surveys suggest that with current standards of practice and even in cases in which PCA is used, a considerable percentage of patients with vaso-occlusive episodes continue to experience severe pain on a regular basis [75,165].

Screaming of unknown origin

Children with neurologic disorders, severe developmental delay, neuro-degeneration, or severe motor impairments who have persistent agitation, distress, or screaming sometimes are admitted to hospital for diagnostic evaluation and therapeutic trials. In some cases, evaluation discloses a specific nociceptive cause (eg, fractures, hip dislocations, esophagitis, ulcers, pancreatitis). In other cases, adjustment of anticonvulsant or antispasm medications may bring relief of apparent distress. In many other cases, these evaluations can be frustrating for patients, families, and clinicians. There is a need for more systematic and evidence-based approaches to these diagnostic and therapeutic interventions.

Recurrent benign pains of childhood

Recurrent headaches, abdominal pains, chest pains, and limb pains are common among children and adolescents. For the most part, diagnostic evaluation and therapeutic trials are managed by community pediatricians and pediatric subspecialists on an outpatient basis. On occasion, patients are admitted to the care of pediatric hospitalists for urgent diagnostic evaluation or when the severity of pain or distress in the family prompts admission for pain treatment. In considering hospital admission for these conditions, it is often helpful to engage primary clinicians and families in a discussion before admission regarding realistic goals of a hospital stay. Clinicians should be wary of promising either complete pain relief or a final diagnostic answer in many of these situations.

Recurrent abdominal pain (RAP) is a common problem that occurs in school-aged children and is frequently encountered by primary care physicians who care for children. Apley and colleagues [166,167] reported that 10% to 25% of all school-aged children experience RAP. An organic cause for RAP is rarely found in most cases. Some studies have attempted to identify a specific cause for RAP in selected children, however. For example, some children with RAP improve with dietary fiber supplementation, even without underlying symptoms of constipation [168]. Other studies support that children without a clear history of lactose intolerance have positive findings on lactose breath hydrogen testing and experience improvement in RAP symptoms when placed on a lactose-restricted diet [169], although this remains an area of controversy [117]. In some cases, RAP evolves into irritable bowel syndrome in adolescence and adulthood [170,171].

There are common features of RAP with respect to clinical characteristics. Most children with RAP are between the ages of 4 and 16 and report episodic, periumbilical pain. The pain is nonradiating, and children are typically medically well without signs of systemic illness. A thorough history and physical examination are essential in distinguishing RAP from other types of abdominal pain. A psychosocial history is also essential for understanding how the family and child cope with pain and identifying behaviors that suggest disability (ie, school avoidance) [171–175]. The history and physical examination should serve as a guide to diagnostic testing. Extensive testing is generally not helpful and may heighten parental and patient anxiety. Reasonable screening tests include a complete blood count, stool guaiac, and urinalysis. Children who have fevers, weight loss, pain that is not periumbilical, or a family history of inflammatory bowel disease require further evaluation. Abnormalities on physical examination or laboratory testing may guide additional investigation. In children who experience chronic persistent abdominal pain rather than the more characteristic episodic pain of RAP, one study found that laparoscopy identified treatable conditions in a surprisingly high percentage of cases [176].

Treatment of RAP should emphasize improved coping skills through cognitive-behavioral therapy [117,177]. Regular school attendance and participation in family and social activities are essential. Reassurance and education to families and patients also are helpful in reducing pain behaviors. Although tricyclic antidepressants are often tried, limited data are available on their efficacy in the treatment of RAP.

Chest pain frequently is experienced by children and adolescents and accounts for at least 65,000 physician visits annually. It is often a source of significant worry for patients and parents because of ominous signs associated with chest pain in adult patients with cardiac disease. Chest pain in children and adolescents is rarely caused by underlying cardiac etiologies, however. In a study by Fyfe and Moodie [178], only 6% of patients who were referred to a pediatric cardiologist for the evaluation of chest pain were diagnosed with cardiac diseases that typically result in chest pain. The most common causes include musculoskeletal conditions, such as costrochondritis and muscle strain from coughing. No specific causes are found in a significant number of children and adolescents. Other causes include slipping rib syndrome, asthma, and esophageal reflux or spasm. In a 2-year follow-up study by Selbst and colleagues [179], new organic pathology was rarely uncovered in most cases and 53% of patients had resolution of their symptoms.

Neuropathic pain refers to pain caused by abnormal excitability in peripheral or central nerves, as contrasted with nociceptive pain, which involves the more common process of detection and afferent signaling of tissue injury or inflammation. Common causes of neuropathic pain in children include complex regional pain, peripheral nerve injuries as a result of extremity trauma, and surgery. Other causes include tumor involvement of nerves and plexuses, metabolic disorders, and chemotherapeutic drugs, such as vincristine. Some causes of neuropathic pain that are relatively common in adults, including postherpetic neuralgia, trigeminal neuralgia, and diabetic neuropathy, are relatively less common in children.

Diagnosis of neuropathic pain is based on a thorough history and physical examination, including a neurologic examination, which also may help to detect underlying associated disease processes. Many children have difficulty describing the pain associated with neuropathic conditions, and they may or may not use terms commonly chosen by adults, including burning, shooting, pins and needles, or tingling. Characteristic physical examination findings include allodynia and dysesthesia. Allodynia describes pain associated with light touch of the skin and suggests abnormalities in sensory processing. In selected cases, nerve conduction velocity and electromyographic studies may help to confirm or refute proposed diagnoses. These studies can be painful, and nerve conduction velocities detect compound action potentials in large fibers but not in the smaller, slower-conducting C-fibers and A-delta fibers that are sometimes involved in painful neuropathies. Quantitative sensory testing is a noninvasive method to determine vibration and thermal detection and pain thresholds and sensory abnormalities. Quantitative sensory testing is well tolerated by children and does not require sedation [180]. In selected cases, quantitative sensory testing may complement information derived from nerve conductive velocity and electro-myographic studies.

The use of drugs for the treatment of neuropathic pain in children is extrapolated from adult studies since there are few prospective pediatric trials. Tricyclics and anticonvulsants are often the first line drugs used. Tricyclics can be also beneficial in improving sleep disturbances. Nortriptyline and amitrip-tyline are most commonly used, usually in twice daily dosing with a larger portion of the dose given before bedtime. A baseline screening ECG is recom-mended prior to intitiation of tricyclics. Anticonvulsants such as gabapentin and carbamezepine, and trileptal have been shown to be effective for some neuro-pathic pain conditions in adults. Gabapentin is widely used in children, partly due to its better safety profile as compared to other anticonvulsants and to tricyclics. Most frequent side effects are somnolence and dizziness. There is no evidence to suggest that anticonvulsants are more effective than tricyclics in treating neuropathic pain in children. Additional prospective pediatric studies are needed. The use of opioids in the treatment of nonmalignant neuropathic pain is somewhat controversial. In some cases, opioids do provide good analgesia but at does that produce excessive and intolerable sedation and other side effects. Opioids are more often used in combination with other drugs such as tricyclics or anticonvulsants for treatment of neuropathic pain due to cancers. In these cases, opioid side effects should be anticipated and managed aggressively.

Complex Regional Pain Syndrome Type 1 (CRPS1), also known as Reflex Sympathetic Dystrophy or Reflex Neurovascular Dystrophy, is a group of conditions characterized by limb pain with neuropathic descriptors, especially allodynia, associated temperature changes, swelling, cyanosis, mottling, in-creased sweating, or other signs of autonomic/neurovascular dysfunction. Where these findings occur along with signs of partial or complete injury in the distribution of a specific peripheral nerve, the terms causalgia or CRPS2 are used. In a majority of cases, some type of initiating event can be identified; these may range from major fractures or surgeries to a minor bump or sprain. A majority of children and adolescents with CRPS are female with a lower limb affected. In about 25% of cases, a second limb becomes affected without associated injury. CRPS is rare in children younger than 8 years of age. The degree of dysfunction varies widely among patients with CRPS. The predomi-nant treatment of pediatric CRPS involves a program of patient and parent education, intensive physical therapy, and cognitive-behavioral treatment [118,181]. For a selected subgroup of patients, a course of epidural analgesia or peripheral nerve blockade may produce initial reduction in pain, improvements in limb perfusion, and increases in limb motion. However, for the majority of pediatric patients, the predominant emphasis should be on active mobilization of the limb and restoration of normal activities. Pediatric hospitalists may become involved in care of these patients during intensive rehabilitation admissions.

Summary

Pediatric hospitalists should make pain assessment and treatment a high priority and a central part of their daily practice. Efforts at improving pain treatment in pediatric hospitals should be multidisciplinary and should involve combined use of pharmacologic and non-pharmacologic approaches. While available information can permit effective treatment of pain for a majority of children in hospitals, there is a need for more research on pediatric analgesic pharmacology, on a variety of non-pharmacologic treatments, and on different models of delivery of care.

References

[1] Beyer JE, Denyes MJ, Villarruel AM. The creation, validation, and continuing development of the Oucher: a measure of pain intensity in children. J Pediatr Nurs 1992;7(5):335–46.

[2] Bieri D, Reeve RA, Champion GD, et al. The Faces Pain Scale for the self-assessment of the severity of pain experienced by children: development, initial validation, and preliminary investigation for ratio scale properties. Pain 1990;41(2):139–50.

[3] Chambers CT, Craig KD. An intrusive impact of anchors in children's faces pain scales. Pain 1998;78:27–37.

[4] McGrath P, Seifert C, Speechley K, et al. A new analogue scale for assessing children's pain: an initial validation study. Pain 1996;64:435–43.

[5] Merkel SI, Voepel-Lewis T, Shayevitz JR, et al. The FLACC: a behavioral scale for scoring postoperative pain in young children. Pediatr Nurs 1997;23:293–7.

[6] Stevens B, Johnston C, Petryshen P, et al. Premature infant pain profile: development and initial validation. Clin J Pain 1996;12:13–22.

[7] Beyer JE, McGrath PJ, Berde CB. Discordance between self-report and behavioral pain measures in children aged 3–7 years after surgery. J Pain Symptom Manage 1990;5(6):350–6.

[8] Schechter NL, Blankson V, Pachter LM, et al. The ouchless place: no pain, children's gain. Pediatrics 1997;99:890–4.

[9] Berde CB, Sethna NF. Analgesics for the treatment of pain in children. N Engl J Med 2002;347:1094–103.

[10] Vane JR, Botting RM. Mechanism of action of nonsteroidal anti-inflammatory drugs. Am J Med 1998;104:2S–8S [discussion 21S–2S].

[11] Needleman P, Isakson PC. The discovery and function of COX-2. J Rheumatol Suppl 1997; 49:6–8.

[12] Warner TD, Vojnovic I, Giuliano F, et al. Cyclooxygenases 1, 2, and 3 and the production

of prostaglandin I2: investigating the activities of acetaminophen and cyclooxygenase-2-selective inhibitors in rat tissues. J Pharmacol Exp Ther 2004;310:642–7.

[13] Sciulli MG, Seta F, Tacconelli S, et al. Effects of acetaminophen on constitutive and inducible prostanoid biosynthesis in human blood cells. Br J Pharmacol 2003;138:634–41.

[14] Davies NM, Good RL, Roupe KA, et al. Cyclooxygenase-3: axiom, dogma, anomaly, enigma or splice error? Not as easy as 1, 2, 3. J Pharm Pharm Sci 2004;7:217–26.

[15] Korpela R, Korvenoja P, Meretoja OA. Morphine-sparing effect of acetaminophen in pediatric day-case surgery. Anesthesiology 1999;91:442–7.

[16] Heubi JE, Barbacci MB, Zimmerman HJ. Therapeutic misadventures with acetaminophen: hepatoxicity after multiple doses in children. J Pediatr 1998;132:22–7.

[17] van Lingen RA, Deinum HT, Quak CM, et al. Multiple-dose pharmacokinetics of rectally administered acetaminophen in term infants. Clin Pharmacol Ther 1999;66:509–15.

[18] Birmingham PK, Tobin MJ, Henthorn TK, et al. Twenty-four-hour pharmacokinetics of rectal acetaminophen in children: an old drug with new recommendations. Anesthesiology 1997;87(2):244–52.

[19] Van Overmeire B, Touw D, Schepens PJ, et al. Ibuprofen pharmacokinetics in preterm infants with patent ductus arteriosus. Clin Pharmacol Ther 2001;70:336–43.

[20] Olkkola KT, Maunuksela EL. The pharmacokinetics of postoperative intravenous ketorolac tromethamine in children. Br J Clin Pharmacol 1991;31:182–4.

[21] Tramer MR, Williams JE, Carroll D, et al. Comparing analgesic efficacy of non-steroidal anti-inflammatory drugs given by different routes in acute and chronic pain: a qualitative systematic review. Acta Anaesthesiol Scand 1998;42:71–9.

[22] Vetter T, Heiner E. Intravenous ketorolac as an adjuvant to pediatric patient-controlled analgesia with morphine. J Clin Anesth 1994;6:110–3.

[23] Lesko SM, Mitchell AA. Renal function after short-term ibuprofen use in infants and children. Pediatrics 1997;100:954–7.

[24] Lesko S, Mitchell A. An assessment of the safety of pediatric ibuprofen: a practitioner-based randomized clinical trial. JAMA 1995;273(12):929–33.

[25] Tramer MR, Moore RA, Reynolds DJ, et al. Quantitative estimation of rare adverse events which follow a biological progression: a new model applied to chronic NSAID use. Pain 2000;85:169–82.

[26] Giannini EBE, Brewer EJ, Miller ML, et al. Ibuprofen suspension in the treatment of juvenile rheumatoid arthritis. J Pediatr 1990;117:645–52.

[27] Burd RS, Tobias JD. Ketorolac for pain management after abdominal surgical procedures in infants. South Med J 2002;95:331–3.

[28] Lago P, Bettiol T, Salvadori S, et al. Safety and efficacy of ibuprofen versus indomethacin in preterm infants treated for patent ductus arteriosus: a randomised controlled trial. Eur J Pediatr 2002;161:202–7.

[29] Rusy LM, Houck CS, Sullivan LJ, et al. A double-blind evaluation of ketorolac tromethamine versus acetaminophen in pediatric tonsillectomy: analgesia and bleeding. Anesth Analg 1995; 80:226–9.

[30] Moiniche S, Romsing J, Dahl JB, et al. Nonsteroidal antiinflammatory drugs and the risk of operative site bleeding after tonsillectomy: a quantitative systematic review. Anesth Analg 2003;96:68–77.

[31] Krishna S, Hughes LF, Lin SY. Postoperative hemorrhage with nonsteroidal anti-inflammatory drug use after tonsillectomy: a meta-analysis. Arch Otolaryngol Head Neck Surg 2003;129:1086–9.

[32] Gerstenfeld LC, Thiede M, Seibert K, et al. Differential inhibition of fracture healing by non-selective and cyclooxygenase-2 selective non-steroidal anti-inflammatory drugs [see comment]. J Orthop Res 2003;21:670–5.

[33] Goodman SB, Ma T, Mitsunaga L, et al. Temporal effects of a COX-2-selective NSAID on bone ingrowth. J Biomed Mater Res A 2005;72A:279–87.

[34] Harder AT, An YH. The mechanisms of the inhibitory effects of nonsteroidal anti-inflammatory drugs on bone healing: a concise review. J Clin Pharmacol 2003;43:807–15.

[35] Burd RS, Tobias JD. Ketorolac for pain management after abdominal surgical procedures in infants. South Med J 2002;95:331–3.
[36] Laine L, Harper S, Simon T, et al. A randomized trial comparing the effect of rofecoxib, a cyclooxygenase 2-specific inhibitor, with that of ibuprofen on the gastroduodenal mucosa of patients with osteoarthritis. Rofecoxib Osteoarthritis Endoscopy Study Group. Gastroenterology 1999;117(4):776–83.
[37] Goldstein JL, Silverstein FE, Agrawal NM, et al. Reduced risk of upper gastrointestinal ulcer complications with celecoxib, a novel COX-2 inhibitor. Am J Gastroenterol 2000;95(7): 1681–90.
[38] Leese PT, Hubbard RC, Karim A, et al. Effects of celecoxib, a novel cyclooxygenase-2 inhibitor, on platelet function in healthy adults: a randomized, controlled trial. J Clin Pharmacol 2000;40(2):124–32.
[39] Levesque LE, Brophy JM, Zhang B. The risk for myocardial infarction with cyclooxygenase-2 inhibitors: a population study of elderly adults. Ann Intern Med 2005;142:481–9.
[40] Nussmeier NA, Whelton AA, Brown MT, et al. Complications of the COX-2 inhibitors parecoxib and valdecoxib after cardiac surgery. N Engl J Med 2005;352:1081–91.
[41] Pickering AE, Bridge HS, Nolan J, et al. Double-blind, placebo-controlled analgesic study of ibuprofen or rofecoxib in combination with paracetamol for tonsillectomy in children. Br J Anaesth 2002;88:72–7.
[42] Sheeran PW, Rose JB, Fazi LM, et al. Rofecoxib administration to paediatric patients undergoing adenotonsillectomy. Paediatr Anaesth 2004;14:579–83.
[43] Danesh BJ, McLaren M, Russell RI, et al. Comparison of the effect of aspirin and choline magnesium trisalicylate on thromboxane biosynthesis in human platelets: role of the acetyl moiety. Haemostasis 1989;19:169–73.
[44] Schechter N, Allen D, Hanson K. Status of paediatric pain control: a comparison of hospital analgesic usage in children and adults. Paediatrics 1986;77:11–5.
[45] Bouwmeester NJ, van den Anker JN, Hop WC, et al. Age- and therapy-related effects on morphine requirements and plasma concentrations of morphine and its metabolites in postoperative infants. Br J Anaesth 2003;90:642–52.
[46] Bouwmeester NJ, Hop WC, van Dijk M, et al. Postoperative pain in the neonate: age-related differences in morphine requirements and metabolism. Intensive Care Med 2003;29:2009–15.
[47] Kart T, Christrup LL, Rasmussen M. Recommended use of morphine in neonates, infants and children based on a literature review: Part 2. Clinical use. Paediatr Anaesth 1997;7:93–101.
[48] Treluyer JM, Gueret G, Cheron G, et al. Developmental expression of CYP2C and CYP2C-dependent activities in the human liver: in-vivo/in-vitro correlation and inducibility. Pharmacogenetics 1997;7:441–52.
[49] Bhat R, Abu-Harb M, Chari G, et al. Morphine metabolism in acutely ill preterm newborn infants. J Pediatr 1992;120:795–9.
[50] Purcell-Jones G, Dorman F, Sumner E. The use of opioids in neonates: a retrospective study of 933 cases. Anaesthesia 1987;42:1316–20.
[51] Bragg P, Zwass MS, Lau M, et al. Opioid pharmacodynamics in neonatal dogs: differences between morphine and fentanyl. J Appl Physiol 1995;79:1519–24.
[52] Moore A, Collins S, Carroll D, et al. Paracetamol with and without codeine in acute pain: a quantitative systematic review. Pain 1997;70:193–201.
[53] Williams DG, Patel A, Howard RF. Pharmacogenetics of codeine metabolism in an urban population of children and its implications for analgesic reliability. Br J Anaesth 2002; 89:839–45.
[54] Collins JJ, Geake J, Grier HE, et al. Patient-controlled analgesia for mucositis pain in children: a three-period crossover study comparing morphine and hydromorphone. J Pediatr 1996;129(5):722–8.
[55] Coda BA, Donaldson G, Bohl S, et al. Comparative efficacy of patient-controlled administration of morphine, hydromorphone, or sufentanil for the treatment of oral mucositis pain following bone marrow transplantation. Pain 1997;72:333–46.

[56] Holdsworth MT, Raisch DW, Winter SS, et al. Pain and distress from bone marrow aspirations and lumbar punctures. Ann Pharmacother 2003;37:17–22.

[57] Ginsberg B, Howell S, Glass PS, et al. Pharmacokinetic model-driven infusion of fentanyl in children. Anesthesiology 1996;85:1268–75.

[58] Kapila A, Glass PS, Jacobs JR, et al. Measured context-sensitive half-times of remifentanil and alfentanil. Anesthesiology 1995;83:968–75.

[59] Egan TD, Minto CF, Hermann DJ, et al. Remifentanil versus alfentanil: comparative pharmacokinetics and pharmacodynamics in healthy adult male volunteers. Anesthesiology 1996;84:821–33.

[60] Scholz J, Steinfath M, Schulz M. Clinical pharmacokinetics of alfentanil, fentanyl and sufentanil: an update. Clin Pharmacokinet 1996;31:275–92.

[61] Fahnenstich H, Steffan J, Kau N, et al. Fentanyl-induced chest wall rigidity and laryngospasm in preterm and term infants. Crit Care Med 2000;28:836–9.

[62] Collins JJ, Dunkel IJ, Gupta SK, et al. Transdermal fentanyl in children with cancer pain: feasibility, tolerability, and pharmacokinetic correlates. J Pediatr 1999;134(3):319–23.

[63] Schechter NL, Weisman SJ, Rosenblum M, et al. The use of oral transmucosal fentanyl citrate for painful procedures in children. Pediatrics 1995;95(3):335–9.

[64] Payne R. Factors influencing quality of life in cancer patients: the role of transdermal fentanyl in the management of pain. Semin Oncol 1998;25:47–53.

[65] Fine P, Marcus M, De Boer A, et al. An open label study of oral transmucosal fentanyl citrate (OTFC) for the treatment of breakthrough cancer pain. Pain 1991;45:149–53.

[66] Portenoy RK, Payne R, Coluzzi P, et al. Oral transmucosal fentanyl citrate (OTFC) for the treatment of breakthrough pain in cancer patients: a controlled dose titration study. Pain 1999;79:303–12.

[67] Ross AK, Davis PJ, Dear GL, et al. Pharmacokinetics of remifentanil in anesthetized pediatric patients undergoing elective surgery or diagnostic procedures. Anesth Analg 2001; 93:1393–401.

[68] Berde CB, Beyer JE, Bournaki MC, et al. Comparison of morphine and methadone for prevention of postoperative pain in 3- to 7-year-old children. J Pediatr 1991;119(1 Pt 1):136–41.

[69] Davis AM, Inturrisi CE. d-Methadone blocks morphine tolerance and N-methyl-D-aspartate-induced hyperalgesia. J Pharmacol Exp Ther 1999;289(2):1048–53.

[70] Mercadante S, Casuccio A, Fulfaro F, et al. Switching from morphine to methadone to improve analgesia and tolerability in cancer patients: a prospective study. J Clin Oncol 2001; 19(11):2898–904.

[71] Ripamonti C, De Conno F, Groff L, et al. Equianalgesic dose/ratio between methadone and other opioid agonists in cancer pain: comparison of two clinical experiences. Ann Oncol 1998;9:79–83.

[72] Ripamonti C, Groff L, Brunelli C, et al. Switching from morphine to oral methadone in treating cancer pain: what is the equianalgesic dose ratio? J Clin Oncol 1998;16:3216–21.

[73] Olkkola KT, Leijala MA, Maunuksela EL. Paediatric ventilatory effects of morphine and buprenorphine revisited. Paediatr Anaesth 1995;5:303–5.

[74] Woods GM, Parson PM, Strickland DK. Efficacy of nalbuphine as a parenteral analgesic for the treatment of painful episodes in children with sickle cell disease. J Assoc Acad Minor Phys 1990;1:90–2.

[75] Beyer JE. Judging the effectiveness of analgesia for children and adolescents during vaso-occlusive events of sickle cell disease. J Pain Symptom Manage 2000;19:63–72.

[76] Cohen SE, Ratner EF, Kreitzman TR, et al. Nalbuphine is better than naloxone for treatment of side effects after epidural morphine. Anesth Analg 1992;75:747–52.

[77] Wang JJ, Ho ST, Tzeng JI. Comparison of intravenous nalbuphine infusion versus naloxone in the prevention of epidural morphine-related side effects. Reg Anesth Pain Med 1998;23: 479–84.

[78] Lynn AM, Nespeca MK, Bratton SL, et al. Intravenous morphine in postoperative infants: intermittent bolus dosing versus targeted continuous infusions. Pain 2000;88:89–95.

[79] Esmail Z, Montgomery C, Courtrn C, et al. Efficacy and complications of morphine infusions in postoperative paediatric patients. Paediatr Anaesth 1999;9:321–7.

[80] Lynn A, Nespeca MK, Bratton SL, et al. Clearance of morphine in postoperative infants during intravenous infusion: the influence of age and surgery. Anesth Analg 1998;86(5): 958–63.

[81] Koren G, Butt W, Chinyanga H, et al. Postoperative morphine infusion in newborn infants: assessment of disposition characteristics and safety. J Pediatr 1985;107:963–7.

[82] Farrington EA, McGuinness GA, Johnson GF, et al. Continuous intravenous morphine infusion in postoperative newborn infants. Am J Perinatol 1993;10:84–7.

[83] Lynn AM, Nespeca MK, Opheim KE, et al. Respiratory effects of intravenous morphine infusions in neonates, infants, and children after cardiac surgery. Anesth Analg 1993; 77:695–701.

[84] Berde CB, Lehn BM, Yee JD, et al. Patient-controlled analgesia in children and adolescents: a randomized, prospective comparison with intramuscular administration of morphine for postoperative analgesia. J Pediatr 1991;118:460–6.

[85] Mackie AM, Coda BC, Hill HF. Adolescents use patient-controlled analgesia effectively for relief from prolonged oropharyngeal mucositis pain. Pain 1991;46:265–9.

[86] Pillitteri LC, Clark RE. Comparison of a patient-controlled analgesia system with continuous infusion for administration of diamorphine for mucositis. Transplantation 1998;22(5):495–8.

[87] Peters JW, Bandell Hoekstra IE, Huijer Abu-Saad H, et al. Patient controlled analgesia in children and adolescents: a randomized controlled trial. Paediatr Anaesth 1999;9:235–41.

[88] Kanagasundaram SA, Cooper MG, Lane LJ. Nurse-controlled analgesia using a patient-controlled analgesia device: an alternative strategy in the management of severe cancer pain in children. J Paediatr Child Health 1997;33:352–5.

[89] Monitto CL, Greenberg RS, Kost-Byerly S, et al. The safety and efficacy of parent-/nurse-controlled analgesia in patients less than six years of age. Anesth Analg 2000;91:573–9.

[90] McNeely JK, Trentadue NC. Comparison of patient-controlled analgesia with and without nighttime morphine infusion following lower extremity surgery in children. J Pain Symptom Manage 1997;13:268–73.

[91] Sykes NP. The relationship between opioid use and laxative use in terminally ill cancer patients. Palliat Med 1998;12(5):375–82.

[92] Wolff BG, Michelassi F, Gerkin TM, et al. Alvimopan postoperative ileus study: alvimopan, a novel, peripherally acting mu opioid antagonist. Results of a multicenter, randomized, double-blind, placebo-controlled, phase III trial of major abdominal surgery and postoperative ileus. Ann Surg 2004;240:728–34.

[93] Paulson DM, Kennedy DT, Donovick RA, et al. Alvimopan: an oral, peripherally acting, mu-opioid receptor antagonist for the treatment of opioid-induced bowel dysfunction. A 21-day treatment-randomized clinical trial. J Pain 2005;6:184–92.

[94] Taguchi A, Sharma N, Saleem RM, et al. Selective postoperative inhibition of gastrointestinal opioid receptors. N Engl J Med 2001;345:935–40.

[95] Yuan CS, Foss JF, O'Connor M, et al. Effects of intravenous methylnaltrexone on opioid-induced gut motility and transit time changes in subjects receiving chronic methadone therapy: a pilot study. Pain 1999;83:631–5.

[96] Yuan CS, Foss JF, O'Connor M, et al. Methylnaltrexone prevents morphine-induced delay in oral-cecal transit time without affecting analgesia: a double-blind randomized placebo-controlled trial. Clin Pharmacol Ther 1996;59:469–75.

[97] Yuan CS, Foss JF, Osinski J, et al. The safety and efficacy of oral methylnaltrexone in preventing morphine-induced delay in oral-cecal transit time. Clin Pharmacol Ther 1997;61: 467–75.

[98] Cepeda MS, Alvarez H, Morales O, et al. Addition of ultralow dose naloxone to postoperative morphine PCA: unchanged analgesia and opioid requirement but decreased incidence of opioid side effects. Pain 2004;107:41–6.

[99] Maxwell LG, Kaufmann SC, Bitzer S, et al. The effects of a small-dose naloxone infusion

on opioid-induced side effects and analgesia in children and adolescents treated with intravenous patient-controlled analgesia: a double-blind, prospective, randomized, controlled study. Anesth Analg 2005;100:953–8.

[100] Crain SM, Shen KF. Antagonists of excitatory opioid receptor functions enhance morphine's analgesic potency and attenuate opioid tolerance/dependence liability. Pain 2000;84:121–31.

[101] Crain SM, Shen KF. Modulatory effects of Gs-coupled excitatory opioid receptor functions on opioid analgesia, tolerance, and dependence. Neurochem Res 1996;21:1347–51.

[102] Hockenberry-Eaton M, Hinds PS, Alcoser P, et al. Fatigue in children and adolescents with cancer. J Pediatr Oncol Nurs 1998;15(3):172–82.

[103] Hinds PS, Hockenberry-Eaton M, Quargnenti A, et al. Fatigue in 7- to 12-year-old patients with cancer from the staff perspective: an exploratory study. Oncol Nurs Forum 1999;26(1):37–45.

[104] Wolfe J, Grier HE, Klar N, et al. Symptoms and suffering at the end of life in children with cancer. N Engl J Med 2000;342:326–33.

[105] Bruera E, Chadwick S, Brenneis C, et al. Methylphenidate associated with narcotics for the treatment of cancer pain. Cancer Treat Rep 1987;71:67–70.

[106] Breitbart W, Rosenfeld B, Kaim M, et al. A randomized, double-blind, placebo-controlled trial of psychostimulants for the treatment of fatigue in ambulatory patients with human immunodeficiency virus disease. Arch Intern Med 2001;161:411–20.

[107] Homsi J, Nelson KA, Sarhill N, et al. A phase II study of methylphenidate for depression in advanced cancer. Am J Hosp Palliat Care 2001;18:403–7.

[108] Tyler DC, Woodham M, Stocks J, et al. Oxygen saturation in children in the postoperative period. Anesth Analg 1995;80:14–9.

[109] Berde C. Local anesthetics in infants and children: an update. Paediatr Anaesth 2004;14:387–93.

[110] Mazoit JX, Dalens BJ. Pharmacokinetics of local anaesthetics in infants and children. Clin Pharmacokinet 2004;43:17–32.

[111] Zelikovsky N, Rodrigue JR, Gidycz CA, et al. Cognitive behavioral and behavioral interventions help young children cope during a voiding cystourethrogram. J Pediatr Psychol 2000;25:535–43.

[112] LaMontagne LL, Hepworth JT, Cohen F, et al. Cognitive-behavioral intervention effects on adolescents' anxiety and pain following spinal fusion surgery. Nurs Res 2003;52:183–90.

[113] Scharff L, Marcus DA, Masek BJ. A controlled study of minimal-contact thermal biofeedback treatment in children with migraine. J Pediatr Psychol 2002;27:109–19.

[114] McGrath PJ, Humphreys P, Goodman JT, et al. Relaxation prophylaxis for childhood migraine: a randomized placebo-controlled trial. Dev Med Child Neurol 1988;30:626–31.

[115] McGrath PJ, Humphreys P, Keene D, et al. The efficacy and efficiency of a self-administered treatment for adolescent migraine. Pain 1992;49:321–4.

[116] Walker LS. Commentary: empirical foundations for the development of behavioral interventions for recurrent abdominal pain. J Pediatr Psychol 1999;24:129–30.

[117] Weydert JA, Ball TM, Davis MF. Systematic review of treatments for recurrent abdominal pain. Pediatrics 2003;111:e1–11.

[118] Lee BH, Scharff L, Sethna NF, et al. Physical therapy and cognitive-behavioral treatment for complex regional pain syndromes. J Pediatr 2002;141:135–40.

[119] Sugarman LI. Hypnosis in a primary care practice: developing skills for the "new morbidities." J Dev Behav Pediatr 1996;17:300–5.

[120] Sugarman LI. Hypnosis: teaching children self-regulation. Pediatr Rev 1996;17:5–11.

[121] American Academy of Pediatrics, Committee on Hospital Care. Child life services. Pediatrics 2000;106:1156–9.

[122] Rusy LM, Weisman SJ. Complementary therapies for acute pediatric pain management. Pediatr Clin North Am 2000;47:589–99.

[123] Kemper KJ. Complementary and alternative medicine for children: does it work? Arch Dis Child 2001;84:6–9.

[124] Kehlet H, Wilmore DW. Multimodal strategies to improve surgical outcome. Am J Surg 2002;183:630–41.

[125] Murrell D, Gibson PR, Cohen RC. Continuous epidural analgesia in newborn infants undergoing major surgery. J Pediatr Surg 1993;28:548–52.

[126] Dalens B, Vanneuville G, Tanguy A. Comparison of the fascia iliaca compartment block with the 3-in-1 block in children. Anesth Analg 1989;69:705–13.

[127] Duflo F, Qamouss Y, Remond C, et al. Patient-controlled regional analgesia is effective in children: a preliminary report. Can J Anaesth 2004;51:928–30.

[128] Dadure C, Raux O, Troncin R, et al. Continuous infraclavicular brachial plexus block for acute pain management in children. Anesth Analg 2003;97:691–3.

[129] Dadure C, Raux O, Gaudard P, et al. Continuous psoas compartment blocks after major orthopedic surgery in children: a prospective computed tomographic scan and clinical studies. Anesth Analg 2004;98:623–8.

[130] De Negri P, Ivani G, Visconti C, et al. The dose-response relationship for clonidine added to a postoperative continuous epidural infusion of ropivacaine in children. Anesth Analg 2001;93:71–6.

[131] Bösenberg AT, Bland BA, Schulte SO, et al. Thoracic epidural anesthesia via caudal route in infants. Anesthesiology 1988;69:265–9.

[132] Desparmet J, Meistelman C, Barre J, et al. Continuous epidural infusion of bupivacaine for postoperative pain relief in children. Anesthesiology 1987;67:108–10.

[133] Giaufre E, Dalens B, Gombert A. Epidemiology and morbidity of regional anesthesia in children: a one-year prospective survey of the French-Language Society of Pediatric Anesthesiologists. Anesth Analg 1996;83:904–12.

[134] Bosenberg A. Pediatric regional anesthesia update. Paediatr Anaesth 2004;14:398–402.

[135] Annequin D, Carbajal R, Chauvin P, et al. Fixed 50% nitrous oxide oxygen mixture for painful procedures: a French survey. Pediatrics 2000;105(4):E47.

[136] Kennedy RM, Luhmann JD, Luhmann SJ. Emergency department management of pain and anxiety related to orthopedic fracture care: a guide to analgesic techniques and procedural sedation in children. Paediatr Drugs 2004;6:11–31.

[137] Marx CM, Stein J, Tyler MK, et al. Ketamine-midazolam versus meperidine-midazolam for painful procedures in pediatric oncology patients. J Clin Oncol 1997;15:94–102.

[138] Pena BM, Krauss B. Adverse events of procedural sedation and analgesia in a pediatric emergency department. Ann Emerg Med 1999;34:483–91.

[139] Taddio A, Ohlsson A, Einarson TR, et al. A systematic review of lidocaine-prilocaine cream (EMLA) in the treatment of acute pain in neonates. Pediatrics 1998;101:E1.

[140] Bishai R, Taddio A, Bar-Oz B, et al. Relative efficacy of amethocaine gel and lidocaine-prilocaine cream for Port-a-Cath puncture in children. Pediatrics 1999;104(3):e31.

[141] Kim MK, Kini NM, Troshynski TJ, et al. A randomized clinical trial of dermal anesthesia by iontophoresis for peripheral intravenous catheter placement in children. Ann Emerg Med 1999;33:395–9.

[142] Bryan HA, Alster TS. The S-Caine peel: a novel topical anesthetic for cutaneous laser surgery. Dermatol Surg 2002;28:999–1003 [discussion 1003].

[143] Wall VJ, Womack W. Hypnotic versus active cognitive strategies for alleviation of procedural distress in pediatric oncology patients. Am J Clin Hypn 1989;31:181–91.

[144] Zeltzer L, LeBaron S. Hypnosis and nonhypnotic techniques for reduction of pain and anxiety during painful procedures in children and adolescents with cancer. J Pediatr 1982;101(6):1032–5.

[145] Dial S, Silver P, Bock K, et al. Pediatric sedation for procedures titrated to a desired degree of immobility results in unpredictable depth of sedation. Pediatr Emerg Care 2001;17:414–20.

[146] Litman RS, Berkowitz RJ, Ward DS. Levels of consciousness and ventilatory parameters in young children during sedation with oral midazolam and nitrous oxide. Arch Pediatr Adolesc Med 1996;150:671–5

[147] Maxwell LG, Yaster M. The myth of conscious sedation. Arch Pediatr Adolesc Med 1996;150:665–7.

[148] Lalwani K, Michel M. Pediatric sedation in North American children's hospitals: a survey of anesthesia providers. Paediatr Anaesth 2005;15:209–13.

[149] Miser AW, McCalla J, Dothage JA, et al. Pain as a presenting symptom in children and young adults with newly diagnosed malignancy. Pain 1987;29(1):85–90.

[150] Berde C, Billett A, Collins JJ. Symptom management and supportive care. In: Pizzo PA, Poplack DG, editors. Principles and practice of pediatric oncology. 5th edition. Philadelphia: Lippincott Williams & Wilkins; 2005 [in press].

[151] Aley KO, Levine JD. Different peripheral mechanisms mediate enhanced nociception in metabolic/toxic and traumatic painful peripheral neuropathies in the rat. Neuroscience 2002; 111:389–97.

[152] Polomano RC, Bennett GJ. Chemotherapy-evoked painful peripheral neuropathy. Pain Med 2001;2:8–14.

[153] Clarkson JE, Worthington HV, Eden OB. Interventions for preventing oral mucositis for patients with cancer receiving treatment. Cochrane Database of Systemic Reviews 2003; 3:CD000978.

[154] Worthington HV, Clarkson JE, Eden OB. Interventions for treating oral mucositis for patients with cancer receiving treatment. Cochrane Database of Systemic Reviews 2004;2:CD001973.

[155] Vielhaber A, Portenoy RK. Advances in cancer pain management. Hematol Oncol Clin North Am 2002;16:527–41.

[156] Zech DF, Grond S, Lynch J, et al. Validation of World Health Organization guidelines for cancer pain relief: a 10-year prospective study. Pain 1995;63:65–76.

[157] Collins JJ, Grier HE, Kinney HC, et al. Control of severe pain in children with terminal malignancy. J Pediatr 1995;126(4):653–7.

[158] Wolfe J, Grier HE, Klar N, et al. Symptoms and suffering at the end of life in children with cancer. N Engl J Med 2000;342:326–33.

[159] Hunt A, Joel S, Dick G, et al. Population pharmacokinetics of oral morphine and its glucuronides in children receiving morphine as immediate-release liquid or sustained-release tablets for cancer pain. J Pediatr 1999;135:47–55.

[160] Collins JJ, Grier HE, Sethna NF, et al. Regional anesthesia for pain associated with terminal pediatric malignancy. Pain 1996;65:63–9.

[161] Truog RD, Berde CB, Mitchell C, et al. Barbiturates in the care of the terminally ill. N Engl J Med 1992;327:1678–82.

[162] Quill TE, Dresser R, Brock DW. The rule of double effect: a critique of its role in end-of-life decision making. N Engl J Med 1997;337:1768–71.

[163] Dougherty M, DeBaun MR. Rapid increase of morphine and benzodiazepine usage in the last three days of life in children with cancer is related to neuropathic pain. J Pediatr 2003;142: 373–6.

[164] Berde C, Wolfe J. Pain, anxiety, distress, and suffering: interrelated, but not interchangeable. J Pediatr 2003;142:361–3.

[165] Jacob E, Miaskowski C, Savedra M, et al. Management of vaso-occlusive pain in children with sickle cell disease. J Pediatr Hematol Oncol 2003;25:307–11.

[166] Apley J, Hale B. Children with abdominal pain. How do they grow up? BMJ 1973;3:7–9.

[167] Apley J, Naish N. Recurrent abdominal pains: a field survey of 1,000 school children. Arch Dis Child 1958;33:165.

[168] Feldman W, McGrath P, Hodgson C, et al. The use of dietary fiber in the management of simple, childhood, idiopathic, recurrent, abdominal pain: results in a prospective, double-blind, randomized, controlled trial. Am J Dis Child 1985;139:1216–8.

[169] Barr RG, Watkins JB, Levine MD. Recurrent abdominal pain (RAP) of childhood due to lactose intolerance: a prospective study. N Engl J Med 1979;300:1449–52.

[170] Hyams JS, Hyman PE, Rasquin-Weber A. Childhood recurrent abdominal pain and subsequent adult irritable bowel syndrome. J Dev Behav Pediatr 1999;20:318–9.

[171] Walker LS, Guite JW, Duke M, et al. Recurrent abdominal pain: a potential precursor of irritable bowel syndrome in adolescents and young adults. J Pediatr 1998;132:1010–5.

[172] Walker LS, Garber J, Greene JW. Psychosocial correlates of recurrent childhood pain: a comparison of pediatric patients with recurrent abdominal pain, organic illness, and psychiatric disorders. J Abnorm Psychol 1993;102:248–58.

[173] Walker LS. Pathways between recurrent abdominal pain and adult functional gastrointestinal disorders. J Dev Behav Pediatr 1999;20:320–2.

[174] Walker LS, Garber J, Greene JW. Somatization symptoms in pediatric abdominal pain patients: relation to chronicity of abdominal pain and parent somatization. J Abnorm Child Psychol 1991;19:379–94.

[175] Claar RL, Walker LS, Smith CA. Functional disability in adolescents and young adults with symptoms of irritable bowel syndrome: the role of academic, social, and athletic competence. J Pediatr Psychol 1999;24:271–80.

[176] Stylianos S, Stein JE, Flanigan LM, et al. Laparoscopy for diagnosis and treatment of recurrent abdominal pain in children. J Pediatr Surg 1996;31:1158–60.

[177] Schwarz SP, Taylor AE, Scharff L, et al. Behaviorally treated irritable bowel syndrome patients: a four-year follow-up. Behav Res Ther 1990;28:331–5.

[178] Fyfe DA, Moodie DS. Chest pain in pediatric patients presenting to a cardiac clinic. Clin Pediatr (Phila) 1984;23:321–4.

[179] Selbst SM, Ruddy R, Clark BJ. Chest pain in children: follow-up of patients previously reported. Clin Pediatr (Phila) 1990;29:374–7.

[180] Meier PM, Berde CB, DiCanzio J, et al. Quantitative assessment of cutaneous thermal and vibration sensation and thermal pain detection thresholds in healthy children and adolescents. Muscle Nerve 2001;24:1339–45.

[181] Sherry DD, Wallace CA, Kelley C, et al. Short- and long-term outcomes of children with complex regional pain syndrome type I treated with exercise therapy. Clin J Pain 1999;15:218–23.

ELSEVIER
SAUNDERS

PEDIATRIC CLINICS
OF NORTH AMERICA

Pediatr Clin N Am 52 (2005) 1029–1046

Pediatric Palliative, End-of-Life, and Bereavement Care

Tammy Kang, MD[a], K. Sarah Hoehn, MD, MBE[b],
Daniel J. Licht, MD[a], Oscar Henry Mayer, MD[a],
Gina Santucci, RN, BSN[c], Jean Marie Carroll, RN, BSN[c],
Carolyn M. Long, MSW[d], Malinda Ann Hill, MA[d],
Jennifer Lemisch, ATR, BC, LPC[e], Mary T. Rourke, PhD[a],
Chris Feudtner, MD, PhD, MPH[a],*

[a]Department of Pediatrics, The Children's Hospital of Philadelphia,
34th Street and Civic Center Boulevard North, Philadelphia, PA 19104, USA
[b]Department of Anesthesia and Critical Care Medicine, The Children's Hospital of Philadelphia,
34th Street and Civic Center Boulevard North, Philadelphia, PA 19104, USA
[c]Department of Nursing, The Children's Hospital of Philadelphia,
34th Street and Civic Center Boulevard North, Philadelphia, PA 19104, USA
[d]Department of Social Work and Family Services, The Children's Hospital of Philadelphia,
34th Street and Civic Center Boulevard North, Philadelphia, PA 19104, USA
[e]Department of Child Life, Education, and Creative Arts Therapy,
The Children's Hospital of Philadelphia, 34th Street and Civic Center Boulevard North,
Philadelphia, PA 19104, USA

Each year in the United States, approximately 50,000 children die, mostly in hospitals, and many more confront life-threatening conditions. Most—if not all—of these children and their families would benefit from timely, comprehensive, compassionate, continuous, and developmentally appropriate supportive care services, including a mixture of palliative, end-of-life, and bereavement care. [1,2]

Palliative care aims to relieve suffering and improve quality of life for patients with advanced illnesses and their families. Effective palliative care includes communicating with patients and family members, managing pain and other symptoms, providing psychosocial, spiritual, and bereavement support, and

* Corresponding author. General Pediatrics, 3535 Market Street, Room 1523, Children's Hospital of Philadelphia, Philadelphia, PA 19104.
E-mail address: Feudtner@email.chop.edu (C. Feudtner).

0031-3955/05/$ – see front matter © 2005 Elsevier Inc. All rights reserved.
doi:10.1016/j.pcl.2005.04.004
pediatric.theclinics.com

coordinating various medical and social services. For dying people of all ages, care should be directed toward relieving symptoms and suffering. For children, such care can be instituted in conjunction with curative therapy. Palliative care is appropriate for children with a wide range of conditions, even when cure remains a distinct possibility. The American Academy of Pediatrics supports the concepts of palliative care, stating that "the components of palliative care are offered at diagnosis and continued throughout the course of illness, whether the outcome ends in cure or death. Palliative care should be accessible in any setting, including home, hospital, and school" [3]. End-of-life care is more narrowly conceived as a phase of palliative care that is provided to patients who are manifesting the signs and symptoms of dying or who require certain procedures to be performed, such as the medical task of ceasing mechanical ventilation or the religious ceremony of last rites. Bereavement care addresses the experience and consequences of grief, which can be manifest before a child dies (so-called anticipatory grief) and after a child's death. Although these three modes of care can be discussed as if they were distinct, in practice they are inexorably entwined.

Historically, children with advanced illness and their families have not received adequate palliative, end-of-life, and bereavement care, partly because of a medical philosophy focused on cure rather than quality of life and a tendency to focus on quality of life only when death is imminent. We realize, however, that children benefit most from care that includes a combination of life-prolonging treatment, palliation of symptoms, rehabilitation, and support for caregivers.

The pediatric hospitalist plays an integral role in providing palliative, end-of-life, and bereavement care for children and families. This article focuses on a multifaceted approach to palliative, end-of-life, and bereavement care, in which the physician is a key member of an interdisciplinary team. We believe that we can improve quality of life and relieve suffering only by paying attention to the medical, emotional, spiritual, and practical needs and goals of dying children and their loved ones [4,5].

Talking to families

Communication, the great facilitator of human relationships, is the foundation of palliative care [6]. Good communication enables patients and family members to collaborate effectively with health care providers and allows these providers to support patients and family as they make decisions and confront the reality of their circumstances. Conversely, bad communication impairs the quality of care and can create negative memories that linger in the minds of family members for years.

Parents of sick children value health care providers who communicate clearly, accurately, and empathically. Importantly, these characteristics are based in part on attributes that individual health care providers possess. Not only is a solid font of knowledge essential but also the provider must be mentally and emotionally prepared for and focused on the task. Equally essential is the ability to devise personal ways to "step out of" the hectic pace of hospital practice and enter a quieter and more intimate mode of relating to other people.

Clarity, accuracy, and empathy in communication also result from specific techniques or habits of how to have difficult discussions. Table 1 outlines steps that are useful when the principal task involves breaking bad news [7]. One must realize that "bad" news can range from the diagnosis of a fatal condition to the message that discharge to home will be delayed because of difficulty staffing home nursing. Once a family has assimilated the news and its implications,

Table 1
Breaking bad news

Steps	Comment
Make a plan	Providers too often initiate a conversation or family meeting without a clear concept of what they hope to achieve; before the discussion, take a minute to mentally rehearse the steps outlined later
Getting the setting and people right	A quiet, private room is best; make sure that all the necessary people — as defined by the family — are present and that you allot enough time
Briefly recap the situation	Confirm that all the people assembled have the same understanding of the situation; state the fundamental issues confronting the child and any pending test results or other events that have prompted the meeting
Provide a warning shot	Before delivering the bad news, allow the parents a few seconds to prepare themselves by uttering a short phrase, such as "I wish the results were different, but . . ." or "I am afraid that what we were worried about has happened, and . . ."
State the bad news simply	Deliver the bad news in plain, straightforward language: ". . . but the test shows that the cancer has come back" or "and our effort to use the machine to breathe for your child is no longer working"
Allow silence	After the news is delivered, silence often fills the room; avoid the temptation to fill the silence immediately with talk; be quiet for a minute
Acknowledge emotion	A simple, humble statement, such as "I can't imagine what you are feeling," can be helpful in addressing one of the most palpable aspects of this experience
Answer questions	Minds often go blank after receiving bad news; solicit questions after recognizing this reality: "I realize that this news is overwhelming. I'm dedicated to helping you understand what it means to your child. If you have questions now or later, once you've thought about this for a while, I'm here and will be here to answer those questions."
Formulate a next-step plan	Depending on how unexpected the news is, now may or may not be the time to discuss elaborate treatment plans; at a minimum, plans can be made to meet again at a specific time: "Let's take a break so that we can consider what this news means and plan on meeting again in an hour [or tomorrow, or next week] to discuss what to do."
Leave but do not abandon	Be clear about leaving and about the plans to return: "I'm going to go now, and will be back to see you again in an hour."
Debrief	Discussing bad news is remarkably demanding and difficult work; a quick debriefing with another staff member who was present during the discussion can be useful in considering how effective the discussion was, how your technique might be improved, and what emotional impact the discussion has had on you

another kind of conversation focuses on defining new goals and plans that confront the reality of the bad news. These and other conversations strive to deepen the therapeutic alliance among patient, family, and health care team. A framework for therapeutic planning discussions, based on a simple yet powerful model of decision making, is outlined in Table 2.

Table 2
Framework for therapeutic planning conversations

Steps	Comment
Review the major problems	Develop with the family a shared understanding of the major problems confronting them and their child: "I think we all find it useful to hear what each of us think are the most important problems and challenges that we need to confront."
Discuss goals, objectives, hopes	The compass by which the course of therapy will be set depends on a clear sense of purpose and the values that underlie that purpose; you can initiate this phase of the discussion with the following question: "Given the problems and challenges, I am thinking about how we can best care for your child. What are your major hopes or goals?" Encourage each participant to state all of their hopes or goals, which may not be entirely consistent (such as "to be cured by a miracle" and "to not suffer before dying"); the aim of this phase is simply to air all of the hopes, goals, or objectives and summarize them for the group when everyone has spoken
Spell out alternative actions	In as nonjudgmental and succinct a manner as possible, clarify the main alternative ways of caring for the child, such as: "I feel that we have two major ways we can proceed, namely, continue to have your child stay in the hospital or work to have your child go home with the help of hospice or home-care nursing." Check to see if anyone has another major option
Examine consequences of options	Typically, no therapeutic option is perfect; once the main options are spelled out, explore as a group the pros and cons of each alternative. "If we keep your child in the hospital, there are some good and not-so-good things I can foresee happening, such as …" The judgments of "good and not-so-good" should refer back to the discussion regarding hopes and goals; solicit other participants' perspectives
Explore tradeoffs	Often a central pattern of tradeoffs between two goals emerges in the discussion of options; addressing this tradeoff explicitly can be helpful: "We seem to be struggling with the problem that the goal of feeling secure, a sense of which the hospital provides, is at odds with the goal of being at home." Stating these tradeoffs can help people clarify which goal is more important or devise new alternatives to accomplish both goals (eg, enhancing the sense of security at home by augmenting the nursing coverage)
Formulate a plan	By this point, the broad elements of a plan typically have emerged by consensus; if so, spell it out and assess whether everyone agrees; if not, acknowledge the disagreement and seek agreement to continue to work together to formulate a mutually acceptable plan
Specify next steps and follow-up assessment	Before ending the conversation, clarify who will do what next and when the next discussion will occur

The first five steps of this framework can be remembered with the mnemonic 'PrOACT' (as in, be proactive): PRoblem, Objectives, Alternatives, Consequences, Tradeoffs.

Involving the family

When the goal of care shifts from cure to providing comfort, a family often looks to the health care team for guidance regarding how to provide the best care for their child. Family-centered care is an underlying principle of palliative and end-of-life-care. Families should be encouraged to maintain their lifestyle to the best of their ability and ensure that their belief system is respected. In discussing quality end-of-life care, the health care team must recognize a family's cultural values and traditions.

Conversations with families should emphasize the importance of improving the quality rather than the quantity of a child's days. There are many ways to maximize quality of life for dying children. Because time is of paramount consideration, the focus should be on making each day meaningful. Health care providers should encourage a child and family to make memories of moments big and small and to celebrate "milestones" (eg, first tooth, first words, birthdays, graduations, religious ceremonies) while the child is still able to participate. Activities such as keeping a journal, making a photo album, videotaping special occasions, making imprints of the child's hands or feet, sharing stories, and keeping locks of hair all help create memories for the whole family.

Families also may look to the health care team for advice on how to communicate with their children about death. Although a child may be acutely aware of his or her condition, parents may have difficulty talking with the child about death. It may be helpful for families to know that studies have shown that children are aware of their condition and impending death even when no "official" conversation has taken place. Although we may believe that children have the right to honest answers about their illness, we also recognize that parents are the fundamental decision makers. Often religious, spiritual, and family traditions play an important role in how parents communicate with their children. One way to help parents with these difficult conversations is to ask them what worries them when answering their child's questions about death or illness. One may consider involving the family's spiritual advisor or another member of the health care team (eg, the hospital chaplain, social worker, or child-life specialist) to facilitate such conversations.

Psychosocial and spiritual needs

Dying children and their families have a host of concerns—psychological, financial, spiritual, cultural, and ethical—that good palliative care should address. Psychosocial interventions seek to provide families with a safe environment to express and process the intense emotions during times of crisis, including fear, grief, anger, loneliness, stress, and isolation, and cope with the challenges as successfully as possible [8]. Each member of a palliative care team, including mental health care and medical professionals, can play a role in these interventions. Whereas all psychosocial professionals, including psychologists, social workers, child-life specialists, and pastoral care workers, tend to focus on issues of adjustment, communication, and making meaning, there is typically a degree of specialization of duty by profession.

Social work with patients at the end of life is multidimensional and can include case management, counseling, advocacy, and acting as a liaison between the patient, family, medical team, and hospice agency [9]. Palliative care social workers can act as a repository for the family's normal but overwhelming feelings of suffering, fear, and loss while facilitating communication between the dying child and his or her family. They also can help families navigate the complex medical and social service systems and access financial support resources while a child is in the hospital and once the child is home. Above all, social workers support and advocate the hopes and wishes of the child and family and remain present with the dying child and family to acknowledge their suffering and help create an environment of hope and healing.

Psychologists can contribute expertise in the areas of formal assessment and intervention, particularly when normal means of coping that usually enable people to adjust to difficult situations become maladaptive. The world of the seriously ill child is often filled with high levels of anxiety and other distress that frequently go untreated in the face of medical needs, which are often seen as more pressing [10]. Psychologists can assess a child's anxiety and distress and then implement formal interventions to reduce troubling symptoms, including serving as a coordinating liaison with psychiatrists. The same kind of assessment can take place on a family level, with psychologists working to assess family needs and provide interventions when distress diverts a family from a more adaptive coping and grieving process. Whereas psychologists are most often called on when psychopathology is noted, psychologists can provide interventions for all families who are confronting serious or terminal illness with the goal of supporting positive or adaptive coping over time [11].

In the hospital setting, child-life specialists and creative arts therapists often function as translators of a child's experience. They search, with the patient and family, for play or art modalities that stimulate imagination and create a bridge or transitional space between a child's inner and outer worlds [12]. Allowing the opportunity for choices in art and play may provide control to patients when they have little choice about being ill or needing medical care at the end of life. Although children and adolescents are not always able to communicate their feelings, art and play can assist them in finding words to describe their experiences and work through traumatic experiences associated with hospitalization, illness, and dying. Creative therapeutic expression can promote a sense of independence and control, facilitate positive self-esteem, and encourage self-expression of thoughts and feelings. By communicating to a patient that all feelings are acceptable, child-life specialists and creative arts therapists develop a therapeutic relationship in which a patient feels accepted and safe. At a time when feelings may be difficult to put into words, art and play can help a child and other family members to express the experience of approaching death and their feelings of impending loss, which provides support to the whole family.

Spiritual support, a critical component of palliative care, is most often the province of pastoral care workers but should be considered by all members of the team. One goal of spiritual care for dying children and their families is to help them find meaning in living and dying. Structured spiritual assessments of a child or family's formal religious and spiritual affiliations, beliefs, practice, and rituals can provide powerful insights, which often lead to intense conversations with the dying patient and family about their search for meaning and what occurs after death. Supportive discussions can help build meaning, offer comfort before and after a child has died, and provide strength during the grieving process. Many dying children and their families wish to have prayers or other spiritually significant rituals occur in the hospital, and pastoral care workers can assist in achieving these goals. Pastoral care workers and social workers also can act as liaisons between the family and outside resources, such as funeral homes, churches, and temples, to ensure that the family's funeral and burial wishes are fulfilled.

Specialization across the psychosocial professions is helpful and necessary. In a mature and effective palliative care team, however, the psychosocial professionals are interdependent, with some overlapping responsibilities and with each professional supporting the roles and responsibilities of the other.

Symptom management

A cornerstone of good palliative and end-of-life care is the alleviation of suffering by the skillful management of symptoms. Several core principles underlie all symptom management strategies. First, patients must be assessed actively and frequently in a comprehensive manner for distressing or bothersome symptoms, including the assessment of "total" pain, which encompasses not only physical pain but also emotional, psychological, social, and spiritual suffering. Second, neither evaluating nor treating the symptom should be more distressing or bothersome than the symptom itself. Finally, if one treatment method is not successful, several different modes of treatment often work synergistically to control a symptom.

Most children experience pain at some point during their illness. Pain is a subjective symptom that is physically and emotionally distressing for a child and the caregiver. Pain can be somatic, visceral, or neuropathic and can be caused by disease-related, treatment-related, or psychological distress. The key to effective pain control is frequent, detailed assessment that includes location, duration, and possible causes. The current standard for pain management in children who have cancer and children who are receiving palliative care consists of four concepts developed by the World Health Organization: (1) by the ladder, (2) by the clock, (3) by the mouth, and (4) by the child. That is, treatment should be escalated according to the World Health Organization Analgesic Step Ladder approach outlined in Table 3, be administered on a scheduled basis, be given by the least invasive route, and be tailored to an individual child's circumstance and needs

Table 3
Escalation of therapy to control pain

Step of therapy	Indication	Guidance

1	Mild pain	Nonopioid analgesics:
		  acetaminophen, ibuprofen, naproxen
		+/− adjuvants:
		  anticonvulsants for neuropathic pain
		  and antidepressants or anxiolytics
		  for coexisting mood disturbances

2	Moderate pain or mild pain not relieved by step 1	Opioid analgesics for step 2: codeine, oxycodone, morphine +/− nonopioid analgesics +/− adjuvants
3	Severe pain or mild-to-moderate pain not relieved by steps 1 or 2	Opioid analgesics for step 3: hydromorphone, fentanyl, patient-controlled analgesic delivery of intravenous narcotic +/− non-opiod analgesics +/− adjuvants

Based on the World Health Organization "ladder" approach to cancer pain management.

[13]. In addition to pain medications, supportive, behavioral, and cognitive methods for alleviating pain may be appropriate for children.

Many parents fear the use of narcotics and need reassurance from their child's medical team. Physicians also must anticipate and manage side effects of narcotics, such as fatigue, constipation, and nausea. If side effects become intolerable, opioids can be rotated; that is, the patient is switched from one opiate to another opiate, with often a slight reduction in the equianalgesic dosage, so that pain is still controlled but side effects are diminished. Table 4 contains equianalgesic opiate doses.

Table 4
Equianalgesic narcotic dosing

Medication	Parenteral dose (mg)	Oral or rectal dose (mg)
Morphine	1	3
Codeine	12	20
Hydromorphone	0.3	0.8
Hydrocodone	NA	3
Oxycodone	NA	2
Fentanyl patch	1.5 μg/h[a]	NA
Methadone	NA	Variable[b]

[a] Fentanyl patches are available in 25-, 50-, 75-, and 100- μg/h doses. Given individual variability in conversion, underestimating the initial fentanyl patch dose is appropriate, augmented with rescue doses of oral morphine if pain is not controlled. The dose of 1.5 μg/h is equianalgesic to 1 mg of oral morphine taken every 4 hours; a dose of 25 μg/h would be equianalgesic to 15 mg of oral morphine taken every 4 hours. Patches take 18 to 24 hours to achieve steady-state serum levels of fentanyl and once removed have a half-life of another 18 hours.

[b] Methadone offers remarkably effective pain relief but should be prescribed by a physician familiar with this medication and the management of pain.

Nausea and vomiting are a common set of symptoms at the end of life. Causes are multifactorial and can include chemotherapy, central nervous system triggers, and gastrointestinal abnormalities. Because being unable to eat or drink as the result of nausea or vomiting has a significant impact on a patient's quality of life, assessment and treatments should be instituted quickly. Treatment is based on likely cause and can include pharmacologic and nonpharmacologic methods. In cases of chemotherapy-induced nausea and vomiting, medications such as prochlorperazine, ondansetron, scopolamine, and metaclopramide can be effective, as can 5-HT3 receptor antagonists (eg, granisetron and ondansetron). One small study showed ondansetron to be effective in the palliative care setting for adults admitted with the chief complaint of nausea and vomiting [14]. Multiple agents often are necessary for effective symptom relief. Nonpharmacologic methods include providing smaller, frequent meals, taking medications after meals if possible, and avoiding smells and tastes that exacerbate the symptoms.

Fatigue, one of the most prevalent symptoms in children at the end of life, is generally defined as the subjective feeling of being tired and lacking energy, which can be caused by depression, anxiety, pain, poor nutrition, medication side effects, hypoxia, infection, and dehydration. Although there are several assessment tools for fatigue in children, diagnosis is based on subjective report by the patient or parent [15,16]. As with nausea and vomiting, treatment seeks first to remedy any possible underlying causes. Maximizing a patient's rest also is important and may involve the use of sleep agents. Pharmacologic and nonpharmacologic interventions have been used in managing cancer-related fatigue in adults. Psychostimulants have been used in patients who have cancer and patients who do not have cancer patients for the treatment of fatigue, especially in patients who have been sedated with opioids. Amphetamines have been used in multiple trials in adult patients who have cancer, HIV, chronic fatigue syndrome, and multiple sclerosis. In adults, psychostimulants, such as methylphenidate or dextroamphetamine or corticosteroids, may alleviate fatigue [17–20]. Although psychostimulants are generally well tolerated and may improve mood, energy, and cognition, in children they can cause jitteriness, insomnia, and decreased appetite. In general it is best to give the medication in the morning and early afternoon rather than in the late afternoon or evening. Nonpharmacologic methods include eliminating sedating medications; establishing a sleep schedule with rest periods throughout the day; maximizing nutrition and hydration by means that accord with patient wishes; and engaging in mild exercise as tolerated.

Anxiety, which is commonly experienced by children who have life-shortening conditions, can be a normal response to several factors: painful procedures, uncomfortable symptoms, undesirable medication side effects, the progression of disease or worsening impairment, diminished choices or loss of control, separation from friends or family environment, and other predicaments that arise in the course of their illnesses. Sometimes, the specific causes of a child's anxiety can be identified and treated effectively. When no specific treatable cause can be uncovered, the most common therapeutic approach involves either an oral or an intravenous benzodiazepine, such as lorazepam, diazepam, or midazolam. This class of medication is known to cause sedation, however, and there is little evidence that the medications effectively diminish anxiety per se.

Constipation, although subsequently recalled by parents of dying children as one of the major bothersome symptoms, is often underrecognized and treated ineffectively by physicians. Reduced oral intake of food or liquid, diminished physical activity, and the use of constipating drugs such as morphine or the other opiates, along with potential gastrointestinal dysmotility as a result of the disease lead to constipation. Prevention of constipation is ideal, with daily attention to whether a patient has had a recent bowel movement combined with daily administration of a stool softener (eg, polyethylene glycol or docusate) and a bowel stimulant (eg, senna). Despite best efforts, constipation sometimes may require treatment with an enema, but such events should prompt a thorough re-evaluation of the preventive medication regimen and possible escalation of dosages.

Dyspnea is the sensation of breathlessness that occurs when the body is unable to meet its ventilatory need. A difficult complaint to quantify accurately, dyspnea is important to recognize and treat, because it can be uncomfortable and herald the onset of respiratory failure [21]. Treatment first should target any and all underlying causes and seek to rebalance ventilatory capacity and metabolic demand. Obstructive airway disease or restrictive lung disease can burden the respiratory system, and respiratory muscle fatigue or limitation because of pain can diminish ventilation to the point at which the respiratory system no longer satisfies the body's basic metabolic needs. Alternatively, the body's metabolic demand may increase beyond what the ventilatory capacity of the lungs can support. For patients with significant tachypnea and obstructive lung disease, bronchodilation and anti-inflammatory therapy should be the first line of treatment. If the dyspnea continues, the physician is obliged to discuss goals of care with the patient and family, explaining possible levels of intervention, such as noninvasive continuous positive airway pressure, bilevel positive airway pressure, or mechanical ventilation. Supplying continuous positive airway pressure may help to prevent premature airway closure during exhalation and increase inspiratory flow, thus alleviating a patient's sensation of not being able to inhale deeply enough. Inspiratory pressure augmentation using bilevel positive airway pressure can help to expand the chest wall, decrease the work of breathing, and improve ventilation in patients with restrictive lung disease, thus reducing dyspnea. Oral and parenteral opiates (eg, morphine) and anxiolytic agents (eg, benzodiazepines) can be titrated upward until the sensation of dyspnea is relieved. Although inhaled narcotics and analgesics have been used to palliate dyspnea in an attempt to minimize the respiratory depression and sedation that systemic opiate treatment can cause [22], the results are mixed [23]. Nebulized morphine has been used in most of the published studies, although nebulized fentanyl has been used successfully [24]. Finally, calming techniques, hypnosis, and the use of fans blowing air across a patient's bed may help increase comfort and minimize dyspnea [25].

Seizures, which are common at the end of life, occur as a result of progression of the primary central nervous system disease or of progression of the primary disease to the central nervous system. Seizures also can result from high fever or metabolic derangement (most frequently hypoglycemia, dysregulated sodium homeostasis, and hypocalcemia). Managing seizures at the end of life is critical, because they can create a barrier between a patient and the family. Parents who have witnessed a child convulsing commonly state that they never want to see their child go through a seizure again [26–28]. Although patients seem to be in agony during a seizure, they report few physical symptoms— confusion, muscle aches and pain from local traumas—after an episode. They are more likely to fear future mental handicap [29] and embarrassment about losing control of consciousness and especially bladder or bowel function in front of friends and family during a seizure [30].

In general, identifying the cause of the seizure is of paramount importance, because some metabolic causes cannot be treated until the underlying cause is corrected. In cases in which a patient is being cared for at home or on whom blood draws have been limited, seizures may be the life-ending event. Various factors influence clinical decisions regarding medications for treating seizures: the acuity of presentation, the presence of other organ damage or malfunction, and, in the context of end-of-life care, the wish to preserve or cloud patient consciousness.

For the acute treatment of a seizure, intravenous benzodiazepines are the therapeutic mainstay. Rectal valium is an excellent alternative when the therapeutic aim is to stop a seizure. For the ongoing management or suppression of a seizure disorder, benzodiazepines can be given on a scheduled basis, but this practice should be avoided unless death is imminent because benzodiazepines cause substantial sedation and may depress respiration. Valproic acid causes negligible sedation but should not be used in patients with mitochondrial defects or other inborn errors of energy metabolism, in children who are younger than 2 years who may have unrecognized metabolic disease, patients who have bleeding diatheses (because it interferes with platelet function), or patients who have liver dysfunction. The best long-term nonsedating options may be the newer anticonvulsant agents, such as levetiracetam or oxcarbazepine. Both medications are available only in oral formulations (liquid and tablet) and achieve good serum concentrations after only two doses, with good overall tolerance. The primary side effect of levetiracetam is behavioral change [31]. Oxcarbazepine, which may cause some initial sleepiness, is also effective for neuropathic pain [32].

Hospice and home nursing care

Not all families choose to care for their dying child at home. For families who do, however, having their child at home during their final days or months can give them a sense of fulfillment and comfort. When discussing the option of pediatric hospice with families, it is helpful to dismantle some misconceptions and answer any questions the family may have regarding hospice service.

The decision to go home on hospice care requires advanced planning and coordination with the health care team, the hospice provider, and the family. To make the transition as seamless as possible, the health care team must have a well-organized plan that is communicated to everyone involved. As an advocate for the child and family, the health care team can help identify appropriate services and providers and clarify the treatment plan and patient needs with the third-party payer to maximize the child's health care benefits.

Although hospices were developed using an adult model of care, many hospices have the capacity, skill, and desire to care for children. The appropriateness of a particular hospice agency can be determined by asking certain questions:

- Has the agency had experience in caring for pediatric patients?
- If so, what was the experience like?
- Do they have staff who have been trained in end-of-life care for children?
- Are they available to come to the hospital to meet the family before discharge?
- Can they provide ongoing bereavement services after the child dies?

Once a hospice program has been identified, it is valuable to discuss with the family their fears and concerns about hospice. Because many families equate hospice with "going home to die" or "giving up hope," they need to know that choosing hospice does not mean forgoing options, such as returning to the hospital or continuing care with their primary physician. Most pediatric hospices do not require parents to sign a do-not-resuscitate order. Any conversations the primary care physician has had with the family about limits of care should be shared with the hospice provider, however.

The main goal of pediatric hospice is to enhance a child's quality of life in his or her final journey. We must remember that the journey belongs to the child and family and that the job of the multidisciplinary health care team—and the partnership between hospital and hospice—is to support them on that journey.

Bereavement

Although the generic process and parameters of grief are well established in the literature [33], the actual experience of loss and adjustment takes different forms. The process of grief is not linear and never fits neatly into predetermined categories and time scales. The way in which support services are provided to families affected by the death of a child and the way in which they are involved before and after the death is crucial to how they experience the loss, are able to accept it and, subsequently, work through the bereavement process. When medical care can extend life for increasingly longer periods between diagnosis of a terminal illness and the actual death, families often have time to anticipate the loss of their child and experience anticipatory grief. This is an important part of the grieving process, one in which family members should be encouraged to acknowledge their feelings and speak openly about the imminent death.

Soon after a child dies, the family members left behind experience acute grief. A health care professional's presence during this time is an important way to offer support and comfort. Most families express the feeling that it helps when people acknowledge the significance of their loss. The health care providers who treated the child should share memories with the family and thank them for the opportunity to have participated in the child's care. They should focus the discussion on the sadness of the death rather than the clinical details of the illness and death. They can provide the family with printed information on grief or refer to community organizations or agencies for support and counseling. By giving family members the information they need, an opportunity to talk about their feelings, and suggestions for coping, the pediatrician can help everyone concerned cope somewhat better with the tragedy of a child's death.

Many physicians and other health care professions experience caregiver grief, which is expressed as feelings of failure, sadness, or frustration, when a child they are caring for dies. Honesty and genuine expression of emotion to others allows a health care provider to be more sensitive to those in your care. By being able to recognize your own grief and responses to grief, you will be able to seek support yourself and be more effective in offering support to others.

A comprehensive bereavement program helps families start on the painful journey of grief. Bereavement services should be tailored to meet the unique needs of families. Grieving families should be provided with alternatives and encouraged to choose which services, if any, suit their needs. Bereavement follow-up services may include individual counseling, support groups, memorial events, written resources, and education. Grief counseling can be helpful for people who are grieving or anticipating the death of a loved one. Professional counseling provides a safe place for expressing and normalizing feelings of grief. Although the journey is arduous, offering support and guidance can help families begin the necessary process of healing.

When parents who have had a child die meet together in a grief support group, a sense of peace and healing can result. Many parents find comfort knowing that they are not alone in their grief. Various types of community-based grief support groups are available. Many hospices, hospitals, religious institutions, and funeral homes offer bereavement support groups that are open to all members of the community.

Ethically problematic situations

Pediatric hospitalists must be able to recognize and manage ethically problematic situations, often by drawing on other personnel and resources at their hospitals. This section presents three common situations encountered in the realm of palliative and end-of-life care [34].

Scenario 1: truth telling

You are caring for a 12-year-old girl with rapidly progressive glioblastoma multiforme who presented with a right hemipareis. Unfortunately, she is not a candidate for any curative treatment and has a poor prognosis. Every time you see her, she asks what is wrong with her and when she will be able to walk again. Her parents prefer to let her think she has a virus rather than telling her the reality of her diagnosis and prognosis.

In pediatrics, most decisions are guided by the best interest principle [35]. This situation presents a challenging conflict between truth telling and denial because there are reasons to justify both courses of action [36]. Arguably, the child's parents think her interests are best served in not knowing that she has a terminal, rapidly progressive illness. From the child's viewpoint, however, she might want to be informed so that she can express her feelings openly and have an honest conversation about dying. This kind of situation is particularly challenging because health care providers often feel a duty to the patient to be honest. They should not, however, disclose her illness and prognosis to her without the family's knowledge. Although there is a paucity of data about the benefits of truth telling with terminally ill children, the American Academy of Pediatrics reports that children and adolescents who know that they have HIV have greater self-esteem than do those who do not know their status [37].

In this case, it is best to counsel the family on the importance of telling their daughter the truth, especially in light of her repeated questions. Child-life services and psychosocial support should be offered to the patient and family. If a conflict between the health care team and the parents persists, any member of the health care team may bring the case before the institutional ethics committee for help in resolving the issue.

Scenario 2: futility

You are the pediatrician on call in a level II neonatal intensive care unit when a full-term baby with a prenatal diagnosis of trisomy 18 is born. Over the ensuing days, the baby has multiple episodes of apnea that require resuscitation with bag mask ventilation. You talk to the family about possible do-not-attempt-resuscitation status and present the option of providing the baby with feeds and palliative care but not cardiopulmonary resuscitation. The parents state that they want everything done because the baby's grandparents told them that was the law.

The grandparents likely recall the outcry over the federal Baby Doe regulations, which were promulgated in 1982 after a baby with Down syndrome and a tracheoesophageal fistula died without surgical intervention [38]. The regulations required that all newborns, even those with terminal illnesses, receive maximal life-prolonging treatment. A hotline phone number was established for hospital staff to report cases anonymously in which care did not conform to the rules. In reality, however, these regulations (currently codified in the federal Child

Abuse and Neglect Act) never have been enforced, nor do they have the power of law or regulation to affect individual level decision making.

The fundamental conflict lies in the parents' insistence that the baby receive cardiopulmonary resuscitation and the health care team's perception that this intervention cannot succeed and represents futile treatment [39]. Currently, however, there are no universally accepted guidelines regarding what constitutes futile treatment, and unilateral do-not-attempt-resuscitation orders are not acceptable. Instead of arguing about whether a treatment is futile, alternative avenues to resolve disputes about limiting resuscitation should be pursued, including perhaps an ethics committee consultation or mediation regarding a do-not-attempt-resuscitation decision [40].

In this case, the primary physician should arrange a family meeting to clarify the parents' goals and hopes for their baby. Perhaps the parents want the baby resuscitated so he can live just long enough to partake in a religious ceremony or meet an important family member. Perhaps they want the baby to live for months or years and will pursue a tracheotomy and mechanical ventilation to care for the baby at home. Clarification of these goals or hopes can help health care professionals understand and empathize with patients or families and move from conflict to collaboration.

Scenario 3: withdrawal of artificial fluids and nutrition

A 10-year-old girl with progressive neurologic failure from an underlying metabolic disorder is admitted with increasingly frequent seizures. Over the last 6 months, she has lost her ability to take anything orally. During her hospitalization, the parents tell you that they feel they are only prolonging their child's suffering. They have talked to their pastor and have decided they would like to stop gastrostomy tube feeds and want their daughter to receive seizure medication and comfort measures only.

This is a challenging situation, because the withdrawal of fluids and nutrition delivered by "artificial means" is emotionally, morally, and politically charged. Ethically, fluids and nutrition provided by intravenous administration or delivered by a feeding tube are considered a form of life-sustaining medical treatment. With parental agreement, physicians may forgo giving hydration and nutrition in cases in which they believe such measures are not "appropriate" [41]. In this case, the physician should try to involve health care providers who have had a long-term relationship with the family to explore whether the parents' decision is based on their concerns about prolonging suffering and inadequate seizure management or whether it is a result of their own exhaustion and need for respite. The family and the health care team must believe that this decision is in the child's best interests. If, after consulting with the primary pediatrician and neurologist, the consensus is that continuation of artificial fluids and nutrition is only prolonging the patient's suffering, then withdrawing artificial fluids and nutrition and instituting aggressive comfort-care measures would be appropriate.

Improving end-of-life care

Regardless of one's degree of experience in pediatric palliative care, improvement is always possible and imperative. Individual health care providers and teams of providers can gain a clearer sense of how to improve the care that they provide by periodically undertaking a self-assessment that considers the major quality-of-palliative-care domains. Table 5 presents a framework for this self-assessment, along with sample questions.

After identifying domains in which significant improvement is possible, individuals or teams should target one area at a time for study (various excellent resources are available in print and on the worldwide web) or discussion and planning with other members of the hospital staff (eg, physician colleagues, nurses, chaplains, psychologists, or members of the hospital administration). Step by step, we can improve the care received by dying children and their families.

Table 5
Framework for assessing and improving quality of care

Quality-of-care domain	Self-assessment questions
Collaborate, communicate, and support decision making	How competent do I feel in these areas? What feedback can other staff members give me about how I am performing?
Minimize bothersome symptoms	Am I doing a good job of pain assessment and control? Is there a particular symptom that I feel uncomfortable managing?
Provide emotional and spiritual support	Whom should I ask to help me provide these kinds of support? Social worker? Child-life specialist? Psychologist? Pastoral care staff?
Maximize other quality-of-life enhancers	Do I have a sufficiently clear sense of what this child and family value most to make sure that our plans support these values? Have I forged ties with all possible allies, from the child's friends to school or wish-granting organizations?
Institute palliative care in a timely manner	Can I raise the issue of symptom management and quality-of-life enhancement earlier in the course of illness to prepare for subsequent conversations?
Visualize and address the full population at need	Are all the children I care for who might die as likely to receive quality end-of-life care? If not, why not?
Provide a continuum of care across multiple sites	How can I improve communication and transitions of care between in-patient and out-patient settings?
Appreciate and manage tradeoffs adroitly	Am I sensitive to the various difficult tradeoffs that patients or parents struggle with or that I am struggling with? How well am I recognizing and managing ethical dilemmas when they arise?
Operate in accord with an evidence base to maximize safety and effectiveness	What do I know about the drugs or other interventions that I am using? Can I find published systematic reviews to enhance my understanding of effective treatment?
Practice the art of individualization	How can I forge more effective therapeutic alliances with specific children and their families?
Provide self-care	Am I acknowledging the impact that caring for dying children has on me? What am I doing to care for myself in this role?

References

[1] Field MJ, Behrman RE, Committee on Palliative and End-of-Life Care for Children and Their Families. When children die: improving palliative and end-of-life care for children and their families. Washington, DC: National Academy Press; 2003.

[2] Feudtner C. Perspectives on quality at the end of life. Arch Pediatr Adolesc Med 2004; 158(5):415–8.

[3] American Academy of Pediatrics, Committee on Bioethics and Committee on Hospital Care. Palliative care for children. Pediatrics 2000;106(2 Pt 1):351–7.

[4] Morrison RS, Meier DE. Clinical practice: palliative care. N Engl J Med 2004;350(25):2582–90.

[5] Himelstein BP, Hilden JM, Boldt AM, et al. Pediatric palliative care. N Engl J Med 2004; 350(17):1752–62.

[6] Hays RM, Haynes G, Geyer JR, et al. Communication at the end of life. In: Carter BS, Levetown M, editors. Palliative care for infants, children, and adolescents: a practical handbook. Baltimore (MD): Johns Hopkins University Press; 2004. p. 112–40.

[7] Buckman R, Kason Y. How to break bad news: a guide for health care professionals. Baltimore (MD): Johns Hopkins University Press; 1992.

[8] Cincotta N. Psychosocial issues in the world of children with cancer. Cancer 1993;71(10): 3251–60.

[9] Zilberfein F, Hurwitz E. Clinical social work practice at the end of life: living with dying. New York: Columbia University Press; 2004.

[10] Wolfe J, Grier HE, Klar N, et al. Symptoms and suffering at the end of life in children with cancer. N Engl J Med 2000;342(5):326–33.

[11] Kazak AE, Noll RB. Child death from pediatric illness: conceptualizing intervention from a family/systems and public health perspective. Professional Psychology: Research Practice 2004; 35(3):219–26.

[12] Rode D. Building bridges within the culture of pediatric medicine: the interface of art therapy and child life programming. Art Therapy: Journal of the American Art Therapy Association 1995;12(2):104–10.

[13] McGrath PA. Development of the World Health Organization guidelines on cancer pain relief and palliative care in children. J Pain Symptom Manage 1996;12(2):87–92.

[14] Currow DC, Coughlan M, Fardell B, et al. Use of ondansetron in palliative medicine. J Pain Symptom Manage 1997;13(5):302–7.

[15] Clarke-Steffen L. Cancer-related fatigue in children. J Pediatr Oncol Nurs 2001;18(2 Suppl 1): 1–2.

[16] Hinds PS, Hockenberry-Eaton M, Gilger E, et al. Comparing patient, parent, and staff descriptions of fatigue in pediatric oncology patients. Cancer Nurs 1999;22(4):277–88.

[17] Breitbart W, Rosenfeld B, Kaim M, et al. A randomized, double-blind, placebo-controlled trial of psychostimulants for the treatment of fatigue in ambulatory patients with human immunodeficiency virus disease. Arch Intern Med 2001;161(3):411–20.

[18] Sarhill N, Walsh D, Nelson KA, et al. Methylphenidate for fatigue in advanced cancer: a prospective open-label pilot study. Am J Hosp Palliat Care 2001;18(3):187–92.

[19] Wagner GJ, Rabkin JG, Rabkin R. Dextroamphetamine as a treatment for depression and low energy in AIDS patients: a pilot study. J Psychosom Res 1997;42(4):407–11.

[20] Wagner GJ, Rabkin R. Effects of dextroamphetamine on depression and fatigue in men with HIV: a double-blind, placebo-controlled trial. J Clin Psychiatry 2000;61(6):436–40.

[21] Carrieri-Kohlman V, Stulbarg MS. Dyspnea: assessment and management. In: Hodgkin JE, Celli BR, Connors GL, editors. Pulmonary rehabilitation: guidelines to success. 3rd edition. Philadelphia: Lippincott Williams & Wilkins; 2000. p. xvii, 57–89.

[22] Cohen SP, Dawson TC. Nebulized morphine as a treatment for dyspnea in a child with cystic fibrosis. Pediatrics 2002;110(3):e38.

[23] Polosa R, Simidchiev A, Walters E. Nebulized morphine for severe interstitial lung disease. Cochrane Database Syst Rev 2002;3:CD002872.

[24] Graff GR, Stark JM, Gueber R. Nebulized fentanyl for palliation of dyspnea in a cystic fibrosis patient. Respiration (Herrlisheim) 2004;71:646–9.

[25] Carrieri-Kohlman V, Stulbarg MS. Dyspnea: assessment and management. In: Hodgkin JE, Connors GL, editors. Pulmonary rehabilitation: guidelines to success. 3rd edition. Philadelphia: Lippincott Williams & Wilkins; 2000. p. 57–89.

[26] Freeman JM, Vining EPG. Seizures and epilepsy in childhood: a guide for parents. 2nd edition. Baltimore (MD): Johns Hopkins University Press; 1997.

[27] van Stuijvenberg M, de Vos S, Tjiang GC, et al. Parents' fear regarding fever and febrile seizures. Acta Paediatr 1999;88(6):618–22.

[28] Baumer JH, David TJ, Valentine SJ, et al. Many parents think their child is dying when having a first febrile convulsion. Dev Med Child Neurol 1981;23(4):462–4.

[29] Fernandes PT, Souza EA. Identification of family variables in parents' groups of children with epilepsy. Arq Neuropsiquiatr 2001;59(4):854–8.

[30] Arunkumar G, Wyllie E, Kotagal P, et al. Parent- and patient-validated content for pediatric epilepsy quality-of-life assessment. Epilepsia 2000;41(11):1474–84.

[31] Mula M, Trimble MR, Sander JW. Psychiatric adverse events in patients with epilepsy and learning disabilities taking levetiracetam. Seizure 2004;13(1):55–7.

[32] Royal M, Wienecke G, Movva V, et al. Open label trial of oxcarbazepine in neuropathic pain. Pain Med 2001;2(3):250–1.

[33] Worden JW. Grief counseling and grief therapy: a handbook for the mental health practitioner. 2nd edition. New York: Springer-Verlag; 1991.

[34] Strong C, Feudtner C, Carter BS, et al. Goals, values, and conflict resolution. In: Carter BS, Levetown M, editors. Palliative care for infants, children, and adolescents: a practical handbook. Baltimore (MD): Johns Hopkins University Press; 2004. p. 23–43.

[35] American Academy of Pediatrics Committee on Bioethics. Guidelines on foregoing life-sustaining medical treatment. Pediatrics 1994;93(3):532–6.

[36] Tuckett AG. Truth-telling in clinical practice and the arguments for and against: a review of the literature. Nursing Ethics: an International Journal for Health Care Professionals 2004;11(5): 500–13.

[37] American Academy of Pediatrics Committee on Pediatrics AIDS. Disclosure of illness status to children and adolescents with HIV infection. Pediatrics 1999;103(1):164–6.

[38] Frader JE. Bay doe blinders. JAMA 2000;284:1143.

[39] Clark PA. Building a policy in pediatrics for medical futility. Pediatr Nurs 2001;27(2):180–4.

[40] Casarett D, Siegler M. Unilateral do-not-attempt-resuscitation orders and ethics consultation: a case series. Crit Care Med 1999;27(6):1116–20.

[41] American Academy of Pediatrics Committee on Bioethics. Ethics and the care of critically ill infants and children. Pediatrics 1996;98(1):149–52.

ELSEVIER
SAUNDERS

PEDIATRIC CLINICS
OF NORTH AMERICA

Pediatr Clin N Am 52 (2005) 1047–1057

Bronchiolitis: In-Patient Focus

Susan E. Coffin, MD, MPH[a,b,*]

[a]Division of Infectious Diseases, University of Pennsylvania School of Medicine, 3400 Spruce Street,
Philadelphia, PA 19104, USA
[b]Department of Infection Prevention and Control, Children's Hospital of Philadelphia,
3561 Civic Center Boulevard, Room 9ST52, Philadelphia, PA 19104, USA

Bronchiolitis is among the most common and serious lower respiratory tract syndromes that affects young children. In developed countries, the case fatality rate among previously healthy children remains low; in contrast, infants with underlying medical conditions, such as immunodeficiency or chronic lung disease, are at risk of prolonged illness and death. Bronchiolitis is associated with significant morbidity among healthy young children. During the winter season, bronchiolitis is the most common cause of hospitalization among infants. Each year in the United States, approximately 2 per 100,000 infants die as a result of complications associated with bronchiolitis [1].

Definition

Bronchiolitis is a clinical syndrome characterized by the acute onset of respiratory symptoms in a child younger than 2 years of age. Typically, the initial symptoms of upper respiratory tract viral infection, such as fever and coryza, progress within 4 to 6 days to include evidence of lower respiratory tract involvement with the onset of cough and wheezing.

Epidemiology

Bronchiolitis occurs most frequently among children younger than 12 months of age. Infants younger than 6 months are at highest risk of clinically significant

---

* Department of Infection Prevention and Control, Children's Hospital of Philadelphia, 3561 Civic Center Boulevard, Room 9ST52, Philadelphia, PA 19104.
    E-mail address: coffin@email.chop.edu

disease [2]. Bronchiolitis is a seasonal disease that coincides with outbreaks of infections secondary to viral respiratory pathogens (see later discussion). In temperate climates, hospital admissions because of bronchiolitis are most common from December to May.

In the United States, as many as 1% of infants are hospitalized for bronchiolitis, and the annual hospital charges associated with bronchiolitis exceed $800 million [3]. The burden of disease related to respiratory syncytial virus (RSV)–associated bronchiolitis recently was assessed. Analyses of national data revealed that more than 700,000 infants visit US emergency departments each year because of RSV-associated bronchiolitis; approximately one third of these infants are admitted to the hospital [4].

Environmental and genetic factors contribute to the severity of disease. Day-care attendance, exposure to passive smoke, and household crowding are associated with an increased risk of bronchiolitis-related hospitalization [5,6]. Race and poverty also have been associated with severe disease [4]. Other studies have suggested that there might be a genetic predisposition to bronchiolitis. For example, infants with bronchiolitis were more likely to have a family member with asthma or other wheezing illness [7].

Over the past 20 years, the rate of hospitalization for bronchiolitis has increased markedly [8]. Recent studies estimated that 2% to 3% of affected children required hospital admission [9]. Some authors have suggested that the widespread adoption of pulse oximetry monitoring in primary care practices and emergency departments might have contributed to this trend. Other factors, however, such as increased daycare attendance and the increase in the number of medically fragile infants, might have led to real increases in the incidence of serious disease [10].

Etiology

Bronchiolitis is usually a consequence of a viral respiratory tract infection (Table 1). RSV is the most common underlying viral infection and has been isolated from 50% to 75% of children younger than 2 years of age hospitalized with bronchiolitis [11]. Other common respiratory viral pathogens, such as influenza, parainfluenza, and adenovirus, have been isolated from children with bronchiolitis [12–14]. Recent investigations have demonstrated that some infants with bronchiolitis also may be infected with rhinovirus [15] or human metapneumovirus [16,17]. Finally, several investigators have reported the recovery of *Mycoplasma pneumoniae* from children with bronchiolitis, although this agent is not commonly recognized as a significant cause of disease in young children [12].

Pathogenesis

Bronchiolitis is a result of progressive infection and inflammation of the respiratory mucosa in a young child. The clinical symptoms of obstructive lower

Table 1
Infectious agents associated with acute bronchiolitis

Infectious agent	Relative frequency (%)	Total frequency
Respiratory syncytial virus		50
Parainfluenza viruses		25
Type 1	(8)	
Type 2	(2)	
Type 3	(15)	
Adenoviruses		5
Mycoplasma pneumoniae		5
Rhinoviruses		5
Influenza viruses		5
Type A	(3)	
Type B	(2)	
Enteroviruses		2
Herpes simplex virus		2
Mumps virus		<1

Data from Feigin, Cherry, editors. Textbook of pediatric infectious diseases. 5th edition. p. 274.

respiratory tract infection are a consequence of the partial occlusion of the distal airways. Histologic examination of the lungs of affected children often reveals necrosis of the respiratory epithelium, monocytic inflammation with edema of the peribronchial tissues, and obstruction of the distal airways with mucus and fibrin plugs. Infants are predisposed to develop wheezing and other symptoms of airway obstruction because of the small caliber of their distal airways and the absence of active immunity to RSV and other respiratory viruses.

Viral replication and virally induced production of inflammatory mediators by respiratory epithelial cells contribute to the pathogenesis of disease. After initial infection of the respiratory epithelium of the upper airway in an immunologically naïve child, viral replication can progress to the mucosal surfaces of the lower respiratory tract. Desquamation of respiratory epithelial cells, edema of the mu-

Table 2
Factors associated with an increased risk and severity of bronchiolitis and postbronchiolitis morbidity

	Increase in frequency	Increase in severity	Increase in later morbidity
Crowding	+++	+++	?
Passive smoking	+++	+++	++
Male gender	+	++	++
Absence of breast feeding	+	+	?
Family history of asthma	±	±	±
Personal atopy	−	−	+++
Congenitally small airways	++	?	−
Airway reactivity	−	+	++
RSV-specific IgE response	++	++	++

+++ implies strong relationship; ++ implies moderate relationship; + implies weak relationship; ± implies controversial relationship; − implies no relationship; ? implies unknown relationship.
Data from Feigin, Cherry, editors. Textbook of pediatric infectious diseases. 5th edition. p. 277.

cosal surface, and enhanced reactivity of airway smooth muscle lead to the respiratory symptoms that characterize bronchiolitis. Some investigators have reported that the clinical spectrum of disease varies somewhat in association with the underlying viral pathogen [15] and that these differences might reflect differences in the profile and extent of inflammatory mediators (such as leukotrienes and cytokines) produced by infected respiratory epithelial cells [18]. The relationship between severe disease and co-infection with multiple respiratory viral pathogens remains unclear.

Environmental factors also play a role in the development of bronchiolitis (Table 2). It is unclear, however, how passive smoke exposure might mediate an increased risk of disease or how household crowding might be associated with an increased disease severity.

Clinical presentation

An infant with bronchiolitis typically presents with illness during the winter months, although sporadic cases appear throughout the year. More than half of affected children are between 2 and 7 months of age [19,20]. Parents often report that a child attends daycare or has a household contact with cold-like symptoms. Early in the illness, infants usually experience copious rhinorrhea. Typically, infants develop a tight cough associated with poor feeding 4 to 6 days after the initial onset of symptoms. The proportion of infants with fever seems to vary by underlying pathogen. Overall, infants with RSV-associated bronchiolitis are often febrile at the time of presentation for medical care; in patients with adenovirus- or influenza-associated bronchiolitis, however, fever is often higher than 39°C.

Infants with bronchiolitis often present for medical care with significant tachypnea, mild-to-moderate hypoxia, and visible signs of respiratory distress, such as nasal flaring and retractions [19,20]. Upon examination, infants typically have audible wheezing, rales or rhonchi, and poor air movement, and the expiratory phase is usually prolonged. Other findings commonly observed in infants hospitalized with bronchiolitis include conjunctivitis, rhinitis, and otitis media. Many infants have a distended abdomen caused by hyperinflation of the lungs.

Respiratory viral pathogens often can be isolated from children hospitalized with bronchiolitis; however, the proportion of disease attributable to specific virus varies by season and year. Viruses can be detected in nasal wash specimens by enzyme-linked immunosorbent assays, indirect fluorescent antibody detection, polymerase chain reaction, or viral culture. The results of viral diagnostic testing can be used to limit the inappropriate use of antibacterial therapy. Knowledge of a specific viral diagnosis also can facilitate appropriate cohorting of patients and staff to prevent nosocomial transmission of these viruses. For example, RSV is transmitted largely through direct and indirect contact, whereas influenza is passed person to person by respiratory droplets. Health care workers who provide care to an infant with RSV-related bronchiolitis compared with influenza-related bronchiolitis should use different personal protective equipment.

Infants with bronchiolitis often have mildly elevated total white blood cell counts, although the differential white blood cell count is typically normal [19]. Hypoxia is often observed on pulse oximetry or analysis of arterial blood samples. Retention of carbon dioxide can be seen in severe cases.

The radiographic findings of bronchiolitis include hyperinflation, patchy infiltrates that are typically migratory and attributable to postobstructive atelectasis, and peribronchial cuffing [19]. Because bronchiolitis is not a disease of the alveolar spaces, a secondary bacterial pneumonitis should be suspected if a true alveolar infiltrate is seen on chest radiograph.

Differential diagnosis

The absence of antecedent upper respiratory tract symptoms should suggest to clinicians that an infant with the acute onset of wheezing might not have bronchiolitis. In newborns, congenital anomalies, such as a vascular ring or congenital heart disease, should be considered. Gastroesophageal reflux, aspiration pneumonia, or foreign body aspiration can mimic the symptoms of bronchiolitis.

Treatment

Supportive care is the mainstay of therapy for infants with bronchiolitis. Moderately ill infants often require supplemental oxygen [21]. Because of tachypnea, partial nasal obstruction, and feeding difficulties, young infants sometimes need intravenous fluids to correct mild-to-moderate dehydration. The role of bronchodilators in the care of infants with bronchiolitis remains controversial [9,21–23]. The inclusion of patients with a history of recurrent wheezing has introduced bias into some studies and might have resulted in an overestimation of the potential benefit of bronchodilators. A recent meta-analysis found that in eight trials that included 394 children, 54% of patients treated with bronchodilators compared with 25% who received a placebo had an improved clinical score (odds ratio for no improvement 0.29; 95% confidence interval, 0.19–0.45). Bronchodilator therapy was not associated with a reduced need for or duration of hospitalization, however [24]. Similarly, a recent randomized, double-blinded, placebo-controlled trial demonstrated that nebulized epinephrine did not shorten the duration of hospitalization [25]. A meta-analysis conducted by Hartling et al [26] also found insufficient evidence to support the use of nebulized epinephrine among hospitalized children.

The role of steroids in the treatment of children with bronchiolitis also has been controversial [27]. A meta-analysis of six placebo-controlled trials demonstrated that corticosteroid therapy was associated with a significant reduction in the length of hospitalization stay (0.43 days; 95% confidence interval, 0.05–0.81); however, if the studies that included patients with a history of wheezing were omitted from the analysis, this difference was no longer significant [28]. Dexamethasone also had no beneficial effect in infants with respiratory failure caused by RSV bronchiolitis [29]. In contrast, some studies have demonstrated that the use of steroids may be of benefit to patients with bronchiolitis if given before hospitalization [30,31]. In a randomized, placebo-controlled trial, Csonka et al demonstrated that infants treated with oral prednisolone upon initial evaluation and during the first 3 hospital days had a 1-day reduction in the duration of symptoms and length of hospital stay. Some clinicians have concluded that early treatment with steroids might shorten the duration of illness.

RSV is the most common cause of bronchiolitis; however, specific antiviral therapy of symptomatic infants has been of limited value. Aerosolized ribavirin treatment of mild-to-moderately ill infants with laboratory-confirmed RSV bronchiolitis does not prevent the need for mechanical ventilation or reduce the length of hospital stay. The American Academy of Pediatrics does not recommend the routine use of ribavirin but suggests that ribavirin might be administered based on specific clinical circumstances and physician experience [31]. Patients who are at risk of persistent viral replication might benefit from ribavirin therapy; some experts recommend that ribavirin be considered when caring for severely immunocompromised patients who develop laboratory-confirmed RSV-associated bronchiolitis, such as children undergoing bone marrow transplantation [32]. Experts debate the role of ribavirin therapy for severely ill infants who require mechanical ventilation. In a single placebo-controlled study, investigators found that infants treated with aerosolized ribavirin had a shorter duration of ventilation and of hospital stay [33]. Finally, investigators have yet to demonstrate that other therapies, including interferon, surfactant, vitamin A, mist therapy, or anticholinergics, have any measurable clinical effect.

Complications and outcomes

The case fatality rate for bronchiolitis is highest among young infants between 1 and 3 months of age. Former premature infants with birth weights less than 1500 g have a bronchiolitis mortality rate of 30 per 100,000 live births [1]. The presence of underlying medical conditions, such as congenital heart disease or chronic lung disease, is another important predictor of poor outcome [34]. In these high-risk children, the case fatality rate may be as high as 5%.

Serious complications, including respiratory failure, apnea, and pneumothorax, occur among infants hospitalized with bronchiolitis, more commonly among former premature infants and infants with congenital abnormalities. Overall, serious complications are associated with prolonged hospital stay and increased direct health care costs. The association between early RSV infection and asthma has been debated hotly [35,36]. Up to 50% of children with a history of bronchiolitis develop recurrent wheezing [36,37]. Some investigators have suggested that a family history of allergic or atopic disease correlates with the subsequent development of asthma; however, this association is incompletely understood [38,39]. Among healthy former premature infants, hospitalization for RSV bronchiolitis has been associated with an increase in subsequent use of health care resources, particularly those associated with respiratory conditions [40]. Subsequent health care visits for respiratory symptoms occurred in 64% of infants previously hospitalized, compared with 13% in infants not hospitalization for RSV bronchiolitis.

For unclear reasons, secondary bacterial infections of the lower respiratory tract are unusual in children with bronchiolitis [41]. Serious bacterial infections, which are identified as bacteremia, urinary tract infection, or meningitis, are another concern for febrile infants with bronchiolitis. It is estimated that one half to two thirds of infants and young children hospitalized for RSV bronchiolitis are febrile. Investigators in Texas demonstrated that children younger than 2 years of age hospitalized with RSV bronchiolitis have a low rate of concurrent serious bacterial infections. In that study of 2396 children admitted with RSV bronchiolitis or pneumonia, the rate of serious bacterial infections was 1.6%, of which 1.1% involved urinary tract infections and 0.5% involved positive blood culture results. All organisms isolated from the positive blood culture were consistent with contaminants. There were no positive cerebrospinal fluid culture results [42]. Two studies compared febrile RSV-positive and RSV-negative infants younger than 8 weeks of age. The rates of serious bacterial infections in the RSV-positive groups ranged from 1.1% to 7%, whereas the rate among RSV-negative infants was 12.5% in both studies. None of the RSV-positive infants had bacterial meningitis, and the predominant serious bacterial infection in these groups was urinary tract infection [43,44]. Of note, infants younger than 28 days had rates of serious bacterial infections of 13.3%, regardless of RSV status [44]. Most children older than 1 month with typical signs and symptoms of bronchiolitis, especially children who are RSV positive, may not warrant full evaluation for invasive bacterial infection and may not require empiric antibiotic therapy at the time of hospitalization. The risk of urinary tract infection remains significant. In the first month of life, the risk of serious bacterial infections remains unchanged regardless of whether an infant is RSV positive or negative.

Prevention

A vaccine to prevent RSV infection in young infants is needed. Despite several decades of effort, however, vaccine development has been slow [45]. Several obstacles to the successful development of a safe and effective RSV vaccine have been identified. First, an ideal RSV vaccine would provide immunologic protection to infants younger than 2 months of age. This challenge has led some investigators to advocate maternal immunization as a potential strategy. Next, natural infection with RSV does not induce complete and durable immunity. An RSV vaccine would be unlikely to induce long-lasting immunity, but a reasonable goal might be for an RSV vaccine to protect the most vulnerable (ie, children younger than 2 years) from serious disease. Finally, the potential for immuno-enhancement upon second exposure to RSV antigens has been a serious obstacle to the successful development of an RSV vaccine.

Recently, the Centers for Disease Control and Prevention recommended that all healthy infants aged 6 to 23 months receive the influenza vaccine [46]. Recent issues with the vaccine supply have limited the early adoption of this recommendation, so the magnitude of its impact remains unknown.

Currently, pediatricians rely on passive immunization to prevent serious RSV-related infections in high-risk infants. Monthly administration of paluvizumab (a monoclonal antibody directed against a key viral surface protein) or hyper-immune immunoglobulin is associated with a significant reduction in the rate of hospitalization for respiratory illnesses among children younger than 2 years of age with a history of prematurity, chronic lung disease, and hemodynamically significant congenital heart disease [47–49] (Table 3). RSV prophylaxis should be administered once per month during the RSV season. Because high-risk infants can develop two severe RSV infections within the same season, prophylaxis should be continued throughout the RSV season even in an infant who develops a documented RSV infection while receiving immunoprophylaxis.

Table 3
Recommendations for the use of respiratory syncytial virus prophylaxis[a]

	First year of life	Second year of life
Infants <2 y	Chronic lung disease requiring medical therapy within 6 months of start of RSV season	Same
	Hemodynamically significant congenital heart disease[b]	Same
Infants born at ≤32 wk EGA	Regardless of the presence of chronic lung disease	Only if other risk factors are present
Infants born at 32–35 wk EGA	Recommendations should be individualized based on the presence of environmental or physiologic risk factors[c]	Not routinely recommended

[a] Either RSV immunoglobulin or palivizumab.

[b] Infants most likely to benefit include those who are receiving medication for congestive heart failure, infants who have moderate-to-severe pulmonary hypertension, infants with cyanotic heart disease.

[c] Environmental risk factors include daycare attendance, school-aged siblings, and exposure to cigarette smoke. Physiologic risk factors include congenital abnormalities of the airways or severe neurologic diseases.

References

[1] Holman RC, Shay DK, Curns AT, et al. Risk factors for bronchiolitis-associated deaths among infants in the United States. Pediatr Infect Dis J 2003;22:483–90.

[2] Henderson FW, Clyde WA, Collier AM, et al. The etiologic and epidemiologic spectrum of bronchiolitis in pediatric practice. J Pediatr 1979;95:183–90.

[3] Kim HW, Arrobio JO, Brandt DC, et al. Epidemiology or respiratory syncytial virus infection in Washington, DC. Am J Epidemiol 1973;98:216–25.

[4] Leader S, Kohlhase K. Recent trends in severe respiratory syncytial virus (RSV) among US infants, 1997 to 2000. J Pediatr 2003;143(5 Suppl):S127–S32.

[5] Reese AC, James IR, Landau LI, et al. Relationship between urinary cotinine level and diagnosis in children admitted to hospital. Am Rev Respir Dis 1992;146:66–70.

[6] Panitch HB, Callahan CW, Schidlow DV. Bronchiolitis in children. Clin Chest Med 1993;14:715–31.

[7] Camilli AE, Holberg CJ, Wright AL, et al. Parental childhood respiratory illness and respiratory illness in their infants. Pediatr Pulmonol 1993;16:275–80.

[8] Anderson LJ, Parker RA, Strikas RA, et al. Daycare center attendance and hospitalization for lower respiratory tract illness. Pediatrics 1988;82:300–8.

[9] Perlstein PH, Kotagal UR, Boling C, et al. Evaluation of an evidence-based guideline for bronchiolitis. Pediatrics 1999;104:1334–41.

[10] Deshpande SA, Northern V. The clinical and health economic burden of respiratory syncytial virus disease among children under 2 years of age in a defined geographical area. Arch Dis Child 2003;88:1065–9.

[11] Glezen WP, Taber LH, Frank AL, et al. Risk of primary infection and reinfection with respiratory syncytial virus. Am J Dis Child 1986;140:543–6.

[12] Loda FA, Clyde WAJ, Glezen WP, et al. Studies on the role of viruses, bacteria, and M. pneumoniae as causes of lower respiratory tract infections in children. J Pediatr 1968;72:161–76.

[13] Foy HM, Cooney MK, Maletzky AJ, et al. Incidence and etiology of pneumonia, croup and bronchiolitis in preschool children belonging to a prepaid medical care group over a four-year period. Am J Epidemiol 1973;97:80–92.

[14] Glezen WP, Loda FA, Clyde WA, et al. Epidemiologic patterns of acute lower respiratory disease of children in a pediatric group practice. J Pediatr 1971;78:397–406.

[15] Korppi M, Kotaniemi-Syrjanen A, Waris M, et al. Rhinovirus-associated wheezing in infancy: comparison with respiratory syncytial virus bronchiolitis. Pediatr Infect Dis J 2004;23:995–9.

[16] Freymouth F, Vabret A, Legrand L, et al. Presence of the new human metapneumovirus in French children with bronchiolitis. Pediatr Infect Dis J 2003;22:92–4.

[17] Williams JV, Harris PA, Tollefson SJ, et al. Human metapneumovirus and lower respiratory tract disease in otherwise healthy infants and children. N Engl J Med 2004;350:443–50.

[18] Sznajer Y, Westcott JY, Wenzel SE, et al. Airway eicosanoids in acute severe respiratory syncytial virus bronchiolitis. J Pediatr 2004;145:115–8.

[19] Ackerman BD. Acute bronchiolitis: a study of 207 cases. Clin Pediatr 1962;1:61–81.

[20] Wohl MEB, Chernick V. Treatment of acute bronchiolitis. N Engl J Med 2003;349:82–3.

[21] Shay DK, Holman RC, Newman RD, et al. Bronchiolitis-associated hospitalizations among US children, 1980–1996. JAMA 1999;282:1440–6.

[22] Mallory MD, Shay DK, Garrett J, et al. Bronchiolitis management preferences and the influence of pulse oximetry and respiratory rate on the decision to admit. Pediatrics 2003;111:E45–51.

[23] Patel H, Platt RW, Pekeles GS, et al. A randomized, controlled trial of the effectiveness of nebulized therapy with epinephrine compared with albuterol and saline in infants hospitalized for acute viral bronchiolitis. J Pediatr 2002;141:818–24.

[24] Kellner JD, Ohlsson A, Gadomski AM, et al. Bronchodilators for bronchiolitis. Cochrane Database Syst Rev 2000;(2):CD001266.

[25] Wainwright C, Altamirano L, Cheney M, et al. A multicenter, randomized, double-blind, controlled trial of nebulized epinephrine in infants with acute bronchiolitis. N Engl J Med 2003;349:27–35.

[26] Hartling L, Wiebe N, Russell K, et al. A meta-analysis of randomized controlled trials evaluating the efficacy of epinephrine for the treatment of acute viral bronchiolitis. Arch Pediatr Adolesc Med 2003;157:957–64.

[27] Springer C, Bar-Yishay E, Uwayyed K, et al. Corticosteroids do not affect the clinical or physiological status of infants with bronchiolitis. Pediatr Pulmonol 1990;9:181–5.

[28] Garrison MM, Christakis DA, Harvey E, et al. Systemic corticosteroids in infant bronchiolitis: a meta-analysis. Pediatrics 2000;105:E44.

[29] van Woensel JB, van Aalderen WM, de Weerd W, et al. Dexamethasone for treatment of patients mechanically ventilated for lower respiratory tract infection caused by respiratory syncytial virus. Thorax 2003;58:383–7.

[30] Weinberger M. Corticosteroids for first-time young wheezers: current status of the controversy. J Pediatr 2003;143:700–2.

[31] American Academy of Pediatrics Committee on Infectious Diseases. Reassessment of the indications for ribavirin therapy in respiratory syncytial virus infections. Pediatrics 1996;97:137–40.

[32] Moscona A. Management of respiratory syncytial virus infections in the immunocompromised child. Pediatr Infect Dis J 2000;19:253–4.

[33] Smith DW, Frankel LR, Mathers LH, et al. A controlled trial of aerosolized ribavirin in infants receiving mechanical ventilation for severe respiratory syncytial virus infection. N Engl J Med 1991;325:24–9.

[34] Grimaldi M, Gouyon B, Michaut F, et al. Severe respiratory syncytial virus bronchiolitis: epidemiologic variations associated with the initiation of palivizumab in severely premature infants with bronchopulmonary dysplasia. Pediatr Infect Dis J 2004;23:1081–5.

[35] Korppi M, Piippo-Savolainen E, Korhonen K, et al. Respiratory morbidity 20 years after RSV infection in infancy. Pediatr Pulmonol 2004;38:155–60.

[36] Hegele RG, Ahmad HY, Becker AB, et al. The association between respiratory viruses and symptoms in 2-week-old infants at high risk for asthma and allergy. J Pediatr 2001;138:831–7.

[37] Bont L, Steijn M, van Aalderen WM, et al. Impact of wheezing after respiratory syncytial virus infection on health-related quality of life. Pediatr Infect Dis J 2004;23:414–7.

[38] Lemanske RF. Viruses and asthma: inception, exacerbation, and possible prevention. J Pediatr 2003;142:S3–8.

[39] Gern JE. Mechanisms of virus-induced asthma. J Pediatr 2003;142:S9–14.

[40] Sampalis JS. Morbidity and mortality after RSV-associated hospitalizations among premature Canadian infants. J Pediatr 2003;143(5 Suppl):S150–6.

[41] Melendez E, Harper MB. Utility of sepsis evaluation in infants 90 days of age or younger with fever and clinical bronchiolitis. Pediatr Infect Dis J 2003;22:1053–6.

[42] Purcell K, Fergie J. Concurrent serious bacterial infection in 2396 infants and children hospitalized with respiratory syncytial virus lower respiratory tract infection. Arch Pediatr Adolesc Med 2002;156:322–4.

[43] Titus MO, Wright SW. Prevalence of serious bacterial infection in febrile infants with respiratory syncytial virus infection. Pediatrics 2003;112:282–4.

[44] Levine DA, Platt SL, Dayan PS, et al. Risk of serious bacterial infection in young febrile infants with respiratory syncytial virus infections. Pediatrics 2004;113:1728–34.

[45] Coffin SE, Offit PA. New vaccines against mucosal pathogens: rotavirus and respiratory syncytial virus. Adv Pediatr Infect Dis 1997;13:333–48.

[46] Harper SA, Fukuda K, Uyeki TM, et al, Centers for Disease Control and Prevention (CDC) Advisory Committee on Immunization Practices (ACIP). Prevention and control of influenza. MMWR Morb Mortal Wkly Rep 2004;53(RR-6):1–40.

[47] Navas L, Wang E, deCarvalho V, et al. Improved outcome of respiratory syncytial virus infection in a high-risk hospitalized population of Canadian children. Pediatric Investigators Collaborative Network on Infections in Canada. J Pediatr 1993;121:348–54.

[48] Meissner HC, Long SS, American Academy of Pediatrics Committee on Infectious Diseases and Committee on Fetus and Newborn. Revised indications for the use of palivizumab and respiratory syncytial virus immune globulin intravenous for the prevention of respiratory syncytial virus infections. Pediatrics 2003;112:1447–52.

[49] Willson DF, Landrigan CP, Horn SD, et al. Complications in infants hospitalized for bronchiolitis or respiratory syncytial virus pneumonia. J Pediatr 2003;143:S142–9.

ELSEVIER
SAUNDERS

PEDIATRIC CLINICS
OF NORTH AMERICA

Pediatr Clin N Am 52 (2005) 1059–1081

Pneumonia in Hospitalized Children

Thomas J. Sandora, MD, MPH[a,*], Marvin B. Harper, MD[a,b]

[a]*Division of Infectious Diseases, Children's Hospital Boston, Harvard Medical School,*
300 Longwood Avenue, LO 650, Boston, MA 02115, USA
[b]*Division of Emergency Medicine, Children's Hospital Boston, Harvard Medical School,*
300 Longwood Avenue, Boston, MA 02115, USA

Epidemiology

Pneumonia is one of the most common infections in the pediatric age group and one of the leading diagnoses that results in overnight hospital admission for children. In 2001, 198,000 patients younger than 15 years were discharged from hospitals in the United States with a primary diagnosis of pneumonia [1]. In North America, the annual incidence of pneumonia in children younger than 5 years is 30 to 45 cases per 1000; in children aged 5 years and older, the annual incidence is 16 to 22 cases per 1000 [2,3]. In developing countries, which account for more than 95% of episodes of clinical pneumonia worldwide, researchers estimate that more than 150 million new cases occur annually in children younger than 5 years [4].

Pneumonia can be classified as either community-acquired pneumonia (CAP) or nosocomial pneumonia; hospital-acquired pneumonia may be ventilator-associated pneumonia or may be acquired in the absence of mechanical ventilation. Ventilator-associated pneumonia differs in several respects from CAP and is addressed separately in this article. Although no precise definition is universally applied, CAP is generally defined as an infection of the lungs that is marked by symptoms of acute infection (ie, fever, cough, or dyspnea) and is typically associated with abnormal auscultatory findings (eg, rales or altered breath sounds) or the presence of an acute infiltrate on chest imaging in an

* Corresponding author.
E-mail address: thomas.sandora@childrens.havard.edu (T.J. Sandora).

0031-3955/05/$ – see front matter © 2005 Elsevier Inc. All rights reserved.
doi:10.1016/j.pcl.2005.03.004
pediatric.theclinics.com

individual not hospitalized or residing in a long-term care facility for at least 14 days before onset of symptoms [5].

Etiologic agents

A large number of micro-organisms can cause pneumonia in children. Table 1 lists the most frequent etiologic agents that are identified in each age group. Overall, viruses are responsible for a large percentage of cases of CAP in the pediatric age group, and they are particularly common in children aged 3 weeks to 4 years [6]. In a recent US study of children aged 2 months to 17 years who were hospitalized for pneumonia, 45% were found to have a viral etiology [7]. In general, the most frequently isolated respiratory viruses are respiratory syncytial virus, parainfluenza viruses, influenza A and B, and adenovirus, although other viruses may occur in specific settings (eg, cytomegalovirus or herpes simplex infection in neonates). Most cases of viral pneumonia can be managed without invasive diagnostic testing, and aside from supportive care, no specific antimicrobial therapy is generally required. For these reasons, the remainder of this article focuses on bacterial pneumonia, although important distinctions related to viral etiologies are highlighted when appropriate.

The epidemiology of bacterial CAP differs by age and has been impacted by vaccine strategies. From birth to 3 weeks of age, the most common causes of pneumonia are Group B streptococci and gram-negative rods (particularly enterics such as *Escherichia coli*). Although viruses predominate from 3 weeks to 3 months of age, bacterial pneumonia can occur in this age group. Afebrile pneumonia at this age is frequently caused by *Chlamydia trachomatis*; this agent

Table 1
Common causes of pediatric community-acquired pneumonia by age

Age	Etiologic agent
Birth – 3 weeks	Group B streptococcus (*Streptococcus agalactiae*)
	Gram-negative rods (eg, *Escherichia coli*)
3 wk – 3 mo	Viruses (eg, respiratory syncytial virus, parainfluenza viruses, influenza A and B, adenovirus)
	Chlamydia trachomatis
	Streptococcus pneumoniae
4 mo – 4 y	*Streptococcus pneumoniae*
	Viruses (eg, respiratory syncytial virus, parainfluenza viruses, influenza A and B, adenovirus)
	Haemophilus influenzae
	Group A streptococcus (*Streptococcus pyogenes*)
	Staphylococcus aureus
	Mycoplasma pneumoniae
	Other streptococcal species (eg, *Streptococcus milleri* group)
≥ 5 y	*Mycoplasma pneumoniae*
	Chlamydophila pneumoniae
	Streptococcus pneumoniae

rarely requires hospital admission unless found in combination with another respiratory tract pathogen, such as respiratory syncytial virus or pertussis. *Streptococcus pneumoniae* is the most common bacterial cause of febrile pneumonia among children aged 3 weeks to 4 years. A recent study from Texas found that 60% of children between 2 months and 17 years of age who were admitted with pneumonia had a bacterial pathogen isolated, and *S. pneumoniae* was confirmed in 73% of those cases [7]. Other less commonly isolated bacteria include *Haemophilus influenzae* (historically type b before widespread vaccine use, but currently includes nontypable *H. influenzae*), *Streptococcus pyogenes*, *Staphylococcus aureus*, and other streptococcal species (including the *Streptococcus milleri* group). In children aged 5 years and older, the most common bacterial pathogens are *Mycoplasma pneumoniae* and *Chlamydophila pneumoniae* (previously known as *Chlamydia pneumoniae*). These atypical agents account for nearly one fourth of all cases of bacterial pneumonia among school-aged children and adolescents [7]. Pneumococcus remains high on the list of agents identified

Table 2
Less common causes of pneumonia in children

Organism	Risk factors or clinical scenarios
Human metapneumovirus	Similar in epidemiology and presentation to respiratory syncytial virus
Bordetella pertussis	Peak incidence in infants and adolescents; exposure to adults with cough illness
Mycobacterium tuberculosis	Most common cause in developing world; travel to endemic region or exposure to high-risk individuals
Listeria monocytogenes	Component of early-onset septicemia in infants from birth to 3 weeks of age; in older patients, ingestion of contaminated food or unpasteurized dairy products (disease often seen in pregnant women)
Cytomegalovirus	Infants with congenital/perinatal infection or part of disseminated illness in immunocompromised hosts
Varicella-zoster virus and herpes simplex virus	May cause pneumonia/pneumonitis as part of disseminated disease
Legionella pneumophila	Exposure to contaminated water supply
Coccidioides immitis	Travel to endemic region (southwest United States)
Histoplasma capsulatum	Travel to endemic region (Ohio and Mississippi River valley)
Blastomyces dermatitidis	Travel to endemic region (Ohio and Mississippi River valley)
Chlamydophila psittaci	Exposure to birds (parakeets)
Hantavirus	Exposure to mouse droppings
Coxiella burnetii	Exposure to sheep
Brucella abortis	Exposure to cattle or goats; ingestion of unpasteurized dairy products
Coronavirus	Associated with severe acute respiratory syndrome (SARS); travel to affected region (particularly Asia)
Avian influenza (influenza A: H5, H7, H9)	Exposure to birds; travel to affected region (Asia)
Francisella tularensis	Exposure to animals (rabbits); bioterrorist activity
Yersinia pestis	Exposure to rats; bioterrorist activity
Bacillus anthracis	Exposure to infected animals; bioterrorist activity

among children who are hospitalized for pneumonia. In addition to these common causes of pneumonia, various other micro-organisms can cause pneumonia in particular circumstances. Table 2 provides a list of these less frequent pathogens and the risk factors or clinical situations that should prompt consideration of more unusual infections. Finally, it is important to remember that a significant proportion of cases of pediatric pneumonia represents a mixed infection [8].

Pathogenesis

Pathogen, host, and environmental factors all play a role in the development of pneumonia, which typically begins with tracheal colonization by the infecting micro-organism [9]. The initial line of defense against the establishment of a respiratory pathogen is the barrier defenses of the airway, namely the mucosal barrier of respiratory epithelium and the mucociliary apparatus that is responsible for clearing foreign material and micro-organisms from the airway [10]. Once the lower respiratory tract is inoculated with a sufficient burden of bacteria, the normal inflammatory response that fights infection (which includes components such as antibodies, complement, phagocytes, and cytokines) also results in damage to functioning lung tissue [11]. The bacteria that commonly cause pneumonia also possess specific virulence factors that enhance their survival and propagation while concurrently resulting in injury to the pulmonary host. For example, S. pneumoniae contains pneumolysin, a pore-forming protein that enables the bacterium to kill host cells, which results in complement activation and a vigorous inflammatory response [12]. Pneumonia also may result from direct seeding of the lung tissue after bacteremia, which may be a particularly important mechanism for bacteria such as pneumococcus and S. aureus.

Clinical manifestations

Several studies have evaluated the use of various clinical symptoms and signs in children with pneumonia. Tachypnea widely has been shown to be the most sensitive indicator [13–16]. The World Health Organization defines tachypnea as a respiratory rate (RR) of more than 60 breaths/min in infants younger than 2 months of age, RR of more than 50 breaths/min from ages 2 to 12 months, and RR of more than 40 breaths/min in children older than 12 months [17]. Several studies have found that cutoffs of more than 50 breaths/min in children younger than 12 months and more than 40 breaths/min in children aged 12 to 35 months provide the greatest combination of sensitivity and specificity in identifying children with lower respiratory infections [18–20], although one study showed that a single value of 50 breaths/min for all ages was equally useful [21]. The precise predictive value depends on the underlying prevalence of disease [22], but a diagnosis of pneumonia in the industrialized world rarely would be made based solely on the presence of tachypnea (which is present in many other childhood illnesses, including bronchiolitis and asthma).

Fever and cough are also frequently present in children with pneumonia, and clinical signs may include retractions or abnormal auscultatory findings, such as rales or decreased breath sounds, which tend to be more specific as indicators of lower respiratory tract infection [23–26]. Other less specific indicators that may be seen in children include malaise, emesis, abdominal pain, and chest pain (which is particularly suggestive of bacterial pneumonia as opposed to viral etiologies, especially when pleuritic in nature). Wheezing may be seen in children with bacterial pneumonia [25] but is more suggestive of bronchiolitis or viral lower respiratory tract infection.

Diagnosis

Differential diagnosis

The diagnosis of pneumonia is likely in patients who present with fever, cough, and tachypnea and who have infiltrates on chest radiography. Various other diseases can present with a similar constellation of signs and symptoms, however. The differential diagnosis may include upper respiratory tract infection, bronchiolitis, congestive heart failure, pulmonary embolism, thoracic tumors, or inflammatory disorders (such as systemic vasculitis), among other entities [27]. Table 3 reviews diseases that should be considered when infiltrates are present on chest radiography.

Table 3
Differential diagnosis of radiographic chest infiltrates

Alveolar infiltrates	Interstitial infiltrates
Infection (pneumonia)	Infection (pneumonia)
Atelectasis	Cystic fibrosis
Pulmonary edema	Bronchopulmonary dysplasia
Hyaline membrane disease	Histiocytosis
Aspiration	Collagen-vascular diseases
Hemorrhage	Sarcoidosis
Hypersensitivity reactions	Pulmonary edema
Lymphoma (Hodgkin's or non-Hodgkin's)	Hemorrhage
Leukemia	Metastatic tumors
Sarcoidosis	Irradiation
Pulmonary alveolar proteinosis	Gaucher's disease
Intralobar sequestration	Niemann-Pick disease
Pulmonary contusion	Tuberous sclerosis
Pulmonary eosinophilia	Neurofibromatosis
	Lymphangiectasia
	Interstitial pneumonitis

Laboratory studies

Several laboratory studies may be helpful in establishing a diagnosis of pneumonia in children. Leukocytosis may be present; in one study, 26% of children who presented to the emergency department with fever and a white blood cell count of more than 20,000/mm^3 were found to have occult pneumonia on chest radiography [26]. Pneumonia also has been shown to be the most common diagnosis in children with white blood cell counts of 25,000/mm^3 or more and even in children with white blood cell counts of 35,000/mm^3 or more [28]. Other inflammatory markers, such as C-reactive protein and the erythrocyte sedimentation rate, are generally elevated. One study found that patients with an elevated C-reactive protein were more likely to have pneumonia of proven or probable bacterial cause as opposed to viral or *Mycoplasma* pneumonia [29].

Cultures of the blood for bacteria traditionally have been recommended in consensus guidelines for the diagnosis and management of pneumonia, particularly when a bacterial cause is suspected [30–32]. This recommendation stems from previous work, which suggested that the rate of bacteremia in adults hospitalized for pneumonia was in the range of 10% to 30%. Several more recent studies have attempted to evaluate the use of blood cultures in the diagnosis of pneumonia, however. In these studies, the yield of blood cultures has been lower—generally ranging from 3% to 11%—and the management of pneumonia is rarely altered [33–35]. Various organisms may be detected, but *S. pneumoniae* has been the most frequently isolated pathogen in these studies. It is likely that the current rate of bacteremia will be lower because of the introduction of the pneumococcal conjugate vaccine in the routine childhood immunization schedule. With increasing resistance to antimicrobial agents and limited available data regarding the use of cultures of the blood among children with pneumonia since the widespread use of the conjugate pneumococcal vaccine, we feel that patients with disease severe enough to require hospital admission and parenteral antimicrobial therapy generally should have cultures of blood sent before therapy. Although it is uncommon to identify a pathogen, the identification of a specific organism (such as *S. pneumoniae* or *S. aureus*) and its associated antimicrobial susceptibilities can be helpful (especially in more severe cases or when pleural effusions are present).

Several other microbiologic tests can be considered as diagnostic aids. Culture of the sputum has had variable use in published studies, with yields ranging from 5% to 34% [34,36]. To be considered reliable (ie, bronchial in origin as opposed to oropharyngeal), a sputum sample should contain fewer than ten epithelial cells per low-powered field [37]. It is difficult to obtain a good sputum sample from children, who often have a nonproductive cough. In general, a valuable sample of expectorated sputum is difficult to obtain from a preschool-aged child. Although a sputum Gram stain with a single predominant organism, leukocytes, and few epithelial cells can be helpful, a negative Gram stain result never should exclude pneumonia as a possible diagnosis. Pneumococcal urinary antigen testing is generally not recommended as a diagnostic modality in pediatric pneumonia; despite good sensitivity, the specificity of this test is low (because it is frequently positive in individuals with nasopharyngeal colonization, particularly young children) [38,39]. Viral diagnostics (either culture or antigen detection using direct fluorescent antibodies) are not necessary in most routine pneumonia cases, but they can be useful in certain circumstances (including cases that involve immunocompromised patients or to help guide infection control precautions). *Mycoplasma* infection can be identified using serology (a positive IgM is an indicator of acute infection); polymerase chain reaction testing is also available and has higher sensitivity and specificity [40], but it is rarely necessary outside of the research setting. *C. pneumoniae* may be detected rapidly by direct fluorescent antibodies from a nasopharyngeal specimen or diagnosed by serology. *Legionella* urinary antigen is the diagnostic modality of choice when *Legionella pneumophila* infection is suspected, and the test can remain positive for weeks after acute infection. It is important to remember that the urinary antigen is negative in cases that involve other species of *Legionella*. The decision to perform a skin test with purified protein derivative in patients who present with pneumonia should be based on the presence of risk factors that would increase the likelihood of tuberculosis or when specific radiographic findings suggest mycobacterial disease (such as the presence of mediastinal adenopathy).

Radiology

The diagnosis of pneumonia frequently is made or confirmed by the presence of consolidation or infiltrates on chest radiography. The presence of respiratory signs (eg, cough, tachypnea, and rales) increases the likelihood of a positive chest radiograph, and one meta-analysis suggested that infants younger than 3 months of age with a temperature of 100.5° F or higher but with no clinical findings of pulmonary disease (defined as rales, ronchi, retractions, wheezes, tachypnea, coryza, grunting, stridor, nasal flaring, or cough) do not require routine chest radiography, because the probability of a normal chest radiograph in the absence of these findings is at least 98.98% [41,42]. When chest radiographs are obtained in patients who have pneumonia, various patterns may be seen. Alveolar infiltrates are seen more frequently in bacterial pneumonia, whereas viral infection is more frequently associated with an interstitial pattern [43]. These distinctions are not universal, however, and studies have confirmed that patients with viral pneumonia can present with infiltrates that have a lobar or alveolar appearance [44]. Interobserver agreement among radiologists about the pattern of infiltrates (alveolar versus interstitial) or the presence of air bronchograms also has been demonstrated to be poor [45]. One interesting study showed that radiologists' readings of chest radiographs in febrile children aged 3 to 24 months were biased by the reading of the treating physician (when compared with radiologists who did not have access to that information) [46]. *Mycoplasma* pneumonia appears most commonly as unilateral or bilateral areas of airspace consolidation and can include reticular or nodular opacities. On high-resolution CT, ground-glass opacities, airspace consolidation, nodules, and bronchovascular thickening are common [47]. When children exhibit persistent or progressive symptoms despite seemingly adequate therapy, contrast-enhanced chest CT can be useful in detecting suppurative complications, such as empyema or necrosis, that may require further intervention [48].

Management

Admission criteria

For adults with CAP, a prediction rule (the Pneumonia Severity Index) was developed and validated to identify patients who are at low risk for death and other adverse outcomes and who might be treated successfully as outpatients [49]. A score is created using various criteria that can be assessed at initial presentation, including demographic factors (eg, age, sex, and nursing home residence), coexisting illnesses (eg, neoplastic disease, congestive heart failure, cerebrovascular disease, renal disease, and liver disease), physical examination findings (eg, mental status, RR, heart rate, blood pressure, and temperature), and laboratory and radiographic findings (eg, arterial pH, blood urea nitrogen, sodium, glucose, hematocrit, partial pressure of arterial oxygen, and pleural effusion). Patients are placed into specific risk classes to guide decisions about the need for hospitalization.

A similar tool for pediatric patients would be useful, but no such validated scoring system has been established. Although specific admission criteria for children may vary among institutions, several criteria for admission are widely used, including ill appearance or septic physiology, hypoxia that requires oxygen administration, moderate or severe respiratory distress, inability to tolerate oral fluids or medications, and social factors, such as the absence of a telephone or the inability to follow-up with a pediatrician or return to the emergency department if disease worsens. Neonates with febrile pneumonia generally should be managed as inpatients, although one field study in India suggested that infants could be treated safely in the community after the first month of life [50]. Patients with underlying conditions that could affect their clinical course adversely and children with complicated pneumonias should be admitted for initiation of therapy.

Empiric antibiotic therapy by age group

Because the most likely etiologic agents depend on the age of the child, it is logical to select initial empiric antibiotic regimens according to age. In neonates from birth to 3 weeks of age, in whom Group B streptococcus and gram-negative rods predominate, the initial coverage should be intravenous (IV) ampicillin and gentamicin in most cases; if disease is severe, a third-generation cephalosporin (eg, cefotaxime) may be added (while continuing the ampicillin to cover *Listeria monocytogenes*, another pathogen in this age group). From age 3 weeks to 3 months, if the infant is afebrile, erythromycin (40 mg/kg/d IV divided every 6 hours) is the drug of choice for treatment of *C. trachomatis*. If fever is present or if a child seems ill, ceftriaxone (50 mg/kg/d every 24 hours) should be given. For patients aged 4 months to 4 years, when viral pneumonia (the most common cause) is suspected, no antibiotic therapy should be administered. If bacterial pneumonia is suspected, IV ampicillin (200 mg/kg/d divided every 6 hours) can be used. If the child appears ill, ceftriaxone may be chosen instead to provide broader coverage. Finally, among children aged 5 years or older, azithromycin (one dose of 10 mg/kg, followed by 5 mg/kg/d) or erythromycin can be used in routine cases to provide coverage of atypical organisms (particularly *Mycoplasma*); ampicillin may be added if there is strong evidence of a bacterial etiology, and ceftriaxone (with or without a macrolide) may be used in children who are more ill. In all ages, if features that suggest *S. aureus* are present, oxacillin or vancomycin should be added, depending on the prevalence of methicillin-resistant staphylococcus in the community [6].

Antibiotic therapy for specific pathogens

Once a specific pathogen has been identified, coverage can be narrowed accordingly. For *Chlamydia* and *Mycoplasma* infections, a macrolide (at the doses described previously) is the drug of choice. In patients with suspected pneumococcal pneumonia, therapeutic choices are driven by local antimicrobial susceptibility patterns. When *S. pneumoniae* has been recovered from an appropriate patient specimen, the antibiotic susceptibility pattern can be used to guide therapy. For isolates that are fully susceptible to penicillin (minimal inhibitory concentration < 0.1 μg/mL), ampicillin should be administered (because of its easier dosing schedule as compared with penicillin). Even for isolates with intermediate susceptibility to penicillin (minimal inhibitory concentration 0.1–1 μg/mL), high-dose ampicillin (200 mg/kg/d) provides excellent coverage. When fully nonsusceptible isolates are encountered (minimal inhibitory concentration ≥ 2 μg/mL), ceftriaxone should be used. Unlike the treatment of meningitis, vancomycin is rarely necessary in the treatment of pneumococcal pneumonia, even when a penicillin nonsusceptible strain is the etiologic agent. It should be added only if ceftriaxone resistance (defined for pneumonia as a minimal inhibitory concentration of ≥ 4 μg/mL) is demonstrated. A recent study from Spain suggested that the combination of a beta-lactam plus a macrolide may be superior to a beta-lactam alone for the treatment of pneumococcal pneumonia in adults, but no randomized trial addressing this hypothesis has been published to date [51]. When *H. influenzae* is considered a likely pathogen (such as in children with underlying lung disease), ceftriaxone or ampicillin-sulbactam is preferred rather than ampicillin because of the presence of beta-lactamase–mediated ampicillin resistance among many *H. influenzae* isolates.

The optimal length of antimicrobial therapy for the treatment of uncomplicated or complicated pneumonia has not been well established for most pathogens. There are data to suggest that a 7- to 14-day course of therapy (or a 5-day course of azithromycin) is adequate for the treatment of *C. pneumoniae* [30,52]. For pneumococcal pneumonia, treatment probably should continue until the patient has been afebrile for 72 hours, and the total duration of therapy probably should not be less than 10 to 14 days (or 5 days if using azithromycin because of its long tissue half-life). Fevers may persist for several days after initiation of appropriate therapy, which reflects the resultant inflammatory cascade and tissue damage. No good data are available to support prolonged treatment courses for patients without underlying conditions (eg, cystic fibrosis) who have uncomplicated pneumonia. Some data suggest that shorter courses of therapy may be equivalent to current standards, although more controlled studies are needed before this practice can be recommended routinely [53,54].

Clinical practice guidelines

Several groups have published practice guidelines for the management of CAP in adults [5,30,32]. No analogous clinical practice guideline for pediatric pneumonia has been accepted universally, although several suggested guidelines have been published [8,31]. Despite the differences among various recommendations, these guidelines serve as excellent compilations of the existing evidence regarding multiple aspects of the treatment of pneumonia. The differences in recommended management strategies contribute to variation in care for this diagnosis, however [55]. Published studies of adult patients with CAP have shown that adherence to a treatment guideline results in improvement in several outcomes, including lower costs, decreased length of stay, more appropriate antibiotic usage, and lower mortality rates [56–61]. Even when guidelines are used, physicians' impressions of their adherence to clinical practice guidelines do not always match their actual adherence to the recommendations contained therein, which suggests that awareness does not guarantee familiarity [62].

Bronchoscopy

The causative organism in cases of pneumonia is frequently not identified by sputum examination or blood culture. When symptoms persist despite empiric antibiotic therapy, bronchoscopy with bronchoalveolar lavage (BAL) is a diagnostic option. Several studies have shown that culture of BAL fluid in children with pneumonia can be useful in making a microbiologic diagnosis [63,64]. Although bronchoscopy is not necessary in routine cases, it should be considered when patients fail to improve with standard therapy or when concern about antibiotic resistance or unusual organisms is high and recovery of the causative agents will change management. Early bronchoscopy may be critical for immunocompromised patients, for whom the selection of empiric therapy is difficult because of the expanded list of potential causes.

Discharge criteria

No single set of criteria defining clinical stability for inpatients with pneumonia has gained widespread acceptance, which introduces variability in decisions about discharge. The combination of normalization of vital signs, ability to take oral nutrition, and clear mental status has been shown to predict a low risk of subsequent clinical deterioration among hospitalized adults with pneumonia [65]. Time to clinical stability and 30-day post-admission mortality have been suggested to be the most reliable clinically based outcome measures for CAP (along with process-of-care measures, such as admission-to-antibiotic time, proportion of patients receiving guideline-based antibiotic therapy, and percentage of patients switched from IV to oral therapy within 24 hours of reaching clinical stability) [66].

Recommended follow-up

Follow-up of children with pneumonia after discharge from the hospital should include involvement from their pediatrician or other primary care provider to ensure that clinical stability continues and that antibiotic therapy is completed as prescribed. In otherwise healthy children, follow-up radiographic studies are not necessary after a single episode of pneumonia. Consolidation on chest radiographs can persist for up to 10 weeks, regardless of clinical improvement [67]. Children with *M. pneumoniae* infection have been found to have detectable abnormalities on high-resolution CT scans more than 1 year after the episode [68]. Follow-up radiographs should be reserved for children with underlying conditions, recurrent or persistent symptoms, or recurrent episodes of pneumonia. In these cases, a period of at least 2 to 3 weeks is recommended before obtaining a follow-up radiograph [69].

Prognosis

Although rates of hospitalization for pneumonia among children have been rising, mortality rates from childhood pneumonia in the United States declined by 97% between 1939 (24,637 deaths from pneumonia) and 1996 (800 deaths) [70]. Case fatality rates (not adjusted for underlying comorbidities) from 1995 to 1997 have been estimated to be 4% in children younger than 2 years of age and 2% in children aged 2 to 17 years [71]. Although antibiotic use probably accounted for much of the decrease in mortality rates during the early part of this time period, recent declines are likely attributable in part to improved access to care for poor children [70]. Improvements in critical care medicine also may reduce mortality, which is highest in children with underlying medical conditions.

Most children who develop pneumonia do not have any long-term sequelae. Some data suggest that up to 45% of children may have symptoms of asthma

5 years after hospitalization for pneumonia, however, which may reflect either unrecognized asthma at the time of presentation with CAP or a propensity to develop asthma after CAP [72].

Complications

Pleural effusions and empyema

Parapneumonic effusions are not uncommon with pneumonia and can occur in conjunction with most etiologic agents. Whereas *S. pneumoniae* accounts for most cases with parapneumonic effusions, *S. aureus* and *S. pyogenes* are associated with particularly high rates of effusion and empyema [73]. Tuberculosis is also a common cause in geographic areas with a high prevalence of disease and should be considered in the differential diagnosis of selected patients [74]. Traditionally, the classification of such effusions as transudative versus empyema has been based on laboratory analysis of the pleural fluid. Characteristics that suggest empyema include pH less than 7.1, lactate dehydrogenase more than 1000 IU/mL, and glucose less than 40 mg/dL [75]. Additional data that may be obtained include an elevated pleural fluid white blood cell count (ie, $>50,000/mm^3$) or a positive microbiologic study (including Gram stain, culture, or other diagnostic tests, such as stains or polymerase chain reaction). Pleural fluid cell count has limited predictive value, however [76], and a positive microbiologic diagnosis is made from pleural fluid analysis in less than one third of cases [77]. CT scan findings (such as pleural thickening or enhancement, among others) have been shown to be inaccurate in predicting which effusions meet laboratory criteria for empyema [78].

Several therapeutic options are available for the management of parapneumonic effusions. Antibiotic therapy alone may result in resolution in some cases. Drainage of the fluid by thoracentesis or placement of a drainage tube (large-bore chest tube or pigtail catheter) can remove the effusion. One study found that either needle aspiration alone or catheter drainage resulted in similar complication rates and lengths of stay, but children who underwent primary aspiration without catheter placement had a higher reintervention rate than children who had catheter placement at the time of initial drainage [79]. Lower pH (especially <7.2) and presence of loculations also were independent predictors of reintervention in this study. The natural history of parapneumonic effusions follows several stages, beginning with an exudative phase, during which the fluid is free-flowing and of low cellularity. This stage is followed 24 to 48 hours later by a fibropurulent phase, during which the accumulation of fibrin and neutrophils may result in loculation. Finally, an organizing phase occurs, with fibroblast activity resulting in the formation of a "peel." Thoracoscopy with surgical débridement may be necessary when the effusion has been longstanding enough to have allowed the development of septations, which reduce the feasibility of tube drainage. Surgery has been shown to reduce the length of stay for hospitalized children whose effusions were considered high grade (defined as containing sonographic evidence of organization such as fronds, septation, or loculation) [80]. In particular, video-assisted thoracoscopic surgery has been shown to have numerous advantages compared with open thoracotomy, including fewer lung resections, fewer associated blood transfusions, less postoperative analgesia, shorter length of stay, faster resolution of fever, and shorter time to removal of chest drains [81].

An alternative option for managing loculated parapneumonic effusions is the use of intrapleural fibrinolytic agents (such as tissue plasminogen activator, streptokinase, or urokinase). These agents are used when inadequate drainage is obtained after chest tube insertion. Recent reports of fibrinolytic therapy in children demonstrate that 60% to 70% of effusions in the fibropurulent phase can be drained completely and another 20% to 30% can be drained partially using the technique of daily instillation of streptokinase or urokinase through a chest tube with a dwell time of 4 hours. This technique is ineffective in draining effusions that already have reached the organizing phase, however [82,83]. Increased drainage also has been demonstrated using a 1-hour dwell of tissue plasminogen activator [84]. One randomized trial in children showed that children who received intrapleural urokinase treatment had a shorter length of stay compared with a placebo group [85]. Fibrinolytic therapy has been associated with several rare complications, including allergic reactions (particularly with streptokinase), hemorrhage, and bronchopleural fistula formation. A large, prospective, randomized trial is needed to define better several aspects of this treatment option, including precise indications, optimal dosing and duration of therapy, and complication rates.

Necrotizing pneumonia and lung abscess

Failure to improve despite appropriate antimicrobial therapy should raise the suspicion of complications, such as parenchymal necrosis or abscess. These complications may be identified on contrast-enhanced CT scan when plain films do not reveal the findings [48]. Decreased parenchymal enhancement may herald the development of cavitary necrosis and a prolonged and more intense illness [86]. Most children who develop cavitary necrosis eventually demonstrate resolution of the pulmonary abnormality on follow-up radiography, however, even in the absence of surgical intervention [87]. Interventional procedures (eg, percutaneous catheter placement) should be avoided in children with necrotizing pneumonia, because such procedures may increase the likelihood of complications, such as bronchopleural fistula formation [88].

Lung abscess is an uncommon complication that more frequently occurs in older children. Abscesses may be primary or secondary. Experts have recommended that therapy routinely should include coverage of gram-positive organisms (*S. aureus* and streptococci) and anaerobes, although gram-negative coverage may be required in selected circumstances. Most patients can be treated medically; needle aspiration or percutaneous catheter drainage of an abscess is safe and often provides diagnostic and therapeutic value in cases that fail to resolve on antibiotic therapy alone, without the associated complication rate seen in necrotizing pneumonia [88–90]. In general, percutaneous drainage should be considered if a patient's condition worsens or when clinical status fails to improve after 72 hours of antibiotic therapy. At least 3 weeks of IV antibiotic therapy should be delivered before lobectomy is considered [91].

Topics of particular interest to hospitalists

Recurrent pneumonia

Recurrent pneumonia is generally defined as two episodes in 1 year or more than three episodes in a lifetime. Most children with recurrent pneumonia have an identifiable underlying predisposing factor. In one pediatric study, the most common of these factors was aspiration secondary to oropharyngeal muscular incoordination (eg, in cerebral palsy); other identified illnesses included immune disorders (generally related to malignancy or abnormalities of the humoral immune system, including HIV infection), congenital heart disease, asthma, congenital or acquired anatomic abnormalities (eg, tracheoesophageal fistula), gastroesophageal reflux, and sickle cell anemia [92]. Evaluation of a child with recurrent pneumonia should include a detailed history that focuses on possible indicators of these underlying illnesses combined with a targeted diagnostic evaluation that may include tests such as swallowing studies, serum immunoglobulins, HIV testing, echocardiography, pulmonary function tests, sweat testing, or radiographic studies, such as chest CT.

Hosts with compromised protective mechanisms

Mechanical ventilation

Several underlying abnormalities may result in a predisposition to the development of pneumonia. Patients with endotracheal tubes or tracheostomies are at risk of lower respiratory tract infection because aspiration of contaminated secretions from the oropharynx or stomach is enhanced by several factors, including pooling of secretions above the cuff with subsequent leak and prolonged supine positioning [9]. Intubated patients in an intensive care unit may have fever or respiratory compromise unrelated to lung infection, and distinguishing bacterial colonization in tracheal aspirates from pneumonia can be difficult. Ventilator-associated pneumonia is best identified using a combination of diagnostic modalities. In one study, 90% of ventilated children with bacterial pneumonia met one of the following three criteria: (1) bronchoscopic protected specimen brush culture with 10^3 or more colony-forming units/mL, (2) intracellular bacteria in 1% or more of cells retrieved by BAL, (3) BAL fluid culture with 10^4 or more colony-forming units/mL [93].

Aspiration pneumonia

Patients with gastroesophageal reflux and patients who are unable to control their secretions because of neurologic impairment (underlying or drug induced) or anatomic disruption are at risk of aspiration pneumonia. Aspiration of oropharyngeal contents may produce a chemical pneumonitis, but it is frequently difficult to assess whether the introduction of oral bacteria has resulted in the establishment of a lower respiratory tract infection. Antibiotic therapy is routinely prescribed for presumed aspiration pneumonia, and the administration of either penicillin or clindamycin (which provide reasonable coverage for oral anaerobes) has been shown to be equally effective therapy for this indication [94]. In children who experience an aspiration event after hospitalization or in others in whom infection with *Pseudomonas* or other gram-negative organisms is suspected (eg, patients with cystic fibrosis), a combination agent such as ampicillin or piperacillin and a beta-lactamase inhibitor should be considered.

Immunodeficiency

Any abnormality in the host immune system may predispose a child to develop pneumonia. Some of the more common scenarios seen in hospitalized patients include malignancy (either hematologic or solid tumors), solid organ or stem cell transplant, congenital or acquired immunodeficiencies, and autoimmune disorders or immunosuppressive medications used to treat systemic illnesses. Regardless of cause, the immunocompromised host should be considered high risk for infection and merits a more aggressive diagnostic and therapeutic approach. Table 4 reviews micro-organisms that may be pathogens in immunocompromised patients with pneumonia. In particular, viral infections (especially cytomegalovirus) and fungal infections (including *Candida* and *Aspergillus*) must be considered [95] along with unusual organisms such as *Pneumocystis jaroveci* (formerly known as *Pneumocystis carinii*) or *Cryptococcus neoformans*. Results of chest radiographs in patients with neutropenia may be negative [96], although findings that suggest an infectious cause (such as nodules) may be visible on plain films [97]. Chest CT scan may demonstrate abnormalities that are not detected on routine radiograph and may help localize lesions (particularly nodules) that are amenable to biopsy to aid in diagnosis [98]. MR imaging is another alternative diagnostic modality and may be more sensitive for the detection of necrotizing pneumonia than CT scan [99]. Flexible bronchoscopy can establish a diagnosis in many cases, and several sampling methods are available. In one study of immunocompromised patients, the diagnostic yield was highest using a combination of BAL and transbronchial biopsy (70%), as compared with BAL alone (38%), transbronchial biopsy alone (38%), or protected specimen brush sampling (13%) [100]. Finally, lung biopsy may be considered to assist in making a diagnosis in patients with a concerning

Table 4
Etiologic agents of pneumonia in immunocompromised hosts

Organism	Comment
Pneumocystis jaroveci	Previously called *Pneumocystis carinii*; associated with cellular immune defects, including HIV infection; typically seen when CD4 count is less than 200 cells/mm^3 or in infants from 3 – 6 months of age
Cryptococcus neoformans	Yeast; intrinsically resistant to caspofungin
Candida spp	May be part of disseminated deep-organ infection
Aspergillus spp	Common cause of nodular lung infection
Zygomycetes	Family of fungi that includes *Rhizopus*, *Mucor*, and others; may be resistant to amphotericin B
Nocardia spp	Environmental bacteria; commonly cause infection of lungs, brain, or skin; require long-term therapy
Cytomegalovirus	Pneumonia as part of disseminated disease
Herpes simplex virus and varicella-zoster virus	Pneumonia as part of disseminated disease
Encapsulated bacteria (*S. pneumoniae*, *H. influenzae*, *Salmonella* spp)	Respiratory infections in asplenic hosts or hosts with humoral immune defects
Nosocomial bacteria, including *Pseudomonas* or enteric gram-negative rods	Consider as cause of pneumonia in neutropenic patients; may be seen in association with central venous catheter infections

clinical status in whom noninvasive testing has failed to uncover an etiologic agent [101]. In general, decisions regarding diagnostic testing may need to be accelerated in this population of patients to permit any interventions to be performed before clinical status deteriorates and a patient is unable to tolerate invasive procedures and to allow appropriate therapy to be initiated earlier in the course of disease.

Nosocomial agents

The differential diagnosis of pneumonia in patients who have been hospitalized for any prolonged period should include routine infectious etiologies and hospital-acquired organisms. Failure to improve with appropriate empiric therapy should raise the concern for antimicrobial resistance. Organisms of particular importance in these situations may include methicillin-resistant *S. aureus*, vancomycin-resistant enterococci, and gram-negative rods with resistance to third-generation cephalosporins, among others. Empiric coverage for pneumonia in patients in the intensive care unit or others at risk for nosocomial infections should include broad-spectrum agents that provide coverage for these antibiotic-resistant organisms (and any organisms known to be a frequent cause of hospital-acquired infections in the institution) until a specific diagnosis can be made and antimicrobial susceptibilities are available. The infection control staff and the hospital microbiology laboratory are invaluable resources in determining which organisms should be considered in these circumstances.

Infection control

Isolation precautions are a topic of particular interest to hospitalists who manage patients with pneumonia, particularly when a specific etiologic agent has not been identified. Because pneumonia can be caused by a wide variety of agents, several different infection control precautions may be appropriate. The single most important procedure to prevent the spread of infection in the hospital is hand hygiene (performed either with soap and water or a waterless alcohol-based hand sanitizer). Table 5 reviews the correct precautions for specific organisms that may be encountered in the hospital setting. Two infections that merit specific mention are pertussis and influenza. These organisms are highly infectious, and exposure among hospital staff may require chemoprophylaxis. Patients with pertussis or influenza should be admitted to a single room whenever possible. Staff also should wear masks when entering the room of patients with influenza (despite the fact that droplet transmission precautions usually only require masks within 3 feet), because several reports have suggested a role for airborne transmission [102–104]. When pulmonary tuberculosis is suspected, strict attention to airborne precautions must be followed. In addition to the use of respirators and negative-pressure isolation rooms, visitation should be limited when possible; at our institution, two primary visitors may undergo screening chest radiography to ensure that they do not have active pulmonary infection.

Table 5
Infection control precautions for specific organisms

Organism	Precautions[a]
Respiratory syncytial virus	Contact
Influenza	Droplet plus mask to enter room, single room
Parainfluenza	Contact
Adenovirus	Droplet and contact
Varicella	Airborne (for chickenpox, non-immune individuals should not enter room); precaution room with anteroom or single room with door closed at all times; zoster in an immunocompromised patient requires airborne and contact precautions
Mycoplasma pneumoniae	Droplet
Bordetella pertussis	Droplet (until patient has received 5 days of effective therapy)
Mycobacterium tuberculosis	Airborne; negative-pressure precaution room with anteroom
Multidrug-resistant bacteria (methicillin-resistant *S. aureus*, vancomycin-resistant enterococci, resistant gram-negative rods)	Special organism precautions

[a] Contact refers to gown and gloves; droplet refers to mask within 3 feet; airborne refers to N95 respirator to enter room; special organism precautions refers to gown and gloves and dedicated patient equipment.

SANDORA & HARPER

Outpatient antimicrobial therapy

As medical care for complex patients increasingly shifts from the inpatient to the outpatient arena, a greater number of infections are being treated by continuing the delivery of parenteral antibiotic therapy in the home or at step-down facilities [105–107]. Outpatient parenteral antimicrobial therapy (OPAT) is a reasonable option for patients with pneumonia who have stabilized clinically in the hospital but are judged to require prolonged parenteral treatment. The treatment of lower respiratory tract infections using OPAT has resulted in excellent clinical outcomes and high levels of patient and physician satisfaction [108,109]. Eligibility for OPAT requires a suitable home environment and the selection of an antimicrobial agent with appropriate pharmacokinetic parameters and drug stability to allow a reasonable dosing schedule at home [110]. An infectious diseases specialist (or a physician knowledgeable about the use of antimicrobial agents in OPAT) and a hospital pharmacist should be involved before discharge in planning for the administration of OPAT. The involvement of discharge planning services in the hospital also can facilitate contact with visiting nurse associations, which can arrange to instruct families in the proper techniques for IV infusions in the home. These agencies can make home visits to observe caregivers and answer questions and obtain blood for laboratory monitoring of disease or medication toxicities. The use of these services, in conjunction with careful follow-up by primary care physicians, provides the best continuity of care from the hospital to the outpatient setting and helps to ensure that patients with pneumonia receive the highest quality of care across the health care spectrum.

References

[1] Hall MJ, DeFrances CJ. 2001 National hospital discharge survey. Available at: http://www.cdc.gov/nchs/data/ad/ad332.pdf. Accessed January 13, 2004.

[2] Wright AL, Taussig LM, Ray CG, et al. The Tucson children's respiratory study. II. Lower respiratory tract illness in the first year of life. Am J Epidemiol 1989;129(6):1232–46.

[3] Murphy TF, Henderson FW, Clyde Jr WA, et al. Pneumonia: an eleven-year study in a pediatric practice. Am J Epidemiol 1981;113(1):12–21.

[4] Rudan I, Tomaskovic L, Boschi-Pinto C, et al. Global estimate of the incidence of clinical pneumonia among children under five years of age. Bull World Health Organ 2004;82:895–903.

[5] Bartlett JG, Dowell SF, Mandell LA, et al. Practice guidelines for the management of community-acquired pneumonia in adults: Infectious Diseases Society of America. Clin Infect Dis 2000;31(2):347–82.

[6] McIntosh K. Community-acquired pneumonia in children. N Engl J Med 2002;346(6):429–37.

[7] Michelow IC, Olsen K, Lozano J, et al. Epidemiology and clinical characteristics of community-acquired pneumonia in hospitalized children. Pediatrics 2004;113(4):701–7.

[8] British Thoracic Society. Guidelines for the management of community acquired pneumonia in childhood. Thorax 2002;57(Suppl 1):i1–24.

[9] Cardenosa Cendrero JA, Sole-Violan J, Bordes Benitez A, et al. Role of different routes of

tracheal colonization in the development of pneumonia in patients receiving mechanical ventilation [see comments]. Chest 1999;116(2):462–70.

[10] Berman S. Acute respiratory infections [review]. Infect Dis Clin North Am 1991;5(2):319–36.

[11] Wijnands GJ. Diagnosis and interventions in lower respiratory tract infections. Am J Med 1992;92(4A):91S–7S.

[12] Hirst RA, Kadioglu A, O'Callaghan C, et al. The role of pneumolysin in pneumococcal pneumonia and meningitis. Clin Exp Immunol 2004;138(2):195–201.

[13] Campbell H, Byass P, Lamont AC, et al. Assessment of clinical criteria for identification of severe acute lower respiratory tract infections in children. Lancet 1989;1(8633):297–9.

[14] Palafox M, Guiscafre H, Reyes H, et al. Diagnostic value of tachypnoea in pneumonia defined radiologically. Arch Dis Child 2000;82(1):41–5.

[15] Murtagh P, Cerqueiro C, Halac A, et al. Acute lower respiratory infection in Argentinian children: a 40 month clinical and epidemiological study. Pediatr Pulmonol 1993;16(1):1–8.

[16] Leventhal JM. Clinical predictors of pneumonia as a guide to ordering chest roentgenograms. Clin Pediatr (Phila) 1982;21(12):730–4.

[17] Mulholland EK, Simoes EA, Costales MO, et al. Standardized diagnosis of pneumonia in developing countries. Pediatr Infect Dis J 1992;11(2):77–81.

[18] Cherian T, John TJ, Simoes E, et al. Evaluation of simple clinical signs for the diagnosis of acute lower respiratory tract infection. Lancet 1988;2(8603):125–8.

[19] Singhi S, Dhawan A, Kataria S, et al. Clinical signs of pneumonia in infants under 2 months. Arch Dis Child 1994;70(5):413–7.

[20] Taylor JA, Del Beccaro M, Done S, et al. Establishing clinically relevant standards for tachypnea in febrile children younger than 2 years. Arch Pediatr Adolesc Med 1995;149(3): 283–7.

[21] Harari M, Shann F, Spooner V, et al. Clinical signs of pneumonia in children [see comments]. Lancet 1991;338(8772):928–30.

[22] Lucero MG, Tupasi TE, Gomez ML, et al. Respiratory rate greater than 50 per minute as a clinical indicator of pneumonia in Filipino children with cough. Rev Infect Dis 1990;12(8): S1081–3.

[23] Esposito S, Bosis S, Cavagna R, et al. Characteristics of *Streptococcus pneumoniae* and atypical bacterial infections in children 2–5 years of age with community-acquired pneumonia. Clin Infect Dis 2002;35(11):1345–52.

[24] Singal BM, Hedges JR, Radack KL. Decision rules and clinical prediction of pneumonia: evaluation of low-yield criteria. Ann Emerg Med 1989;18(1):13–20.

[25] Tan TQ, Mason Jr EO, Barson WJ, et al. Clinical characteristics and outcome of children with pneumonia attributable to penicillin-susceptible and penicillin-nonsusceptible *Streptococcus pneumoniae*. Pediatrics 1998;102(6):1369–75.

[26] Bachur R, Perry H, Harper MB. Occult pneumonias: empiric chest radiographs in febrile children with leukocytosis [see comments]. Ann Emerg Med 1999;33(2):166–73.

[27] McIntosh K, Harper M. Acute uncomplicated pneumonia. In: Long S, Pickering LK, Prober CG, editors. Principles and practice of pediatric infectious diseases. 2nd edition. Philadelphia: Churchill-Livingstone; 2003. p. 219–25.

[28] Mazur LJ, Kline MW, Lorin MI. Extreme leukocytosis in patients presenting to a pediatric emergency department. Pediatr Emerg Care 1991;7(4):215–8.

[29] McCarthy PL, Frank AL, Ablow RC, et al. Value of the C-reactive protein test in the differentiation of bacterial and viral pneumonia. J Pediatr 1978;92(3):454–6.

[30] Mandell LA, Bartlett JG, Dowell SF, et al. Update of practice guidelines for the management of community-acquired pneumonia in immunocompetent adults. Clin Infect Dis 2003; 37(11):1405–33.

[31] Jadavji T, Law B, Lebel MH, et al. A practical guide for the diagnosis and treatment of pediatric pneumonia. CMAJ 1997;156(5):S703–11.

[32] Niederman MS, Bass Jr JB, Campbell GD, et al. Guidelines for the initial management of adults with community-acquired pneumonia: diagnosis, assessment of severity, and initial antimicro-

bial therapy: American Thoracic Society. Medical Section of the American Lung Association. Am Rev Respir Dis 1993;148(5):1418–26.

[33] Campbell SG, Marrie TJ, Anstey R, et al. The contribution of blood cultures to the clinical management of adult patients admitted to the hospital with community-acquired pneumonia: a prospective observational study. Chest 2003;123(4):1142–50.

[34] Sanyal S, Smith PR, Saha AC, et al. Initial microbiologic studies did not affect outcome in adults hospitalized with community-acquired pneumonia. Am J Respir Crit Care Med 1999; 160(1):346–8.

[35] Hickey RW, Bowman MJ, Smith GA. Utility of blood cultures in pediatric patients found to have pneumonia in the emergency department. Ann Emerg Med 1996;27(6):721–5.

[36] Theerthakarai R, El-Halees W, Ismail M, et al. Nonvalue of the initial microbiological studies in the management of nonsevere community-acquired pneumonia. Chest 2001;119(1): 181–4.

[37] Morris AJ, Tanner DC, Reller LB. Rejection criteria for endotracheal aspirates from adults. J Clin Microbiol 1993;31(5):1027–9.

[38] Esposito S, Bosis S, Colombo R, et al. Evaluation of rapid assay for detection of *Streptococcus pneumoniae* urinary antigen among infants and young children with possible invasive pneumococcal disease. Pediatr Infect Dis J 2004;23(4):365–7.

[39] Dominguez J, Blanco S, Rodrigo C, et al. Usefulness of urinary antigen detection by an immunochromatographic test for diagnosis of pneumococcal pneumonia in children. J Clin Microbiol 2003;41(5):2161–3.

[40] Ieven M, Ursi D, Van Bever H, et al. Detection of *Mycoplasma pneumoniae* by two polymerase chain reactions and role of *M. pneumoniae* in acute respiratory tract infections in pediatric patients [see comments]. J Infect Dis 1996;173(6):1445–52.

[41] Crain EF, Bulas D, Bijur PE, et al. Is a chest radiograph necessary in the evaluation of every febrile infant less than 8 weeks of age? Pediatrics 1991;88(4):821–4.

[42] Bramson RT, Meyer TL, Silbiger ML, et al. The futility of the chest radiograph in the febrile infant without respiratory symptoms. Pediatrics 1993;92(4):524–6.

[43] Korppi M, Kiekara O, Heiskanen-Kosma T, et al. Comparison of radiological findings and microbial aetiology of childhood pneumonia. Acta Paediatr 1993;82(4):360–3.

[44] Friis B, Eiken M, Hornsleth A, et al. Chest X-ray appearances in pneumonia and bronchiolitis: correlation to virological diagnosis and secretory bacterial findings. Acta Paediatr Scand 1990;79(2):219–25.

[45] Albaum MN, Hill LC, Murphy M, et al. Interobserver reliability of the chest radiograph in community-acquired pneumonia: PORT investigators. Chest 1996;110(2):343–50.

[46] Kramer MS, Roberts-Brauer R, Williams RL. Bias and overcall in interpreting chest radiographs in young febrile children. Pediatrics 1992;90(1 Pt 1):11–3.

[47] Reittner P, Muller NL, Heyneman L, et al. *Mycoplasma pneumoniae* pneumonia: radiographic and high-resolution CT features in 28 patients. AJR Am J Roentgenol 2000;174(1):37–41.

[48] Donnelly LF, Klosterman LA. The yield of CT of children who have complicated pneumonia and noncontributory chest radiography. AJR Am J Roentgenol 1998;170(6):1627–31.

[49] Fine MJ, Auble TE, Yealy DM, et al. A prediction rule to identify low-risk patients with community-acquired pneumonia. N Engl J Med 1997;336(4):243–50.

[50] Bang AT, Bang RA, Morankar VP, et al. Pneumonia in neonates: can it be managed in the community? Arch Dis Child 1993;68(5 Spec No):550–6.

[51] Martinez JA, Horcajada JP, Almela M, et al. Addition of a macrolide to a beta-lactam-based empirical antibiotic regimen is associated with lower in-hospital mortality for patients with bacteremic pneumococcal pneumonia. Clin Infect Dis 2003;36(4):389–95.

[52] Harris JA, Kolokathis A, Campbell M, et al. Safety and efficacy of azithromycin in the treatment of community-acquired pneumonia in children. Pediatr Infect Dis J 1998;17(10): 865–71.

[53] Dunbar LM, Wunderink RG, Habib MP, et al. High-dose, short-course levofloxacin for community-acquired pneumonia: a new treatment paradigm. Clin Infect Dis 2003;37(6): 752–60.

[54] Mandell LA, File Jr TM. Short-course treatment of community-acquired pneumonia. Clin Infect Dis 2003;37(6):761–3.

[55] Ravago TS, Mosniam J, Alem F. Evaluation of community acquired pneumonia guidelines. J Med Syst 2000;24(5):289–96.

[56] Dean NC, Silver MP, Bateman KA, et al. Decreased mortality after implementation of a treatment guideline for community-acquired pneumonia. Am J Med 2001;110(6):451–7.

[57] Gleason PP, Kapoor WN, Stone RA, et al. Medical outcomes and antimicrobial costs with the use of the American Thoracic Society guidelines for outpatients with community-acquired pneumonia. JAMA 1997;278(1):32–9.

[58] Marrie TJ, Lau CY, Wheeler SL, et al. A controlled trial of a critical pathway for treatment of community-acquired pneumonia. CAPITAL study investigators: community-acquired pneumonia intervention trial assessing levofloxacin. JAMA 2000;283(6):749–55.

[59] Malone DC, Shaban HM. Adherence to ATS guidelines for hospitalized patients with community-acquired pneumonia. Ann Pharmacother 2001;35(10):1180–5.

[60] Menendez R, Ferrando D, Valles JM, et al. Influence of deviation from guidelines on the outcome of community-acquired pneumonia. Chest 2002;122(2):612–7.

[61] Capelastegui A, Espana PP, Quintana JM, et al. Improvement of process-of-care and outcomes after implementing a guideline for the management of community-acquired pneumonia: a controlled before-and-after design study. Clin Infect Dis 2004;39(7):955–63.

[62] Marras TK, Chan CK. Use of guidelines in treating community-acquired pneumonia. Chest 1998;113(6):1689–94.

[63] Grigg J, van den Borre C, Malfroot A, et al. Bilateral fiberoptic bronchoalveolar lavage in acute unilateral lobar pneumonia. J Pediatr 1993;122(4):606–8.

[64] Rock MJ. The diagnostic utility of bronchoalveolar lavage in immunocompetent children with unexplained infiltrates on chest radiograph. Pediatrics 1995;95(3):373–7.

[65] Halm EA, Fine MJ, Marrie TJ, et al. Time to clinical stability in patients hospitalized with community-acquired pneumonia: implications for practice guidelines. JAMA 1998;279(18):1452–7.

[66] Barlow GD, Lamping DL, Davey PG, et al. Evaluation of outcomes in community-acquired pneumonia: a guide for patients, physicians, and policy-makers. Lancet Infect Dis 2003;3(8):476–88.

[67] Jay SJ, Johanson Jr WG, Pierce AK. The radiographic resolution of *Streptococcus pneumoniae* pneumonia. N Engl J Med 1975;293(16):798–801.

[68] Kim CK, Chung CY, Kim JS, et al. Late abnormal findings on high-resolution computed tomography after Mycoplasma pneumonia. Pediatrics 2000;105(2):372–8.

[69] Donnelly LF. Maximizing the usefulness of imaging in children with community-acquired pneumonia. AJR Am J Roentgenol 1999;172(2):505–12.

[70] Dowell SF, Kupronis BA, Zell ER, et al. Mortality from pneumonia in children in the United States, 1939 through 1996. N Engl J Med 2000;342(19):1399–407.

[71] Feikin DR, Schuchat A, Kolczak M, et al. Mortality from invasive pneumococcal pneumonia in the era of antibiotic resistance, 1995–1997. Am J Public Health 2000;90(2):223–9.

[72] Clark CE, Coote JM, Silver DA, et al. Asthma after childhood pneumonia: six year follow up study. BMJ 2000;320(7248):1514–6.

[73] Hardie WD, Roberts NE, Reising SF, et al. Complicated parapneumonic effusions in children caused by penicillin-nonsusceptible *Streptococcus pneumoniae*. Pediatrics 1998;101(3 Pt 1):388–92.

[74] Valdes L, Alvarez D, Valle JM, et al. The etiology of pleural effusions in an area with high incidence of tuberculosis. Chest 1996;109(1):158–62.

[75] Light RW, Girard WM, Jenkinson SG, et al. Parapneumonic effusions. Am J Med 1980;69(4):507–12.

[76] Freij BJ, Kusmiesz H, Nelson JD, et al. Parapneumonic effusions and empyema in hospitalized children: a retrospective review of 227 cases. Pediatr Infect Dis 1984;3(6):578–91.

[77] Nagler J, Harper MB, Fleisher GR. Value of thoracentesis in the diagnosis and management of infectious pleural effusions. Pediatr Res 2001;51(4):280A–1A.

[78] Donnelly LF, Klosterman LA. CT appearance of parapneumonic effusions in children: findings are not specific for empyema. AJR Am J Roentgenol 1997;169(1):179–82.

[79] Mitri RK, Brown SD, Zurakowski D, et al. Outcomes of primary image-guided drainage of parapneumonic effusions in children. Pediatrics 2002;110(3):e37.

[80] Ramnath RR, Heller RM, Ben-Ami T, et al. Implications of early sonographic evaluation of parapneumonic effusions in children with pneumonia. Pediatrics 1998;101(1 Pt 1):68–71.

[81] Subramaniam R, Joseph VT, Tan GM, et al. Experience with video-assisted thoracoscopic surgery in the management of complicated pneumonia in children. J Pediatr Surg 2001;36(2): 316–9.

[82] Ozcelik C, Inci I, Nizam O, et al. Intrapleural fibrinolytic treatment of multiloculated post-pneumonic pediatric empyemas. Ann Thorac Surg 2003;76(6):1849–53 [discussion 1853].

[83] Ulku R, Onen A, Onat S, et al. Intrapleural fibrinolytic treatment of multiloculated pediatric empyemas. Pediatr Surg Int 2004;20(7):520–4.

[84] Weinstein M, Restrepo R, Chait PG, et al. Effectiveness and safety of tissue plasminogen activator in the management of complicated parapneumonic effusions. Pediatrics 2004; 113(3 Pt 1):e182–5.

[85] Thomson AH, Hull J, Kumar MR, et al. Randomised trial of intrapleural urokinase in the treatment of childhood empyema. Thorax 2002;57(4):343–7.

[86] Donnelly LF, Klosterman LA. Pneumonia in children: decreased parenchymal contrast enhancement. CT sign of intense illness and impending cavitary necrosis. Radiology 1997; 205(3):817–20.

[87] Donnelly LF, Klosterman LA. Cavitary necrosis complicating pneumonia in children: sequential findings on chest radiography. AJR Am J Roentgenol 1998;171(1):253–6.

[88] Hoffer FA, Bloom DA, Colin AA, et al. Lung abscess versus necrotizing pneumonia: implications for interventional therapy. Pediatr Radiol 1999;29(2):87–91.

[89] Rice TW, Ginsberg RJ, Todd TR. Tube drainage of lung abscesses. Ann Thorac Surg 1987; 44(4):356–9.

[90] Zuhdi MK, Spear RM, Worthen HM, et al. Percutaneous catheter drainage of tension pneumatocele, secondarily infected pneumatocele, and lung abscess in children. Crit Care Med 1996;24(2):330–3.

[91] Emanuel B, Shulman ST. Lung abscess in infants and children. Clin Pediatr (Phila) 1995; 34(1):2–6.

[92] Owayed AF, Campbell DM, Wang EE. Underlying causes of recurrent pneumonia in children. Arch Pediatr Adolesc Med 2000;154(2):190–4.

[93] Labenne M, Poyart C, Rambaud C, et al. Blind protected specimen brush and bronchoalveolar lavage in ventilated children. Crit Care Med 1999;27(11):2537–43.

[94] Jacobson SJ, Griffiths K, Diamond S, et al. A randomized controlled trial of penicillin vs clindamycin for the treatment of aspiration pneumonia in children [see comments]. Arch Pediatr Adolesc Med 1997;151(7):701–4.

[95] Gentile G, Micozzi A, Girmenia C, et al. Pneumonia in allogenic and autologous bone marrow recipients: a retrospective study. Chest 1993;104(2):371–5.

[96] Jochelson MS, Altschuler J, Stomper PC. The yield of chest radiography in febrile and neutropenic patients. Ann Intern Med 1986;105(5):708–9.

[97] Logan PM, Primack SL, Staples C, et al. Acute lung disease in the immunocompromised host: diagnostic accuracy of the chest radiograph. Chest 1995;108(5):1283–7.

[98] Brown MJ, Miller RR, Muller NL. Acute lung disease in the immunocompromised host: CT and pathologic examination findings. Radiology 1994;190(1):247–54.

[99] Leutner CC, Gieseke J, Lutterbey G, et al. MR imaging of pneumonia in immunocompromised patients: comparison with helical CT. AJR Am J Roentgenol 2000;175(2):391–7.

[100] Jain P, Sandur S, Meli Y, et al. Role of flexible bronchoscopy in immunocompromised patients with lung infiltrates. Chest 2004;125(2):712–22.

[101] Deterding RR, Wagener JS. Lung biopsy in immunocompromised children: when, how, and who? [editorial; comment]. J Pediatr 2000;137(2):147–9.

[102] Moser MR, Bender TR, Margolis HS, et al. An outbreak of influenza aboard a commercial airliner. Am J Epidemiol 1979;110(1):1–6.

[103] Riley RL. Airborne infection. Am J Med 1974;57(3):466–75.

[104] Bridges CB, Kuehnert MJ, Hall CB. Transmission of influenza: implications for control in health care settings. Clin Infect Dis 2003;37(8):1094–101.

[105] Bernard L, El H, Pron B, et al. Outpatient parenteral antimicrobial therapy (OPAT) for the treatment of osteomyelitis: evaluation of efficacy, tolerance and cost. J Clin Pharm Ther 2001; 26(6):445–51.

[106] Tice AD, Strait K, Ramey R, et al. Outpatient parenteral antimicrobial therapy for central nervous system infections. Clin Infect Dis 1999;29(6):1394–9.

[107] Nathwani D. The management of skin and soft tissue infections: outpatient parenteral antibiotic therapy in the United Kingdom. Chemotherapy 2001;47(Suppl 1):17–23.

[108] Morales JO, Snead H. Efficacy and safety of intravenous cefotaxime for treating pneumonia in outpatients. Am J Med 1994;97(2A):28–33.

[109] Esposito S. Treatment of lower respiratory tract infections in Italy: the role of outpatient parenteral antibiotic therapy. Chemotherapy 2001;47(Suppl 1):33–40.

[110] Tice AD, Rehm SJ, Dalovisio JR, et al. Practice guidelines for outpatient parenteral antimicrobial therapy: IDSA guidelines. Clin Infect Dis 2004;38(12):1651–72.

ELSEVIER
SAUNDERS

PEDIATRIC CLINICS
OF NORTH AMERICA

Pediatr Clin N Am 52 (2005) 1083–1106

Musculoskeletal Infections in Children

Gary Frank, MD, MS[a,b], Henrietta M. Mahoney, MD[a,c],
Stephen C. Eppes, MD[c,d],*

[a]*Department of Pediatrics, Alfred I. duPont Hospital for Children and Nemours Children's Clinic,
PO Box 269, Wilmington, DE 19899, USA*
[b]*Department of Clinical Informatics, Alfred I. duPont Hospital for Children and
Nemours Children's Clinic, PO Box 269, Wilmington, DE 19899, USA*
[c]*Department of Pediatrics, Jefferson Medical College, Thomas Jefferson University,
Philadelphia, PA 19107, USA*
[d]*Division of Infectious Diseases, Alfred I. duPont Hospital for Children and
Nemours Children's Clinic, Wilmington, DE 19899, USA*

Osteomyelitis

Introduction and epidemiology

Osteomyelitis is an infection of the bone and bone marrow generally of a bacterial origin. In the highly vascular bones of children, the most common form is acute hematogenous osteomyelitis (AHO). Approximately half of pediatric cases occur in children younger than 5 years of age [1–3], and boys are approximately twice as likely to be affected as girls [2,4]. The incidence has not been found to be higher in any one race than another [2,5]. Higher rates are seen in immunocompromised populations such as patients with sickle cell disease. Most cases occur in long bones. In a study of 163 infants and children with osteomyelitis [5], the femur, tibia, and humerus accounted for 68% of infections. Most cases are limited to a single site, with less than 10% involving two or more locations [2].

---

* Corresponding author. Division of Infectious Diseases, Alfred I. duPont Hospital for Children, PO Box 269, Wilmington, DE 19899.

   E-mail address: seppes@nemours.org (S.C. Eppes).

0031-3955/05/$ – see front matter © 2005 Elsevier Inc. All rights reserved.
doi:10.1016/j.pcl.2005.04.003   *pediatric.theclinics.com*

Pathogenesis

Infection of bone may occur in several ways, including hematogenous spread, direct inoculation, and contiguous spread from a local infection [6,7]. In children, most cases result from hematogenous deposition of organisms in bone marrow after a transient episode of bacteremia. Approximately one third of patients report a history of blunt trauma [5], which may injure the bone and increase the likelihood of seeding the bone during bacteremia. Direct inoculation of bacteria into bone may occur during surgery or as a result of penetrating trauma, puncture wounds, or complex fractures.

Osteomyelitis most commonly begins in the metaphysis of long bones [6], which are highly vascular structures. In neonates, the metaphyseal capillaries form a connection with the epiphysial plate. The periosteum is thin and does not adhere tightly to the underlying bone. As a result, the periosteum is more likely to perforate and spread infection into the surrounding tissues. Spread through the epiphysis also may result in septic arthritis and permanent growth plate damage (Fig. 1). The hips and shoulders are common sites of epiphyseal infection. In later infancy, the cortex thickens and the metaphyseal capillaries begin to atrophy, which decreases the risk of epiphyseal involvement and spread to local joint and soft tissue, although subperiosteal abscesses still form. In children and adolescents, the cortex is significantly thicker and infection in these patients rarely extends beyond the cortex.

Virulence factors of certain bacteria also favor the development of hematogenous osteomyelitis. *Staphylococcus aureus* bacteria adhere to bone by ex-

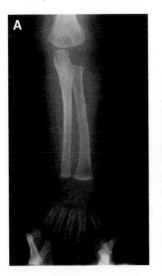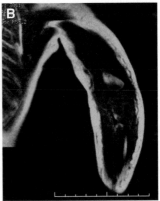

Fig. 1. (*A*) Radiograph of the left elbow of a 9-month-old child admitted for treatment of septic arthritis. The film revealed periosteal elevation in the distal portion of the humerus consistent with osteomyelitis. (*B*) MRI of the same patient revealed increased signal intensity on T2 images in the midpoint of the distal humerus, along with increased signal intensity in the distal humeral epiphysis.

pressing adhesins, which bind to a component of the bone matrix [7]. *S. aureus* also can survive intracellularly once internalized by osteoblasts [7]. Growing colonies of bacteria then surround themselves with a protective biofilm or glyco-calyx, which consists of exopolysaccharide polymers that allow ligand-receptor interaction and bonding of the bacteria to the substrate [8]. As the infection advances, cortical bone is destroyed and infection and inflammation may extend into the subperiosteal space. If the infection is left untreated, chronic osteo-myelitis may develop, which is characterized by extensive tissue destruction caused by inflammatory cytokines that increase osteoclast activity and attract macrophages and monocytes. Necrotic cortical bone may separate and lead to the formation of a sequestrum, and new bone may form an incasing sheath around necrotic bone, known as an involucrum [6]. Inflammation also can lead to significant fibrosis.

Microbiology

In older infants and children, *S. aureus* is the most commonly identified organism and accounts for 61% to 89% of cases of AHO [5,9]. Group A β-hemolytic streptococci (GABHS) are next in frequency, and cause up to 10% of cases [10]. In the past, *Haemophilus influenzae* accounted for 3% to 7% of cases [1,5,9], but the advent of effective immunization has virtually eliminated this cause of osteomyelitis [10,11]. *Streptococcus pneumoniae* is another relatively common organism in patients with AHO. *Kingella kingae* is a common cause of osteomyelitis in the Middle East and is being recognized increasingly in the United States. Osteomyelitis caused by *K. kingae* tends to occur in young children after upper respiratory tract infections and stomatitis in the late summer through early winter [12]. Certain gram-negative bacteria are also known to cause AHO. *Salmonella* spp. are commonly identified in patients with sickle cell disease, and *Pseudomonas aeruginosa* is often identified in cases of osteochon-dritis after puncture wounds of the feet [13,14].

Although *S. aureus* is the most commonly reported organism in the neonatal age group, Group B streptococcus and enteric gram-negatives such as *Escherichia coli* are also common [15]. Mycobacteria and fungi are rare causes of osteomyelitis [14]. *Bartonella henselae* is an atypical cause of osteomyelitis in patients with cat-scratch disease [16,17]. Polymicrobial infection is rare and is seen most commonly in cases of puncture wounds or other trauma.

Clinical presentation

Older children and adolescents often present after days to weeks of symptoms and most commonly complain of pain at the affected site and fever. The pain is typically constant and well localized. Infants and toddlers may present with irritability, refusal to bear weight or use an extremity, or limp. In younger patients, subperiosteal spread may lead to erythema, warmth, and swelling of the affected site. Young patients also may present with fever of unknown origin because they are unable to localize pain.

Neonates with osteomyelitis may present with pseudoparalysis and significant tenderness with palpation of the affected site [15]. They often have a history of a preceding infection, and approximately one third have multiple sites involved [18]. Neonates are also at higher risk of concomitant joint infection compared with older patients [2,18].

Differential diagnosis

The differential diagnosis for osteomyelitis includes cellulitis, septic arthritis, toxic synovitis, thrombophlebitis, trauma, fracture, rheumatologic diseases (eg, juvenile rheumatoid arthritis), pain crisis in sickle cell disease, Ewing's sarcoma, osteosarcoma, and leukemia.

Diagnosis and evaluation

Blood tests are often supportive but not specific for osteomyelitis. A complete blood count may reveal leukocytosis, but it may be normal, especially in chronic cases [6]. In a study of 44 children with AHO, only 35% had leukocytosis at the time of admission [9]. Inflammatory markers, such as the erythrocyte sedimentation rate and C-reactive protein, are elevated in more than 90% of patients [5,9] and can be used to follow response to therapy. The C-reactive protein and erythrocyte sedimentation rate often continue to rise in the first 2 to 5 days after initiation of therapy and return to normal within 1 (C-reactive protein) to 3 (erythrocyte sedimentation rate) weeks [9].

Identification of an organism is critical to confirming the diagnosis and guiding antimicrobial selection. Needle aspiration is likely to yield an organism in approximately two thirds of cases [3,5], whereas blood cultures yield positive results in 36% to 55% of specimens [2,3]. Open procedures that involve metaphyseal drilling may enhance the yield and may be therapeutic.

The value of plain films (Table 1) depends on the duration of active disease, and in most patients the infection is clinically localizable before radiologic

Table 1
Advantages and disadvantages of various imaging modalities for osteomyelitis

Modality	Advantages	Disadvantages
Plain film	Inexpensive, quick, easy	Insensitive in early disease
CT	Improved sensitivity, relatively quick	Radiation exposure, may require sedation
MRI	Very sensitive, even in early disease, may reveal pus collections or extension into adjacent joint or soft tissue	Long study, often requires sedation, expensive
Bone scan	Very sensitive, identifies multifocal disease, may reveal unsuspected sites in preverbal children	Less specific, long study, often requires sedation, expensive, radiation exposure

changes are evident on radiographs [19]. In the first 3 days, plain films may reveal localized soft-tissue swelling. By days 3 to 7, swelling of the surrounding muscle may lead to obliteration of the normally visible fat planes. Osteolytic lesions are generally not apparent until there has been more than 50% loss of bone density [20]—often 2 weeks or more after initial symptoms—and periosteal reaction is not evident until days 10 to 21 of illness [5,21].

Nuclear scintigraphy is helpful in young patients who are unable to verbalize the location of their pain, when multiple sites are suspected, and in differentiating osteomyelitis from cellulitis. The technetium 99m methylene diphosphonate bone scan is the most commonly ordered nuclear imaging procedure (Fig. 2) [21]. After injection, there is immediate distribution to areas of hyperemia; later imaging demonstrates increased uptake in areas of osteoclastic/osteoblastic activity. It is sensitive for the detection of early osteomyelitis [7] but is not specific for infection. Tagged leukocyte scans (eg, indium 111 or technetium 99m) can be used but require special technical skills and may yield false-positive results.

Cross-sectional imaging may be necessary to distinguish associated soft-tissue infection, delineate the extent of bone involvement, and help plan surgical management [22]. CT can reveal areas of cortical bone destruction, periosteal reaction, sequestration, and soft-tissue abscesses. Images should be obtained with and without enhancement.

With a reported sensitivity of 97% [23], MRI is becoming the modality of choice in patients with a strong suspicion of osteomyelitis [24]. The high resolution makes it useful for differentiating between bone and soft-tissue infection [6]. Edema and exudate of the medullary space may be noted in the initial stages of osteomyelitis (Fig. 3), which allows for early diagnosis. Coronal

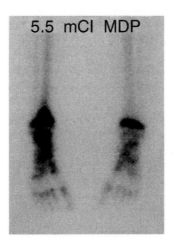

5.5 mCI MDP

Fig. 2. Three-phase bone scan of a 1-year-old boy who presented with fever and a painful right lower extremity. Flow images revealed increased flow to the right lower extremity with increased activity to the distal metaphysis of the right tibia. Blood pool images showed increased radiotracer uptake to the distal metaphysis of the right tibia.

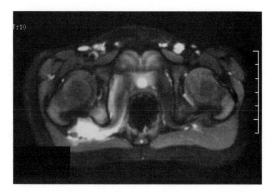

Fig. 3. MRI image of a 1-year-old boy with 3 weeks of right hip pain. There is marked abnormal increased signal intensity in the posterior aspect of the right ischium on the T2-weighted images, compatible with marrow edema and consistent with osteomyelitis. Extensive edema and inflammation also are seen in the right obturator internus muscle and in the gamellus muscles posterolateral to the right ischium.

or sagittal images are especially useful for planning surgical procedures and assessing the growth plates and epiphyses. Gadolinium enhancement is recommended to improve sensitivity [21].

Management

Treatment of osteomyelitis initially requires inpatient management with a combination of antibiotic therapy and possible surgical procedures [1,5–7,20]. Upon admission, an orthopedic surgeon should be consulted, especially if imaging reveals subperiosteal or soft-tissue abscesses, sequestra, or intramedullary purulence. A surgeon's roles include performing diagnostic needle aspiration, decompression and drainage (when necessary), and long-term follow-up in complicated cases. Surgical intervention is reported to be required in approximately 50% of cases [2,5], although some authors recommend a more conservative approach [3].

Empiric medical therapy should cover *S. aureus* and GABHS, and traditionally, a semi-synthetic penicillinase-resistant penicillin was recommended (eg, nafcillin or oxacillin, 150–200 mg/kg/d, divided in four doses). Several recent reports have indicated a sharp increase in the number of cases of community-acquired methicillin-resistant *S. aureus* infections, however [25]. In communities with a high incidence of community-acquired methicillin-resistant *S. aureus*, vancomycin should be considered for empiric therapy of osteomyelitis until sensitivities are available. Alternatively, clindamycin may be effective against community-acquired methicillin-resistant *S. aureus* [26], but inducible resistance may reduce its effectiveness. This resistance can be detected using a D-test performed by the microbiology laboratory. In infants and children up to 5 years of age, a second- or third-generation cephalosporin (eg, cefuroxime, cefotaxime, ceftriaxone) provides coverage against many *S. aureus*, most streptococci, and *K. kingae*.

Empiric therapy in neonates should cover Group B streptococcus and enteric gram-negative bacilli in addition to the pathogens common in older infants and children. In neonates, cefotaxime may be used for empiric therapy, and coverage can be narrowed once culture results and sensitivities are available.

In patients with presumed pseudomonal infection (eg, puncture wound osteochondritis of the foot), one should consider an extended spectrum beta-lactam (eg, ceftazidime, cefepime, piperacillin/tazaobactam) plus an aminoglycoside for at least the first 2 weeks.

Once an organism has been identified, coverage can be narrowed based on results of susceptibility testing. The minimum recommended length of treatment is 3 weeks because of the increased likelihood of developing chronic osteomyelitis if the length of therapy is shortened [27]. Most authors recommend treatment for 4 to 6 weeks [28]. If long-term intravenous antibiotics are administered, placement of a peripherally inserted central catheter should be considered for completion of the regimen as an outpatient. Several studies support switching to an oral antibiotic if there is a high likelihood of compliance, an organism has been identified, clinical improvement is noted, the patient is afebrile, and inflammatory markers have begun to normalize after the first week of parenteral therapy [2,3,29,30].

When changing to oral antibiotics, doses of two to three times those normally recommended are often used. Some authors recommend following weekly serum bactericidal titers to ensure that adequate blood levels are achieved [3]. To measure bactericidal titers, a patient's blood is drawn 1 to 2 hours after administration of the antibiotic and testing is performed to establish the highest dilution of the patient's serum, which kills 99.9% of inoculated bacteria after 18 hours of culture. Dilutions of at least 1:8 are desirable [3]. More recently, Marshall et al [31] questioned the need for serial bactericidal titers in patients treated with oral antibiotics for skeletal infections, and many microbiology laboratories no longer perform this procedure.

Special considerations

Chronic osteomyelitis

Up to 19% of patients with AHO who are inadequately treated may develop chronic osteomyelitis compared with 2% of patients who receive antibiotic therapy for longer than 3 weeks [5]. Chronic osteomyelitis is characterized by a chronic, suppurative course with intermittent acute exacerbations. This may occur after an open fracture or when subperiosteal or metaphyseal pus is not adequately drained. Treatment is often difficult and involves long-term antibiotics, sometimes up to 6 to 12 months, often in combination with one or more surgeries for débridement. The extensive surgical debridement may necessitate reconstructive surgery with bone grafts and muscle flaps [27].

Brodie abscess

A Brodie abscess is a subacute form of osteomyelitis that results in a collection of necrotic bone and pus in a fibrous capsule, which is formed by surrounding granulation tissue [27]. It occurs most commonly in the long bones of adolescents. The defect may be seen on plain film, and on MRI it has a distinctive target appearance. Although the erythrocyte sedimentation rate is usually elevated, it may be normal. Management involves surgical drainage followed by antibiotic therapy. Properly treated patients have a good prognosis.

Osteomyelitis in patients with sickle hemoglobinopathies

Osteomyelitis in patients with sickle cell disease may be difficult to differentiate from a vaso-occlusive crisis. Both syndromes can present with fever, bone pain, and tenderness. Spiking fevers above 39°C, chills, toxic appearance, and leukocytosis are more concerning for osteomyelitis in this population. Infection can be difficult to differentiate from infarction on imaging studies, and needle aspiration or biopsy of the affected site may be required. In addition to S. aureus, Salmonella spp. are common etiologic agents [32], and empiric therapy (eg, a cephalosporin, possibly in combination with vancomycin) should be chosen accordingly. Prolonged parenteral therapy (at least 6–8 weeks) is often required.

Pseudomonas osteochondritis

Up to 2% of nail puncture wounds of the foot are complicated by osteochondritis, and P. aeruginosa is the infecting organism in most cases [14]. P. aeruginosa can be found in the liner of sneakers, although infections may occur after puncture wounds through other types of shoes or even bare feet. Management generally involves surgery to remove necrotic cartilage and obtain specimen for culture. After adequate debridement, an intravenous antibiotic with pseudomonas coverage and coverage of the more common pathogens (eg, cefepime or piperacillin/tazobactam) is generally used for 7 to 14 days. Although adult studies seem to indicate that oral ciprofloxacin for 7 to 14 days is usually adequate [14], some authors believe that intravenous therapy should be used in pediatric cases [33,34]. Anecdotally, the use of prophylactic ciprofloxacin in patients with puncture wounds may prevent the development of osteochondritis.

Spinal osteomyelitis

Osteomyelitis of the spine may be in the form of discitis or vertebral osteomyelitis. Discitis is an inflammatory process, usually of a lumbar disc, that is most common in children younger than 5 years of age (mean age, 2.8 years) [16]. Discitis generally results from low-grade bacterial infection, although some authors believe that it can be noninfectious (eg, after trauma to the spine). Patients may present with a limp, backache, or refusal to walk. Fevers are generally absent or low grade. Plain films may demonstrate narrowing of the disc space. Antibiotic therapy should cover S. aureus and GABHS and may be given orally for the entire course or intravenously for 5 to 7 days followed by oral administration for another 7 to 14 days.

Vertebral osteomyelitis occurs in 1% to 2% of cases of osteomyelitis and tends to occur in slightly older children (mean age, 7.5 years) [16]. It may result from hematologic seeding of the vertebrae or through extension of a local infection, such as discitis. *S. aureus* is the most common organism, but other organisms, including *Bartonella henselae* (cat-scratch disease), have been reported [16]. In some areas of the world, tuberculous spondylitis (Pott disease) is not uncommon [35]. Patients with Pott disease may manifest with kyphosis and neurologic deficits. Diagnosis of vertebral osteomyelitis is often based on MRI. Surgery may be required urgently if there is evidence of spinal cord compression. Antibiotics should be administered for at least 4 weeks.

Chronic recurrent multifocal osteomyelitis

Chronic recurrent multifocal osteomyelitis is characterized by recurrent episodes of bony inflammation, pain, and fever with periodic exacerbations and remissions [27]. Culture results are negative, and antibiotics have not been found to alter the course of the disease. Chronic recurrent multifocal osteomyelitis presents most commonly in children and adolescents, with a mean age at presentation of 14 years [36]. Chronic recurrent multifocal osteomyelitis is associated with Sweet syndrome (ie, acute febrile neutrophilic dermatosis), psoriasis, and pustulosis palmaris et plantaris. Plain films may demonstrate multiple areas of osteolysis and sclerosis, especially in the long bones and clavicles. Treatment generally involves glucocorticoids and nonsteroidal anti-inflammatory drugs. Other reported therapies include immune modulators, antimetabolites, calcium modulators, colchicine, and hyperbaric oxygen.

Septic arthritis

Introduction and epidemiology

Septic arthritis refers to bacterial invasion of the joint space and the subsequent inflammatory response. Septic arthritis is commonly a disease of childhood, with approximately half of all cases occurring in patients younger than 20 years of age [37]. Rates of septic arthritis are estimated to be between 5.5 and 12 cases per 100,000 children [38]. The peak incidence is in children younger than 3 years, and boys are affected approximately twice as often as girls [37–39]. Septic arthritis occurs more commonly in patients with diabetes mellitus, sickle cell disease, and immunodeficiencies. The most commonly affected joints are those of the lower extremities, including knees, hips, and ankles, which account for up to 80% of cases [37,40,41].

Pathogenesis

There are several mechanisms by which bacteria may be introduced into the synovial fluid. Septic arthritis may occur as a result of hematogenous seeding of the synovium during a transient episode of bacteremia, from contiguous spread of an adjacent infection such as osteomyelitis, or by direct inoculation during surgery or as a result of penetrating trauma. Characteristics of the joint, which increase the likelihood of infection during bacteremia (hematogenous spread), include the highly vascular nature of synovium and the lack of a limiting basement membrane, which may allow bacteria to enter the joint space more readily. Several strains of *S. aureus* also have collagen receptors on their surface.

Once the joint space is invaded by bacteria, endotoxins are released. In response to these endotoxins, cytokines, such as tumor necrosis factor and interleukin-1, are released, which in turn stimulate the release of proteolytic enzymes and increase leukocyte migration [42,43]. This combination of factors leads to destruction of the synovium and cartilage matrix. Although cases of septic arthritis rarely have been fatal since the introduction of antibiotics, destruction of the joint space leads to long-term sequelae in a significant percentage of patients [44,45].

Some joints are more susceptible to damage. For example, increased pressure within the hip can interrupt blood flow and lead to avascular necrosis of the femoral head. Prompt recognition and aggressive management are critical.

Microbiology

The specific bacteria isolated from joint fluid in patients with septic arthritis vary with age. In all age groups outside of the neonatal period, *S. aureus* is the most common organism [39,45,46]. Other frequently identified organisms include GABHS and *S. pneumoniae*. In the neonatal period, *S. aureus* remains a common organism, but group B streptococcus is also frequently identified [47,48]. Neonates are also at risk for gram-negative enteric bacilli. Neonates and sexually active adolescents are at risk for infection by *Neiserria gonorrhoeae* [49].

Currently an unusual cause of septic arthritis, *H. influenzae* type B commonly was identified before the introduction of an effective vaccine [41,44,46]. *K. kingae* may be identified in toddlers with a preceding history of an upper respiratory tract infection [50]. In addition to the usual organisms, patients with sickle cell disease are at risk for bone and joint infections by *Salmonella* spp. *Neisseria meningitides* is a rare cause of septic arthritis but is commonly associated with reactive arthritis. *P. aeruginosa* also has been reported as a causative agent [51].

Clinical presentation

Patients with septic arthritis usually present with focal findings at the infected joint. Symptoms include edema, erythema, joint effusion, and tenderness. Patients tend to keep the affected joint in a position that maximizes intracapsular volume and comfort. Knees are held moderately flexed, and hips are kept flexed, abducted, and externally rotated. Refusal to move an affected joint is referred to as pseudoparalysis, and even passive movement may be painful. Systemic symptoms such as fever, malaise, and poor appetite are also seen in most patients. The progression of the disease is rapid, with many patients having symptoms for no more than 72 hours before diagnosis.

Diagnosis in neonates is often more difficult. Inflammation may be less impressive because of an immature immune system. The hip, the most commonly affected joint in neonates [40,44,48], is deep, and any present inflammation may be disguised. Discomfort may be noted with diaper changes and other manipulation of the hip.

In all age groups, approximately 75% to 80% of cases involve joints of the lower extremities, with the knees and the hips being most commonly affected [37,39,40]. Other commonly affected joints include the ankles, wrists, elbows, and shoulders. Small, distal joints are less likely to be involved. Polyarticular joint involvement occurs in less than 10% of patients but is seen in up to 50% of patients with infection caused by *N. gonorrhoeae* [37,40,44,46].

Differential diagnosis

Multiple entities may be confused with septic arthritis, including hemarthrosis, traumatic effusion, transient synovitis, reactive arthritis, Lyme arthritis, juvenile rheumatoid arthritis, arthritis of acute rheumatic fever, osteomyelitis, tumor, slipped capital femoral epiphysis, and Legg-Calvé-Perthes disease. In particular, transient synovitis (also known as toxic synovitis) often mimics septic arthritis. Transient synovitis is presumed to be a postviral phenomenon and often affects the hip in boys between the ages of 3 and 10 years. The arthritis that occurs with Lyme disease is also a great imitator of septic arthritis and must be considered in endemic areas. Multiple bacteria, including *N. meningitidis*, *Streptococcal* spp., *Salmonella* spp., and *Mycoplasma pneumoniae* are associated with postinfectious reactive arthritides. In cases of suspected septic arthritis, concomitant osteomyelitis of an adjacent bone should be suspected.

Diagnosis and evaluation

The cornerstone of diagnosis is the evaluation of aspirated joint fluid. The fluid should be sent for gram stain, aerobic culture, and cell count with differential [52]. Typical findings of aspirated synovial fluid are presented in Table 2. An organism is isolated from culture of joint fluid in approximately 60% of cases [41,45], which allows for definitive diagnosis and narrowing of antibiotic coverage. Synovial fluid should be aspirated into a heparinized syringe. *K. kingae* is a slow-growing fastidious organism. If it is suspected, synovial fluid should be inoculated directly into a blood culture bottle, which increases the yield [50].

Blood cultures produce positive results in one third of cases and may help identify the pathogen in cases where the synovial culture fluid is negative [41,45]. In general, the white blood cell count, C-reactive protein, and erythrocyte sedi-

Table 2
Typical synovial fluid findings

	Septic arthritis	Transient synovitis	Normal joint
Color	Serosanguinous	Yellow	Yellow
Clarity	Turbid	Generally clear, but depends on number of white blood cells	Clear
White blood cells	>50,000–100,000/mm^3	5,000–15,000/mm^3	<200/mm^3
% Polymorphonuclear neutrophils	>75%	<25%	<25%
Culture	Positive in 60%	Negative	Negative
Glucose	<40 mg/dL	Equal to serum	Equal to serum

mentation rate are elevated in patients with septic arthritis, but some patients present with normal inflammatory markers [44,45,53,54].

Imaging studies also may be helpful in making the diagnosis but should not delay aspiration of the joint or the prompt surgical and antibiotic management in cases in which septic arthritis is suspected. Plain films may demonstrate a widened joint space in a patient with a septic hip but are more useful for ruling out other conditions, such as fractures, Legg-Calvé-Perthes disease, and slipped capital femoral epiphysis. Ultrasonography is useful in identifying and quantifying a joint effusion, especially in deeper joints, such as the hips, and may be used to guide needle aspiration of these joints (Fig. 4) [54,55]. Bone scan and MRI are often used and may play a critical role in diagnosing concomitant osteomyelitis [55].

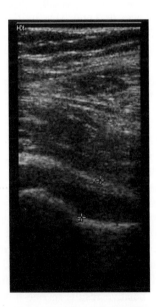

Fig. 4. Sonographic evaluation of the hips in an 11-year-old boy with fever and right hip pain. Moderate effusion of the right joint space that measured 1.3 cm is noted.

Management

Antibiotic therapy should be initiated immediately after blood and synovial fluid cultures have been obtained. Antibiotics have good penetration into the synovial fluid, with several studies finding equal concentrations in the joint fluid and serum 1 hour after administration [56–58]. The gram stain can help guide the initial antibiotic choice; however, the antibiotic therapy should not be delayed if this result cannot be obtained promptly. If gram-positive cocci are seen, empiric therapy with a semi-synthetic, penicillinase-resistant penicillin (eg, oxacillin, 150 mg/kg/d, divided in four doses) is the traditional choice. Vancomycin or clindamycin should be considered in areas with high rates of community-acquired methicillin-resistant *S. aureus,* however (see previous discussion). If Gram stain reveals gram-negative organisms or if no organisms are seen, one should consider a third-generation cephalosporin, such as cefotaxime or ceftriaxone, which covers most gram-positive organisms and *K. kingae*, *Salmonella* spp., and *H. influenzae*. In sexually active adolescents, ceftriaxone or cefotaxime may be used to cover *N. gonorrhoeae*. Neonates are often treated with oxacillin or nafcillin plus cefotaxime or gentamicin, although cefotaxime alone covers the most likely etiologic agents. Coverage can be narrowed once identification of the organism and susceptibilities are available.

Most authors agree that septic arthritis of the hip is a medical emergency that requires immediate surgical drainage. Infants with septic arthritis of the shoulder are also treated with emergent surgical drainage. When other joints are affected, some authors advocate repeated, daily aspiration, which has proved to be superior to surgical drainage in an adult study [59]. If a large amount of fibrin or debris is present, the infection is loculated, or there is a lack of improvement within 3 days, however, then surgical drainage is recommended. Physical therapy may be beneficial as adjunctive management in some cases, especially when a child is hesitant to use the joint.

In uncomplicated cases, the total duration of therapy should be at least 3 weeks, with at least 1 week of antibiotics given intravenously. If a patient improves clinically after 1 week and inflammatory markers are normalizing, then the remaining 2 weeks of antibiotics can be given orally. Despite appropriate management, approximately 40% of patients with hip involvement and 10% of patients with knee involvement suffer significant sequelae, such as growth plate damage and loss of function [44,45,60]. Close follow-up in all patients and physical therapy in selected patients are essential.

Pyomyositis

Introduction and epidemiology

Pyomyositis is a bacterial infection of skeletal muscle with a predilection for large muscle groups, and it often results in localized abscess formation. Although relatively uncommon in more temperate areas, such as North America [61], pyomyositis accounts for up to 4% of surgical admissions in some tropical areas [62]. This geographic distribution has led to the alternative name of pyomyositis tropicans. Within North America, the highest incidence of pyomyositis is in the southernmost regions. In children, the peak incidence seems to occur between 5 and 9 years of age [63].

Pathogenesis

Pyomyositis is believed to occur when a transient bacteremia seeds a site of local muscle trauma or strain [64,65]. Patients with pyomyositis are able to recall a history of trauma in only approximately 25% of cases, however [66,67]. Vigorous exercise, presumably a cause of muscle strain, also may be a causative factor [68,69]. Other authors have suggested that an antecedent viral infection may be a predisposing factor in some cases [66].

Microbiology

S. aureus is the most commonly identified organism; it accounts for approximately 90% of cases of pyomyositis in tropical areas [66,67] and approximately 70% of cases in North America [70]. Box 1 lists other reported causes. Clostridial infections can lead to a fulminant form of myonecrosis, which is often fatal [71].

Box 1. Reported causes of pyomyositis

S. aureus
Group A strepotococcus
Other Staphylococcal and Streptococcal spp.
E. coli
Salmonella enteritidis
Citrobacter freundii
Clostridium spp.
Serratia spp.
Klebsiella spp.
Yersinia spp.
Pasteurella spp.
Mycobacterium tuberculosis
Candida albicans

Data from references [1,3,4,8,13–15].

Clinical presentation

The initial presentation of pyomyositis is often subacute, and initial symptoms may be vague. In a review of 16 cases of pyomyositis in children [72], the mean duration of symptoms before presentation was 8.9 days. Patients presented with pain (100%), fever (93.8%), swelling (62.5%), and limp (100% of lower body abscesses).

Pyomyositis occurs in three stages [70,73,74]. The invasive stage is characterized by low-grade fevers, general malaise, and dull, cramping pain. Although the overlying skin often appears normal, a firm or "woody" texture may be appreciated on deep palpation. Abscess formation occurs during the suppurative stage, and patients tend to have more focal complaints. Often there is increased tenderness with overlying erythema and swelling. During the late stage of pyomyositis, patients develop high fevers, exhibit more local signs of infection, and complain of severe pain. Patients in the late stage of pyomyositis can develop systemic manifestations, including metastatic abscesses, arthritis, and renal failure. Septic shock and toxic shock may ensue if urgent management is not initiated. Although rare, death has been reported after this late stage of pyomyositis [66].

Pyomyositis most commonly affects the quadriceps, gluteal, and iliopsoas muscles [66]. Other affected areas include the paraspinus, psoas, shoulder girdle, extremities (eg, gastrocnemius), chest wall, and abdominal wall [66,72–75]. Patients with psoas muscle involvement may present with limp, hip pain, or back pain. Multiple sites are involved in 11% to 43% of patients [66,67].

More rapidly necrotizing infections of muscle also have been described. Infections with GABHS [76] often occur in patients with a primary varicella infection and can cause a rapidly progressive, necrotizing form of pyomyositis (see the later discussion on necrotizing fasciitis). Within hours of presentation, patients can develop hypotension, oliguria, lethargy, and toxic shock. A scarlatiniform rash may be present.

Clostridial myonecrosis (gas gangrene) generally occurs 2 to 3 days after wound contamination with *Clostridium perfingens* and is characterized by myonecrosis, gas production, and sepsis. Patients may present initially with localized pain and pallor [77]. Subcutaneous emphysema and crepitus may be appreciated. Symptoms may progress rapidly with the appearance of hemorrhagic bullae and the development of cutaneous necrosis, acidosis, coagulopathy, and shock.

Differential diagnosis

In a review of 97 cases of pyomyositis in adults, erroneous diagnoses at admission included thrombophlebitis (7 cases), sarcoma or malignancy (7 cases), cellulitis (3 cases), osteochondritis (1 case), contusion (1 case), and compartment syndrome (1 case) [78]. The broad differential diagnosis of pyomyositis also includes other infectious processes, such as septic arthritis, acute appendicitis, and osteomyelitis. Other inflammatory processes that may mimic pyomyositis include polymyositis, bursitis, and other rheumatic diseases. Pyomyositis also may be confused with muscle strain, viral myositis (eg, influenza, enterovirus), deep venous thrombosis, or hematoma.

Diagnosis and evaluation

Ultrasonography is a quick and inexpensive study that can detect muscle abscesses [79] and may be used to guide percutaneous drainage. Alternatively, CT can provide good delineation of muscle structure and may demonstrate a fluid collection. MRI with gadolinium is the most sensitive study for detecting early inflammatory changes. MRI also can define the extent of muscle involvement and may help identify patients with early disease who do not require surgical intervention [73].

Laboratory studies tend to be nonspecific. A complete blood count generally demonstrates a leukocytosis with a left shift. Eosinophilia is more common in patients from the tropics [73] and may represent concomitant parasitic infection. The erythrocyte sedimentation rate is often elevated [78]. Muscle enzymes, such as creatine kinase and aldolase, are generally normal. In one study, blood cultures yielded positive results in 29% of cases [80]. Fluid aspirated from the site of infection is more likely to yield an organism.

Management

Surgical incision and drainage are generally required, although certain patients who present with muscle inflammation but do not yet have abscess formation may be managed with antibiotic therapy alone [73,74]. CT [81] or ultrasound-guided percutaneous drainage is another alternative to surgical management in some patients.

Because *S. aureus* accounts for most infections, a semi-synthetic penicillinase-resistant penicillin (eg, nafcillin or oxacillin, 150 mg/kg/d, divided every 6 hours) is the traditional choice for empiric therapy. Clindamycin is an alternative, especially in patients with penicillin allergies, and vancomycin should be considered for empiric therapy in areas with a high incidence of community-acquired methicillin-resistant *S. aureus* (see discussion in the section on osteomyelitis).

The optimal length of therapy is not well described. In general, intravenous antibiotics should be continued until clinical improvement is evident. Based on sensitivities, appropriate oral antibiotics should be continued for a total of 2 to 6 weeks [66,73,74].

Necrotizing GABHS infections require immediate surgical exploration/ debridement and possible fasciotomy. Therapy should include clindamycin for the Eagle effect [82] (see the section on necrotizing fasciitis) because most cases of pyomyositis are diagnosed after the organisms have reached a steady-state growth phase.

Necrotizing fasciitis

Introduction and epidemiology

Necrotizing fasciitis (also known as hospital gangrene or hemolytic strep-tococcal gangrene) was described as early as the fifth century BC, when Hippocrates wrote, "flesh, sinews and bones fell away in large quantities. The flux which formed was not like pus but a different sort of putrefaction with a copious and varied flux... There were many deaths" [83]. Necrotizing fasciitis is a rapidly progressive, deep-seated bacterial infection of the subcutaneous soft tissue that may involve any area of the body. It often follows a fulminant course and has a high mortality rate. Estimates of the mortality rate range from 25% to 75% [84,85].

Although more than 500 cases of necrotizing fasciitis have been reported in North America, it is an uncommon disease and the true incidence is not known [86,87]. Men are affected slightly more commonly than women [84,85,88]. An increased frequency is reported in persons with diabetes, intravenous drug users, alcoholics, immunosuppressed patients, and patients with peripheral vascular disease [85,86,88]. Necrotizing fasciitis also occurs in young, previously healthy patients, including children. Mortality rates in children and previously healthy individuals tend to be much lower [86].

Pathogenesis

Necrotizing fasciitis begins with the introduction of bacterial infection. Extension of the infection along fascial planes leads to necrosis of the superficial muscle fascia and the deeper layers of the dermis. Destruction and thrombosis of the small blood vessels in the area lead to necrosis of the surrounding tissues. The extensive tissue damage often leads to systemic symptoms, including multiorgan failure and shock.

Predisposing factors include trauma, surgery, burns, and eczema [84]. In neonates, necrotizing fasciitis may complicate omphalitis or circumcision. Less commonly associated factors include insect bites, perirectal abscesses, incarcerated hernias, and subcutaneous insulin injections. Necrotizing fasciitis has been reported in several cases as a complication of varicella infection [86,89,90]. Necrotizing fasciitis also may occur with a preceding GABHS pharyngitis or without any previous evidence of trauma or infection.

An association between the use of nonsteroidal anti-inflammatory drugs and necrotizing fasciitis has been reported [89,91,92]. Given the frequency of nonsteroidal anti-inflammatory drug use worldwide, however, most authors believe that patients with necrotizing fasciitis are likely to have taken the drugs for their analgesic and anti-inflammatory properties and that a true cause-and-effect relationship is unlikely [92].

Microbiology

Necrotizing fasciitis is often polymicrobial in origin [84,85,93] and involves gram-negative bacilli, enterococci, streptococci, *S. aureus* and anaerobes such as *Bacteroides* spp, *Peptostreptococcus* spp, and *Clostridium* spp (Table 3). This polymicrobial form of the disease is described as necrotizing fasciitis type 1 and is often seen postoperatively or in patients with diabetes mellitus or peripheral vascular disease. Gas gangrene is the result of clostridial infection (*C. perfringens, C. histolyticum, C. septicum*) often secondary to trauma or crush injury. It is a myonecrotic disease that quickly leads to systemic toxicity and shock.

Necrotizing fasciitis type 2 is an infection with GABHS that may occur postoperatively or as a result of penetrating trauma, varicella infection, burns, or minor cuts. It is characterized by rapidly extending necrosis and severe systemic toxicity. Type 2 disease is the most common type in children with necrotizing fasciitis [86,88,94].

Less common than type 1 or type 2, necrotizing fasciitis type 3 is caused by marine *Vibrio* spp., which enter through skin lesions that have been exposed to seawater or marine animals.

Table 3
Bacteria associated with necrotizing fasciitis [84,85,93]

Category	Organism
Gram-positive aerobes	Group A beta-hemolytic streptococcus
	S. aureus
	Other staphylococcal and streptococcal spp.
	Enterococci
Gram-negative aerobes	*E. coli*
	P. aeruginosa
	Enterobacter cloacae
	Klebsiella spp.
	Proteus spp.
	Serratia spp.
	Acinetobacter calcoaceticus
	Citrobacter freundii
	Pasteurella multocida
Anaerobes	*Bacteroides* spp.
	Clostridium spp.
	Vibrio spp.
	Peptostreptococcus spp.

Data from references [84,85,93].

Clinical presentation

Patients may report a history of recent surgery, trauma, omphalitis, or varicella infection [89,90]. In children, necrotizing fasciitis often presents 1 to 4 days after trauma with soft-tissue swelling and pain near the infected area. Patients may appear well at initial presentation. When associated with varicella, the findings typically begin 3 to 4 days after onset of the exanthem [90]. Infants and toddlers may be fussy or irritable. Toddlers and young children may present with a limp or refusal to bear weight. Initially, pain with manipulation of an affected extremity tends to be out of proportion to the cutaneous signs of infection.

Induration and edema are generally apparent within the first 24 hours and are followed rapidly by blistering and bleb formation [95,96]. Infection spreads in the plane between the subcutaneous tissue and the superficial muscle fascia, which results in the progressive destruction of fascia and fat. The skin takes on a dusky appearance, and a thick, foul-smelling fluid is produced. Pain and tenderness in the subcutaneous space is exquisite and often seems out of proportion to the cutaneous appearance, but destruction of the nerves that innervate the skin may lead to anesthesia of the overlying skin. High fevers are common. The rapidly progressing infection can lead to toxic shock syndrome and severe systemic toxicities, including renal and hepatic failure, acute respiratory distress syndrome, and decreased myocardial contractility.

Differential diagnosis

The differential diagnosis of necrotizing fasciitis includes other soft-tissue infections, such as cellulitis, pyomyositis, and gas gangrene. In cases of Fournier's gangrene, hernias, epididymitis, orchitis, and testicular torsion also must be considered.

Diagnosis and evaluation

Although white blood cell counts may be normal or elevated, there is often a pronounced bandemia. Thrombocytopenia and evidence of a coagulopathy also may be apparent. Attempts to identify causative organisms should be made through collection of anaerobic and aerobic blood cultures, although the results are frequently negative [85,90]. Cultures of the wound and surgically debrided tissue also should be taken. Frozen section biopsies can be helpful in making a timely diagnosis.

Radiologic studies may support the diagnosis, but they should not delay surgical intervention. Plain films may show gas or soft-tissue edema but are otherwise nonspecific. Although CT may be useful in defining the extent of soft-tissue involvement, MRI is the preferred modality. MRI may reveal extension of inflammation along the fascial plains.

Management

Emergent, wide surgical debridement is critical and may need to be repeated immediately [84,85,93]. Delays in surgery are associated with increased mortality, and antibiotic therapy in the absence of surgical debridement is ineffective [84,93]. Gram stain of surgical or aspirated material from the infected site may be helpful in guiding antibiotic selection. In patients with suspected GABHS infection, the antibiotic regimen should include intravenous penicillin (150,000 U/kg/d, divided every 4–6 hours) and clindamycin (40 mg/kg/d, divided every 6 hours).

Clindamycin is added for the "eagle effect," which was first described in 1952 in a seminal article by Harry Eagle, MD, who described treatment failure of penicillin in mice injected with GABHS [82]. Eagle noted that "the greatly reduced therapeutic activity of penicillin in the older infections is due to the fact that the organisms are no longer metabolizing as actively as in the inflammatory focus." In other words, GABHS initially proliferate rapidly until a steady state of growth is reached. Beta-lactam antibiotics are less effective during this steady-state phase, because they inhibit cell wall synthesis of actively replicating organisms. Clindamycin, however, is not affected by the decreased growth rate, because it works at the ribosomal level and offers the added benefit of reducing toxin synthesis by the organism [97]. The combination of a penicillin with clindamycin is more effective than either agent alone. In patients with polymicrobial infections, consider a beta-lactam/beta-lactamase inhibitor combination, such as ampicillin/sulbactam or piperacillin/tazobactam.

Supportive therapy includes careful fluid management, pain control, and management of multisystemic organ failure, usually in an intensive care setting. Patients with a GABHS necrotizing fasciitis are at risk for toxic shock syndrome, and many experts recommend intravenous immunoglobulin in this situation [98]. The role of hyperbaric oxygen therapy is controversial. Patients who survive may require amputation, skin grafting, and reconstructive surgery.

Summary

Musculoskeletal infections, including osteomyelitis, septic arthritis, necrotizing fasciitis, and pyomyositis, can occur in previously healthy children and lead to severe long-term morbidity if not recognized and treated promptly. Early diagnosis is crucial, and initial presentation is often to the primary care pediatrician. In addition to making a diagnosis, identification of the causative organism is imperative, especially in light of increasing resistance patterns. Identification may be accomplished through direct culture of debrided or aspirated tissue. Although they often produce negative results, blood cultures should be obtained in all cases because they may yield the pathogen. Initial antibiotic management should cover the most common etiologic organisms, and consideration should be given to local rates of community-acquired methicillin-resistant *S. aureus*.

Radiologic studies may be diagnostic, and the high sensitivity and resolution of MRI often make it the study of choice. In suspected cases of necrotizing fasciitis, prompt surgical management should not be delayed by radiologic evaluation. Although rarely fatal, musculoskeletal infections may be associated with long-term sequelae. Initial management should be aggressive, treatment courses should not be shortened, and long-term follow-up is essential.

References

[1] LaMont RL, Anderson PA, Dajani AS, et al. Acute hematogenous osteomyelitis in children. J Pediatr Orthop 1987;7:579–83.

[2] Nelson JD. Acute osteomyelitis in children. Infect Dis Clin North Am 1990;4(3):513–22.

[3] Vaughan PA, Newman NM, Rosman MA. Acute hematogenous osteomyelitis in children. J Pediatr Orthop 1987;7:652–5.

[4] Gillespie WJ. Epidemiology in bone and joint infection. Infect Dis Clin North Am 1990; 4(3):361–75.

[5] Dich VQ, Nelson JD, Haltalin KC. Osteomyelitis in infants and children. Am J Dis Child 1975; 129:1273–8.

[6] Lazzarini L, Mader J, Calhoun J. Osteomyelitis in long bones. J Bone Joint Surg Am 2004; 86-A(10):2305–18.

[7] Lew DP, Waldvogel FA. Osteomyelitis. N Engl J Med 1997;336(14):999–1007.

[8] Gristina AG. Adherent bacterial colonization in the pathogenesis of osteomyelitis. Science 1985; 228:990–3.

[9] Unkila-Kallio L, Kallio M, Eskola J, et al. Serum C-reactive protein, erythrocyte sedimentation rate, and white blood cell count in acute hematogenous osteomyelitis of children. Pediatrics 1993;92(6):800–4.

[10] Ibia EO, Imoisili M, Pikis A. Group A β-hemolytic streptococcal osteomyelitis in children. Pediatrics 2003;112:22–6.

[11] Bowerman S, Green N, Menicio G. Decline of bone and joint infections attributable to haemophilus influenzae type b. Clin Orthop Relat Res 1997;1(341):128–33.

[12] Yaupsky P, Dagan R, Howard CB, et al. Clinical features and epidemiology of invasive *Kingella kingae* infections in southern Israel. Pediatrics 1993;92(6):800–4.

[13] Fitzgerald RH, Cowan JDE. Puncture wounds of the foot. Orthop Clin North Am 1975; 6(4):965–71.

[14] Raz R, Miron D. Oral ciprofloxacin for treatment of infection following nail puncture wounds of the foot. Clin Infect Dis 1995;21:194–5.

[15] Edwards MS, Baker CJ, Wagner ML, et al. An etiologic shift in infantile osteomyelitis: the emergence of the group B streptococcus. J Pediatr 1978;93(4):578–83.

[16] Fernandez M, Carrol C, Baker C. Discitis and vertebral osteomyelitis in children: an 18-year review. Pediatrics 2000;105(6):1299–304.

[17] Mirakhur B, Shah S, Ratner A, et al. Cat scratch disease presenting as orbital abscess and osteomyelitis. J Clin Microbiol 2003;41(8):3991–3.

[18] Asmar BI. Osteomyelitis in the neonate. Infect Dis Clin North Am 1992;6(1):117–32.

[19] Butt WP. The radiology of infection. Clin Orthop Relat Res 1973;96:20–30.

[20] Darville T, Jacobs R. Management of acute hematogenous osteomyelitis in children. Pediatr Infect Dis J 2004;23:255–7.

[21] Oudjhane K, Azouz M. Imaging of osteomyelitis in children. Radiol Clin North Am 2001; 39(2):251–65.

[22] Struk DW, Munk PL, Lee MJ, et al. Imaging of soft tissue infections. Radiol Clin North Am 2001;39(2):277–302.

[23] Mazur JM, Ross G, Cummings J, et al. Usefulness of magnetic resonance imaging for the diagnosis of acute musculoskeletal infections in children. J Pediatr Orthop 1995;15:144–7.

[24] McAndrew P, Clark C. MRI is best technique for imaging acute osteomyelitis. BMJ 1998; 316(7125):147.

[25] Sattler CA, Mason Jr EO, Kaplan SL. Prospective comparison of risk factors and demographic and clinical characteristics of community-acquired, methicillin-resistant versus methicillin-susceptible Staphylococcus aureus infection in children. Pediatr Infect Dis J 2002;21(10):910–7.

[26] Martinez-Aguilar G, Hammerman WA, Mason Jr EO, et al. Clindamycin treatment of invasive infections caused by community-acquired, methicillin-resistant and methicillin-susceptible Staphylococcus aureus in children. Pediatr Infect Dis J 2003;22(7):593–8.

[27] Ramos OM. Chronic osteomyelitis in children. Pediatr Infect Dis J 2002;21(5):431–2.

[28] Vasquez M. Osteomyelitis in children. Curr Opin Pediatr 2002;14:112–5.

[29] Bryson YJ, Connor JD, LeClerc M, et al. High-dose oral dicloxacillin treatment of acute staphylococcal osteomyelitis in children. J Pediatr 1979;94(4):673–6.

[30] Walker SH. Staphylococcal osteomyelitis in children, success with cephaloridine-cephalexin therapy. Clin Pediatr 1973;12(2):98–100.

[31] Marshall GS, Mudido P, Rabalais GP, et al. Organism isolation and serum bactericidal titers in oral antibiotic therapy for pediatric osteomyelitis. South Med J 1996;89(1):68–70.

[32] Mallouh A, Talab Y. Bone and joint infection in patients with sickle cell disease. J Pediatr Orthop 1985;5(2):158–62.

[33] Jarvis JG, Skipper J. Pseudomonas osteochondritis complicating puncture wounds in children. J Pediatr Orthop 1994;14(6):755–9.

[34] Jacobs RF, McCarthy RE, Elser JM. Pseudomonas osteochondritis complicating puncture wounds of the foot in children: a 10-year evaluation. J Infect Dis 1989;160(4):657–61.

[35] Sternbach G. Percivall Pott: tuberculous spondylitis. J Emerg Med 1996;14(1):79–83.

[36] Stanton RP, Lopez-Sosa FH, Doidge R. Chronic recurrent multifocal osteomyelitis. Orthop Rev 1993;22(2):229–33.

[37] Baitch A. Recent observations of acute suppurative arthritis. Clin Orthop 1962;22:153–65.

[38] Gillespie WJ. Epidemiology in bone and joint infection. Infect Dis Clin North Am 1990; 4(3):361–75.

[39] Chartier Y, Martin WJ, Kelly PJ. Bacterial arthritis: experiences in the treatment of 77 patients. Ann Intern Med 1939;50:1462–73.

[40] Heberling JA. A review of two hundred and one cases of suppurative arthritis. J Bone Joint Surg 1941;23(4):917–21.

[41] Nelson JD. The bacterial etiology and antibiotic management of septic arthritis in infants and children. Pediatrics 1972;50:437–40.

[42] Curtiss P, Klein L. Destruction of articular cartilage in septic arthritis. II. In vitro studies. J Bone Joint Surg Am 1965;47:1595–604.

[43] Fell H, Jubb R. The effect of synovial tissue on the breakdown of articular cartilage in organ culture. Arthritis Rheum 1977;20:1359–71.

[44] Samilson RL, Bersani FA, Watkins MB. Acute suppurative arthritis in infants and children: the importance of early diagnosis and surgical drainage. Pediatrics 1958;21:798–803.

[45] Morrey BF, Bianco AJ, Rhodes KH. Septic arthritis in children. Orthop Clin North Am 1975; 6:923–34.

[46] Luhmann JD, Luhmann SJ. Etiology of septic arthritis in children: an update for the 1990s. Pediatr Emerg Care 1999;15:40–2.

[47] Del Beccaro MA, Champoux AN, Bockers T, et al. Septic arthritis versus transient synovitis of the hip: the value of screening laboratory tests. Ann Emerg Med 1992;21:1418–22.

[48] Obletz BE. Acute suppurative arthritis of the hip in the neonatal period. Am J Orthop 1960; 42(A):23–30.

[49] Kohen DP. Neonatal gonococcal arthritis: three cases and review of the literature. Pediatrics 1974;53:436–40.

[50] De Groot R, Glover D, Clausen C, et al. Bone and joint infections caused by Kingella kingae: six cases and review of the literature. Rev Infect Dis 1988;10:998–1004.

[51] Tindel JR, Crowder JG. Septic arthritis due to *Pseudomonas aeruginosa*. JAMA 1971;218(4): 559–61.

[52] Shmerling RH, Delbanco TL, Tosteson ANA, et al. Synovial fluid tests: what should be ordered. JAMA 1990;264(8):1009–14.

[53] Pioro MH, Mandell BF. Life threatening complications of autoimmune disease. Rheum Dis Clin North Am 1997;23(2):239–58.

[54] Zawin JK, Hoffer FA, Rand FF, et al. Joint effusion in children with an irritable hip: ultrasound diagnosis and aspiration. Radiology 1993;187:459–63.

[55] Greenspan A, Tehranzadeh J. Imaging of musculoskeletal and spinal infections. Radiol Clin North Am 2001;39(2):343–55.

[56] Baciocco EA, Iles RL. Ampicillin and kanamycin concentrations in joint fluid. Clin Pharmacol 1971;12:858–63.

[57] Balboni VG, Shapiro IM, Kydd DM. The penetration of penicillin into joint fluid following intramuscular administration. Am J Med Sci 1945;210:588–91.

[58] Nelson JD. Antibiotic concentrations in septic joint effusions. N Engl J Med 1971;284:349–53.

[59] Goldenberg DL, Brandt KD, Cohen AS, et al. Treatment of septic arthritis: comparison of needle aspiration and surgery as initial modes of joint drainage. Arthritis Rheum 1975;18:83–90.

[60] Betz RR, Cooperman DR, Wopperer JM, et al. Late sequelae of septic arthritis of the hip in infancy and childhood. J Pediatr Orthop 1990;10:365–72.

[61] Gibson RK, Rostnethal SJ, Lukert BP. Pyomyositis: increasing recognition in temperate climates. Am J Med 1984;77:768–72.

[62] Horn CV, Master S. Pyomyositis tropicans in Uganda. East Afr Med J 1968;45:463–71.

[63] Ameh EA. Pyomyositis in children: analysis of 31 cases. Ann Trop Paediatr 1999;19(3):263–5.

[64] Akman I, Ostrov B, Varma BK, et al. Pyomyositis: report of three patients and review of the literature. Clin Pediatr 1996;35(8):397–401.

[65] Ashken MH, Cotton RE. Tropical skeletal muscle abscesses (pyomyositis tropicans). Br J Surg 1963;50:846–52.

[66] Chiedozi LC. Pyomyositis: review of 205 cases in 112 patients. Am J Surg 1979;137(2):255–9.

[67] Chacha PB. Muscle abscesses in children. Clin Orthop 1970;70:174–80.

[68] Jayoussi R, Bialik V, Eyal A, et al. Pyomyositis caused by vigorous exercise in a boy. Acta Paediatr 1995;84:226–7.

[69] Meehan J, Grose C, Soper RT, et al. Pyomyositis in an adolescent female athlete. J Pediatr Surg 1995;30:127–8.

[70] Christin L, Sarosi GA. Pyomyositis in North America: case reports and review. Clin Infect Dis 1992;15(4):668–77.

[71] Abella BS, Kuchinic P, Hiraoka T, et al. Atraumatic clostridial myonecrosis: case report and literature review. J Emerg Med 2003;24(4):401–5.

[72] Gubbay AJ, Isaacs D. Pyomyositis in children. Pediatr Infect Dis J 2000;19:1009–13.

[73] Spiegel DA, Meyer JS, Dormans JP, et al. Pyomyositis in children and adolescents: report of 12 cases and review of the literature. J Pediatr Orthop 1999;19(2):143–50.

[74] Bickels J, Ben-Sira L, Kessler A, et al. Primary pyomyositis. J Bone Joint Surg Am 2002; 84A(12):2277–86.

[75] Patel SR, Olenginski TP, Perruquet JL, et al. Pyomyositis: clinical features and predisposing conditions. J Rheumatol 1997;24(9):1734–8.

[76] Wheeler DS, Vazquez WD, Vaux KK, et al. Streptococcal pyomyositis: case report and review. Pediatr Emerg Care 1998;14(6):411–2.

[77] Hart GB, Lamb RC, Strauss MB. Gas gangrene. J Trauma 1983;23(11):991–1000.

[78] Gomez-Reino JJ, Aznar JJ, Pablos JL, et al. Nontropical pyomyositis in adults. Semin Arthritis Rheum 1994;23(6):396–405.

[79] Yousefzadeh DK, Schumann EM, Mulligan GM, et al. The role of imaging modalities in diagnosis and management of pyomyositis. Skeletal Radiol 1982;8(4):285–9.

[80] Brown JD, Wheeler B. Pyomyositis: report of 18 cases in Hawaii. Arch Intern Med 1984; 144(9):1749–51.

[81] McLoughlin MJ. CT and percutaneous fine-needle aspiration biopsy in tropical myositis. AJR Am J Roentgenol 1980;134(1):167–8.

[82] Eagle H. Experimental approach to the problem of treatment failure with penicillin. I. Group A streptococcal infection in mice. Am J Med 1952;13:389–99.

[83] Descamps V, Aitken J, Lee MG. Hippocrates on necrotising fasciitis. Lancet 1994;344:556.

[84] McHenry CR, Piotrowski JJ, Petrinic D. Determinants of mortalitiy for necrotizing soft-tissue infections. Ann Surg 1995;221:558–65.

[85] Francis KR, LaMaute HR, Davis JM, et al. Implications of risk factors in necrotizing fasciitis. Am Surg 1993;59:304–8.

[86] Davies HD, McGeer A, Schwartz B, et al. Invasive group A streptococcal infections in Ontario, Canada. N Engl J Med 1996;335:547–54.

[87] Editorial CDC. Invasive group A streptococcal infections: United Kingdom, 1994. JAMA 1994; 272:16.

[88] Stevens DL, Tanner MH, Winship J, et al. Severe group A streptococcal infections associated with a toxic shock-like syndrome and scarlet fever toxin A. N Engl J Med 1989;321:1–7.

[89] Zerr DM, Alexander ER, Duchin JS, et al. A case-control study of necrotizing fasciitis during primary varicella. Pediatrics 1999;103:783–90.

[90] Brogan TV, Nizet V, Waldhausen JH, et al. Group A streptococcal necrotizing fasciitis complicating primary varicella: a series of fourteen patients. Pediatr Infect Dis J 1996;15:556–7.

[91] Zerr DM, Rubens CE. NSAIDS and necrotizing fasciitis. Pediatr Infect Dis J 1999;18(8):724–5.

[92] Aronoff DM, Bloch KC. Assessing the relationship between the use of nonsteroidal anti-inflammatory drugs and necrotizing fasciitis caused by group A streptococcus. Medicine 2003; 82:225–35.

[93] Voros D, Pissiotis C, Georgantas D, et al. Role of early and extensive surgery in the treatment of severe necrotizing soft tissue infections. Br J Surg 1993;80(9):1190–1.

[94] Hoge CW, Schwartz B, Talkington DF, et al. The changing epidemiology of invasive group A streptococcal infections and the emergence of streptococcal toxic shock-like syndrome: a retrospective population-based study. JAMA 1993;269:384–9.

[95] Stevens DL. Invasive group A streptococcal infections. Clin Infect Dis 1992;14:2–13.

[96] Stevens DL. Invasive group A streptococcal infections: the past, present and future. Pediatr Infect Dis J 1994;13:561–6.

[97] Stevens DL, Gibbons AE, Bergstrom R, et al. The eagle effect revisited: efficacy of clindamycin, erythromycin, and penicillin in the treatment of streptococcal myositis. J Infect Dis 1988;158: 23–8.

[98] Barry W, Hudgins L, Donta ST, et al. Intravenous immunoglobulin therapy for toxic shock syndrome. JAMA 1992;267(24):3315–6.

ELSEVIER
SAUNDERS

PEDIATRIC CLINICS

OF NORTH AMERICA

Pediatr Clin N Am 52 (2005) 1107–1126

Pediatric Central Nervous System Infections and Inflammatory White Matter Disease

Mary T. Silvia, MD, Daniel J. Licht, MD*

Division of Neurology, The Children's Hospital of Philadelphia, 34th & Civic Center Boulevard, Philadelphia, PA 19104, USA

Pediatric central nervous system (CNS) infections are a common cause of hospitalization, morbidity, and mortality. The evaluation, differential diagnosis, and treatment of children suspected to have CNS involvement continue to change as pediatric medicine evolves. Advances in prenatal and perinatal care, immunizations, and treatment of diseases that result in immunosuppression have particular impact. In addition, parainfections, such as acute disseminated encephalomyelitis (ADEM), acute transverse myelitis, and autoimmune conditions should be considered when evaluating a hospitalized child with symptoms of CNS inflammation in the absence of an isolated bacterial, fungal, or viral etiology. This article briefly explores the immune regulation of the pediatric CNS and how it influences the development and resolution of infections, parainfections, and other inflammatory encephalitides in hospitalized children.

Immunology of the central nervous system

Although challenged more recently, the brain has long been thought of as an immunoprivileged organ with distinctive features such as a tight blood-brain barrier (BBB), endogenous glial cells including microglia and astrocytes, low-level expression of MHC and adhesion molecules, an immunosuppressive microenvironment, activated T-cell immunosurveillance that helps defend against inflammation and infection, limited lymphatic drainage, and specialized cerebrospinal fluid (CSF) circulation [1–6]. The aforementioned features also can

_____
* Corresponding author.
E-mail address: licht@email.chop.edu (D.J. Licht).

0031-3955/05/$ – see front matter © 2005 Elsevier Inc. All rights reserved.
doi:10.1016/j.pcl.2005.03.003   *pediatric.theclinics.com*

result in unique vulnerability to pathologic processes, however, and limited responses to wound and injury healing [7,8].

First, the BBB and the brain capillary endothelial cells are connected by tight junctions and lack the fenestrations that are present on endothelial cells in other organs. This lack of fenestrations limits the size of molecules, proteins, and potential pathogens that can enter the CNS; this results in the presence of more active transport mechanisms operating in the tight barrier of the CNS as opposed to mechanisms of passive transport. The capillary endothelium can be induced to up-regulate the expression of MHC class I and II molecules. Under pathologic conditions, this up-regulation can alter the permeability of the BBB and its susceptibility to infection and inflammation by facilitating adhesion and entry into the brain [9,10]. Second, constitutive and infiltrative cells contribute to the immune response of the CNS. Astrocytes, microglia, and perivascular macrophages are the resident immune effector cells and are involved in normal support functions and reactions to injury, inflammation, and subsequent repair [11].

Astrocyte processes serve many functions. They act as metabolic buffers and suppliers of nutrients when directed toward neuronal layers. They surround capillaries of the BBB contributing to the limited flow of large molecules, secrete cytokines, and present antigens to T cells [12,13]. Astrocyte processes are the primary cells involved in repair and scar formation in the brain and undergo cellular hypertrophy and hyperplasia [8]. They have been thought to help with the removal of myelin and neuronal debris during injury, although there is evidence that under certain circumstances they may interfere with axonal regeneration, remyelination, and function of residual neuronal circuits as well [14]. Microglia are bone marrow–derived cells that serve as macrophages within the CNS. In response to injury, they act as phagocytic cells and often are accompanied by blood-derived macrophages. They react rapidly to pathologic changes within the CNS and are activated early in the course of disease [15], at which time they express MHC molecules.

In addition to microglia and astrocytes, T cells are constitutively present in low levels in the CNS, and their levels can be increased by changes in MHC-molecule expression at the level of the capillary epithelium of the BBB [10]. In the setting of inflammation, adhesion molecules are up-regulated on the BBB by cytokines and other inflammatory mediators, allowing for cell migration. Specifically, interleukins promote adhesion molecule and cytokine expression in T cells, B cells, monocytes, and endothelial cells [16]. Perivascular macrophages, microglia, pericytes, and astrocytes can be induced to present antigens to infiltrating T cells in the inflammatory process, initiating a cascade whereby the immune system tries to clear the antigen. This process does not distinguish between infectious antigen or autoantigen [14]. Although astrocytes and microglia secrete a variety of protective molecules to help the repair of damaged tissue [17], they are thought to help in wound repair via the removal of myelin and other neuronal breakdown products. This process has been postulated to result in further damage via demyelination, axonal damage, neuronal loss, and gliosis [14]. In the setting of the special immunologic features of the CNS described earlier, disease processes such as viral encephalitides and potential postviral complications such as the parainfection ADEM are described in this article.

Viral encephalitides

Viral encephalitides are often in the differential diagnosis of a child with acute mental status change, with symptoms ranging from relatively asymptomatic and mild to severe and life-threatening. The criteria for diagnosis of encephalitis are (1) alteration in consciousness or mental status change with symptoms ranging from irritability to lethargy or coma or (2) focal neurologic findings with or without evidence of meningeal inflammation [18]. Approximately 1000 to 2000 cases of encephalitis are reported to the Centers for Disease Control and Prevention per year.

The pathogenesis of viral encephalitis usually occurs through hematogenous spread to the CNS via the choroid plexus, providing direct entry through vascular endothelium. In a few cases, including herpes simplex encephalitis and rabies, entry to the CNS is via retrograde travel along peripheral axons. The virus often replicates in the neuronal cells. The subsequent injury to the neurons and their specific location, including neuronal cell death, often correlates with severity of the clinical presentation. The relative speed and efficiency of viral replication also help determine illness progression [19]. Viral infection of the CNS requires cell-to-cell spread [19] via four mechanisms. The first mechanism is sequential cellular infection. The second involves movement in the extracellular space. The third mechanism requires axonal transport, and the fourth spreads via lymphocytes or glial cells [19]. When inside the cell by way of various attachment mechanisms, viral genome replication occurs with subsequent exit, through exocytosis or cell rupture, for continued infection and spread. On pathologic specimens, diagnoses are made through the recognition of viral inclusion bodies within the neurons, evidence of astrocytic and glial reaction [20], aggregates of inflammatory cells, immunohistochemistry against viral antigens, polymerase chain reaction (PCR) against specific viral antigens agents, and electron microscopy, which can aid in the visualization of viral structure within CNS tissue.

Epidemiology

Although the causative virus in many cases of encephalitis can be difficult to isolate, most cases can be attributed to enteroviruses and arboviruses [18]. Box 1 lists the most common viruses implicated in viral encephalitis. The viral encephalitides are classified further by their seasonal predilection and their pattern of incidence (Table 1). Viral encephalitides also are categorized by their epidemic status: acute sporadic encephalitis, acute epidemic encephalitis, and subacute/chronic encephalitis. Other groups include encephalitides in the immu-

Box 1. Localization of encephalitis: examples of syndrome and infections

Brainstem
    Polio
    Enterovirus 71
    West Nile virus
    Nipah virus
    ADEM
    Bickerstaff's encephalitis
    HSV
    PML
    VZV
    Rabies
Cerebellar ataxia
    VZV
    Measles
    Mumps
    Epstein-Barr virus
    Measles vaccine
    ADEM
Deafness, vertigo, or cranial nerve palsies
    Mumps
    Cytomegalovirus
    Measles
    Rubella
    HSV
    VZV
    Epstein-Barr virus
    Hepatitis
    Adenovirus
    Influenza
    Parainfluenza
    Enteroviruses
    Yellow fever
    Western equine encephalitis
    Tick-borne encephalitis
    St. Louis encephalitis
    Lymphocytic choriomeningitis
    ADEM
Encephalomyelitis
    Measles
    VZV
    Rubella

Mumps
Epstein-Barr virus
Influenza
Measles vaccine
Smallpox vaccine
Influenza vaccine
Rabies vaccine
ADEM
Myelitis
Measles
Mumps
Influenza
Epstein-Barr virus
HSV
VZV
Rubella
Hepatitis
Enteroviruses
Smallpox vaccine
Rabies vaccine
ADEM
Optic neuritis
Measles
Rubella
Mumps
VZV
Hepatitis
Epstein-Barr virus
Rabies vaccine
ADEM
Parkinsonism and movement disorder
Von Economo's encephalitis
Japanese B encephalitis
Measles
Western equine encephalitis
ADEM

Abbreviations: ADEM, acute disseminated encephalomyelitis; HSV, herpes simplex virus; PML, progressive multifocal leukoencephalopathy; VZV, varicella-zoster virus.

Adapted from Aminoff MJ. Neurology and general medicine. 3rd edition. Philadelphia: Churchill Livingston; 2001. p. 731.

Table 1
Viral causes of encephalitis

	Frequency	Season
Herpes viruses		
Herpes simplex 1 and 2	Common	Any season
Cytomegalovirus	Common	Winter/spring
Varicella-zoster virus	Infrequent	Winter/spring
Epstein-Barr virus	Common	Winter/spring
Simian herpes B virus	Common	
Arthropod-borne viruses (arboviruses)		
California encephalitis virus	Common	Summer/fall
Eastern encephalitis virus	Common	Summer/fall
Western encephalitis virus	Common	Summer/fall
St. Louis encephalitis virus	Common	Summer/fall
West Nile virus	Common	Summer/fall
Other viruses		
HIV	Common	Any season
Rabies virus	Common	Any season
Lymphocytic choriomeningitis virus	Infrequent	
Influenza virus	Infrequent	Winter/spring
Mumps virus	Infrequent	Winter/spring
Measles virus	Rare	Winter/spring

nocompromised patient, encephalitides in the immunocompetent patient, and the prion disorders. Considering the aforementioned epidemiology, the evaluation of a child with acute mental status change and suspected viral encephalitis may be guided by considering many factors, including the age of the patient, vaccination status, season, history of tick exposure, progression of disease, history of recent outbreaks of specific pathogens, geographic location, history of travel, and immunologic status. Table 2 lists the major viruses in the above-mentioned categories.

Diagnostic evaluation

Children who present with viral encephalitis usually present with a prodrome of malaise, fever, irritability, nausea, decreased oral intake, and occasionally neck pain and nuchal rigidity (Fig. 1). A differentiating feature from other CNS diseases, including isolated meningitis, is that there is progression to encephalopathy. This encephalopathy may manifest as confusion or delirium and progressive decline in level of consciousness leading to coma, seizures, aphasia, and focal motor abnormalities [20]. These symptoms overlap with other CNS diseases, including ADEM (see later). It is often necessary to exclude consideration of other CNS pathologies before making a diagnosis of viral encephalitis to determine the appropriate treatment strategy. Table 3 lists presenting symptoms of encephalitis and ADEM.

Table 2
Type of encephalitis

Acute sporadic	
Brain only	HSV
With systematic illness	Adenovirus, EBV, mumps, HHV-6
From animals	Rabies, lymphocytic choriomeningitis
Acute parainfectious postyaccinial	
After childhood illness or vaccination	ADEM, Reye's syndrome, vasculitis
Acute epidemic	
Human to human	Influenza, enterovirus
Insect to human	Japanese/St. Louis/eastern equine Encephalitides, West Nile virus
Animal to human	Rabies, Nipah virus
Unknown	Von Economo's encephalitis
Subacute and chronic	
Epidemic	HIV
Immunocompromised	PML, CMV, VZV, measles EBV, HHV-6
Immunocompetent	SSPE, progressive rubella Panencephalitis, VZV
Prion disorders	CJD, vCJD

Abbreviations: ADEM, acute disseminated encephalomyelitis; CJD, Creutzfeldt-Jakob disease; CMV, cytomegalovirus; EBV, Epstein-barr virus; HHV-6, human herpes virus 6; HSV, herpes simplex virus; PML, Progressive multifocal leukoencephalopathy; SSPE, subacute sclerosing panencephalitis; vCJD, Variant Creutzfeld-Jacob disease; VZV, varicella-zoster virus.
Data from Boos J, Esiri MM. Diagnostic evaluation. In: Viral encephalitis in humans. Washington DC: ASM Press; 2003. p. 24.

Points of history particularly relevant include the age of the patient, immunization status (including any recent immunizations), temporal progression of illness and symptoms, possible antecedent viral infection or systemic symptoms, immunologic status, history of maternal herpesvirus in the perinatal period, history of travel or exposure to ticks or mosquitoes in endemic areas, and potential history of case clusters or other local epidemics. Key aspects of the physical examination include evaluation of mucous membranes, skin, and lymphoid tissue and a complete neurologic examination. Involvement of the peripheral nervous system can help differentiate isolated viral encephalitis from entities such as ADEM and transverse myelitis, which can involve the brain and the spinal cord [20]. Lymphadenopathy, splenomegaly, and tonsillar hypertrophy provide evidence for a systemic lymphoid response. Rashes, including rashes that involve the palms and soles, provide evidence for enteroviral infection. In a patient with suspected viral encephalitis and mental status change, serial examinations are essential because viral injury to neurons may result in cerebral edema and consequent brain herniation syndrome.

Hematologic studies often show leukocytosis with a lymphocytic predominance and an elevated erythrocyte sedimentation rate. A typical pattern of CSF abnormalities is shown in Table 4, which can help differentiate viral encephalitis from ADEM. Glucose is usually normal exception for in mumps and herpes simplex virus (HSV) encephalitis, which has been associated with hypoglycor-

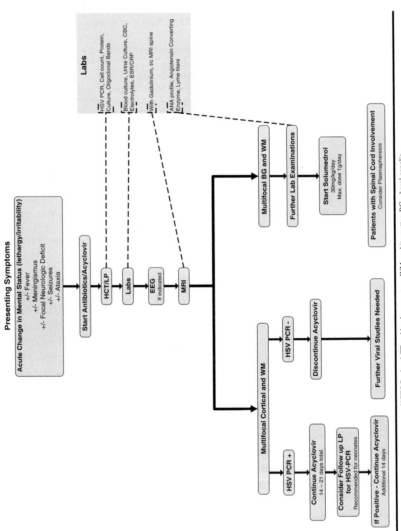

HCT/LP – head CT and lumbar puncture, WM – white matter, BG – basal ganglia

Table 3
Presenting symptoms of acute disseminated encephalomyelitis (ADEM) and encephalitis

Symptom	ADEM	Encephalitis
Fever	+	+++
Meningismus	++	+++
Mental status changes	+++	+++
Seizure	++	+++
Headache/vomiting	++	+++
Focal neurologic deficit	+++	+++
Ataxia	+++	++
Vision changes	++	+
Cranial nerve palsy	++	++
Sensory changes	+	+
Bowel/bladder dysfunction	++	+
Aphasia	++	++

rhachia [18]. In addition to an opening pressure and CSF cell counts, protein, glucose, bacterial culture, and Gram stain, suspected cases of viral encephalitis should have PCR studies sent for enterovirus and HSV. Additional CSF testing should be performed (eg, arbovirus titers) as the history warrants. Serum, urine, and nasal aspirates also should be sent for viral studies because this improves the diagnostic yield for specific viruses.

Because treatable causes of encephalitis (ie, HSV) are often indistinguishable from other causes of encephalitis, an accurate correct diagnosis is essential. In adults with HSV, CSF cultures have a sensitivity of less than 10%. The sensitivity increases for tests that measure HSV antigens or antibodies in the CSF to 75% to 80% with specificities of 60% to 90% [21]. The gold standard for the diagnosis of HSV infection is brain biopsy, but HSV PCR of the CSF has become the test of choice and has been shown to have approximately 98% sensitivity and 94% specificity [22,23].

MRI findings in viral encephalitis

The MRI appearance of viral encephalitis is that of diffuse scattered or confluent areas of T2-weighted hyperintensities that are isointense or hypointense on T1-weighted imaging and exert a variable degree of mass effect and edema. Pathologic changes include evidence of hemorrhage seen best on echo-gradient imaging. Inflammation often involves the meninges as well. Gadolinium en-

Fig. 1. Algorithm for diagnosis and treatment of encephalitis. ANA, antinuclear antibody; BG, basal ganglia; CBC, complete blood count; ESR/CRP, erythrocyte sedimentation rate/C-reactive protein; EEG, electroencephalogram; HCT/LP, head CT and lumbar puncture; WM, white matter.

Table 4
Lumbar puncture results

	ADEM	Encephalitis
Cell count (lymphocytes)	5–200 cells/high power field (typically <100)	5–1000 cells/high power field (typically >100)
Protein	20–500 mg/dL (typically <100)	20–100 mg/dL (typically~20)
Glucose	Normal	Normal

hancement is diffuse and often involves the meninges (Fig. 2A,B). Although these general features apply to most viral encephalitides, certain infections show particular characteristic tropisms for areas of the brain that are helpful in the differential diagnosis. The herpesviruses are a large class of double-stranded DNA viruses that include HSV-1 and HSV-2, varicella-zoster virus, Epstein-Barr virus, cytomegalovirus, and human herpes virus-6 and and human herpes virus-7. Classically, HSV encephalitis has been associated with hemorrhagic inflammation of the temporal lobe and sylvian fissure. These infections are frequently bilateral. In neonates, the areas of inflammation are seldom well defined and manifest with loss of distinction of the gray-white interface on T2-weighted imaging. Echo-gradient imaging reveals the hemorrhagic component, and diffusion-weighted imaging frequently reveals infarction. Varicella-zoster virus seldom causes encephalitis, but is a common pathogen in transverse myelitis and cerebellitis.

Special cases

Neonatal herpes encephalitis

Because of the substantial mortality and morbidity in newborns, early diagnosis of HSV encephalitis and treatment with acyclovir has been shown to be a primary factor affecting clinical outcome [24]. Kimberlin et al [24] looked at the natural history of HSV infections in infants treated in the first 7 years since acyclovir became available and compared it with patients treated in the last 7 years. Mortality and morbidity have been linked to widespread viral replication within the CNS and throughout the major organ systems [25], and early initiation of therapy has been shown to affect outcome positively [26]. Kimberlin et al [24] retrospectively studied the clinical presentations of the study participants to determine symptoms or physical findings that led to earlier diagnosis and treatment of neonatal HSV disease.

Although more recent studies have shown that longer treatment durations (21 days versus 10 days) and higher doses of acyclovir (60 mg/kg/d) have improved outcomes [24,27,28], the mortality and morbidity of this disease remain high. Among neonates with HSV encephalitis, 63% exhibited skin vesicles, 49% were lethargic, 44% had fever, 16% had conjunctivitis, 57% had seizures, 3% had pneumonia, and none had disseminated intravascular coagulation. The absence of fever was common in this population, making the diagnosis of neonatal HSV

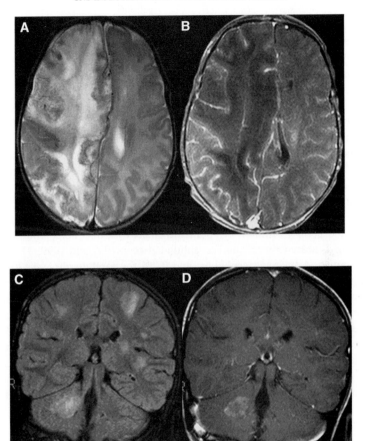

Fig. 2. (*A–B*) HSV encephalitis. (*A*) MRI of the brain shows diffuse gray and white matter involvement with cortical necrosis. (*B*) Postgadolinium T1-weighted image at the same level shows bilateral meningeal and parenchymal enhancement. (*C–D*) ADEM. (*C*) FLAIR MRI shows multifocal white matter, basal ganglia, and cerebellar involvement. (*D*) Postgadolinium T1-weighted image at the same level shows patchy enhancement of only a few lesions.

infection more difficult. Mortality in patients with CNS disease was significantly associated with prematurity ($P = .049$) and trended toward significance in patients who had seizures at initiation of therapy ($P = .064$). Patients with seizures at initiation of therapy were found to have greater mortality and to be at increased risk for abnormal development compared with patients who did not have seizures [24].

Decreasing the time interval between diagnosis of neonatal HSV infection and initiation of treatment is associated strongly with a positive outcome on morbidity and mortality. The Kimberlin et al [24] study suggested that there had not been any significant progress in this parameter, however. The authors concluded that the clinician should have a high index of suspicion for neonatal HSV infection in the differential diagnosis of an acutely ill infant younger than 28 days of age and initiate acyclovir therapy early.

Enterovirus encephalitis

Enteroviruses are the most common cause of meningitis in the United States [29] and an important cause of encephalitis [30]. Although most cases of entero- viral encephalitis are self-limited, a substantial proportion of patients experience either short-term or long-term disability. Enteroviruses are members of the picor- navirus family, which are small RNA viruses. The enterovirus encephalitides include entities caused by coxsackie A and B, echoviruses, and the numbered enteroviruses 68 through 71. The peak incidence of the disease in the United States is in the summer and early fall, but it can occur sporadically throughout the year. Of the 10 to 15 million symptomatic enteroviral infections reported to the Centers for Disease Control and Prevention between 1997 and 1999, 37.6% were for meningitis, 4.1% for encephalitis, and 0.2% for paralytic disease [20].

Hallmark features of enteroviral encephalitis include fever, headache, nausea, vomiting, and nuchal rigidity. Other symptoms include confusion, delirium, leth- argy, and seizures. In general, enteroviral encephalitis seems to involve the entire brain [31,32] as opposed to HSV, which has a predilection for the temporal lobes. In case series of outbreaks of enteroviral meningoencephalitis, most patients recovered completely within 3 weeks. In 1981, the Centers for Disease Control and Prevention reported a mortality rate of 2.5%, although reporting of enteroviral infections is voluntary, which could elevate this number falsely secondary to underreporting of milder cases.

Treatment

Treatment for encephalitis is primarily supportive, unless a treatable etiology is found. Most children with encephalitis require intensive care monitoring, especially for the prompt detection of potential complications, such as respiratory failure, seizures, electrolyte imbalances, and cerebral edema. Seizures resulting from viral encephalitis can be difficult to treat and may require high doses of multiple anticonvulsants, benzodiazepam intravenous infusions, or general anesthesia (e.g., pentobarbital or isoflurane coma) [33]. Extended electroencepha- logram monitoring may be necessary. Medical complications include catheter and respiratory infections, pressure ulcers, joint contractures, corneal abrasions, deep vein thrombosis, and gastrointestinal hemorrhage [20].

Whenever HSV is an etiologic consideration, acyclovir should be started immediately. Initiation of this antiviral therapy should not be delayed to ensure obtaining a pre-acyclovir CSF specimen. Detection of HSV by PCR testing of this fluid likely remains reliable, despite treatment, for several days. Therapy can be discontinued when HSV testing is negative. PCR testing is increasingly avail- able within institutions or at regional laboratories.

Other specific viral encephalitides may respond to other therapies, although most are experimental and are not standard of care. In a critically ill child, use of these agents may be considered for compassionate-use protocols. Varicella-zoster encephalitis involving the brainstem or cerebellitis can be treated with a combination of acyclovir and steroids. In immunocompromised hosts, specific therapies for other viral agents include foscarnet, ganciclovir, or cidofovir for cytomegalovirus or human herpes virus-6. Because of the low incidence of some of these diseases, studies consist primarily of case series, case reports, open-label trials, and anecdotal reports. Care must be taken when considering the aforementioned therapies because many may have significant side effects and lack efficacy in this age group.

Acute disseminated encephalomyelitis

ADEM, although rare (annual incidence of 0.4/100,000), is the most common white matter disease in children. The true incidence is difficult to ascertain because of the rare nature of the disease and the difficulty in determining if the episode is instead a first presentation of multiple sclerosis (MS). In contrast to the viral processes described previously, ADEM is considered a parainfection and is based on the theory of molecular mimicry, which postulates that an antibody response generated against a viral or bacterial antigen cross-reacts with normal host tissue. Although many diseases are associated with autoimmunity, ADEM, acute transverse myelitis, Devic's neuromyelitis optica, optic neuritis, and MS are the most clinically relevant CNS parainfections for practicing clinicians.

In an attempt to separate first attacks of MS from ADEM, a study performed by Leake et al [34] prospectively and retrospectively analyzed 42 children with ADEM to determine the percentage of the study population with an initial diagnosis of ADEM who went on to develop MS. Their results indicated that 9.5% of the study population subsequently were diagnosed with MS after multiple episodes of demyelination.

Clinical features and diagnosis

Although there are no established guidelines for the diagnosis and treatment of ADEM, several features of the history and clinical examination suggest the diagnosis. On presentation, the symptoms that predominate are a reflection of the disseminated involvement of the brain and spinal cord. Initial examinations are a confusion of encephalopathy or delirium with focal or multifocal neurologic deficits. Hemiparesis with bilateral pyramidal tract signs or ataxia is common. Other symptoms on presentation include fever, headache, meningismus, malaise, paresthesias or other sensory abnormalities, seizures (usually partial motor status epilepticus), aphasia, visual disturbances or acute blindness, cranial neuropathies, bowel and bladder dysfunction, parkinsonism, and myoclonus or other movement abnormalities [9,35–37] (Table 3). Specific combinations of symptoms suggest classic named syndromes and can be helpful in guiding an astute clinician to the early and correct diagnosis. A boy who presents with bladder dysfunction and blindness suggests Devic's neuromyelitis optica. A child who presents with acute onset of hemiplegia and contralateral sensory disturbance suggests Brown-Séquard syndrome.

A history of an antecedent viral infection or recent vaccination was found in 54% to 77% of cases. There is a small male predominance (1.8:1). These infections include, but are not limited to, those listed in Table 1. When rash is present as part of a viral exanthem, neurologic symptoms usually appear earlier, most often between 3 and 10 days [9].

The initial workup of a patient with symptoms suggesting ADEM, especially a patient with signs of encephalopathy, usually includes basic laboratory studies such as a complete blood cell count with differential, basic metabolic panel, urine toxicology screen, liver function testing, and an erythrocyte sedimentation rate. Although there are no specific or sensitive tests for ADEM, Anlar et al [35] documented a peripheral leukocytosis greater than 10,000/mm^3 in 50%, thrombocytosis in 19.4%, and an elevated erythrocyte sedimentation rate in 33% of patients presenting with ADEM (Table 4).

A lumbar puncture should be performed for opening pressure, cell counts, protein, glucose, bacterial culture, aqnd viral PCR studies as indicated (HSV with or without enterovirus) and serum titers (ie, Lyme or *Bartonella*) if indicated by history. Although the CSF cell counts can be normal (63%), a mild lymphocytic pleocytosis (100–200 cells/cm^3) is common along with a modest protein elevation (16%) [35]. In addition, the presence of oligoclonal bands, suggesting intrathecal IgG synthesis, was predictive of patients who went on to develop MS [36].

MRI is an important diagnostic tool in ADEM. The lesions are multifocal white matter lesions characterized by perivenous demyelination [38–40]. MRI shows patchy areas of increased signal intensity on T2-weighted and fluid-attenuated inversion recovery (FLAIR) sequences in the deep and subcortical white matter of the cerebral hemispheres and the cerebellar and brainstem white matter [39,41] and spinal cord [42,43]. Typically the lesions are scattered and asymmetric in distribution, and there may be petechial hemorrhage within the lesions in the more severe cases [44]. The location of the lesions on MRI often correlates with the symptoms at presentation (Fig. 2C,D). In a retrospective analysis of 18 patients conducted by Murthy et al [37], lesions were common in the subcortical white matter. In 15 patients in whom imaging was available, imaging showed 100% with lesions in the frontal lobe, 93% in the parietal lobe, 53% in the temporal lobe, and 40% in the occipital lobe; 93% had lesions in the subcortical white matter; 60%, in the periventricular white matter; 13%, in the cerebellum; and 47%, in the brainstem. Each patient had an average of 16.8 lesions. Gray matter lesions also are common, with the most affected being the basal ganglia (20% in this series) and thalamus (27%), likely owing to the high content of white matter tracts within them, followed by the cerebral cortex.

The lesions of ADEM rarely exert mass effect except when located in the brainstem or cerebellum [37,45]. Enhancement is not uniform, and individual lesions in a single patient can show patchy, nodular, gyriform, or no enhancement [39]. Diffusion-weighted imaging most often shows increased diffusion on apparent diffusion coefficient maps, but diffusion can be restricted in more severe cases. Magnetization transfer sequences, which exploit differences in relaxation between water transiently bound to macromolecules and unbound water, are useful in discerning areas of demyelination from areas of edema [46–48].

The differential diagnosis for this MRI appearance includes multiembolic infarction, vasculitis, and MS. ADEM can be distinguished from embolic infarction and vasculitis by the involvement of gray and white matter and restricted diffusion on diffusion-weighted imaging. By definition, the acute MRI studies of MS and ADEM are indistinguishable radiographically because MS remains a clinical diagnosis. Follow-up imaging with the documentation of new lesions favors the diagnosis of MS.

Treatment and prognosis

Although the clinical course of ADEM can be dramatic with rapid progression of neurologic deficits and mental status, with prompt diagnosis and early and aggressive treatment, the overall prognosis of ADEM is good. Treatment for ADEM is based on modulation of a proposed immune-mediated response involving cellular and humoral mechanisms [49,50]. First-line therapy consists of high-dose intravenous methylprednisolone, although the exact dosage used varies by institution; 30 mg/kg/d to a maximum dose of 1 g/d is used for periods ranging from 3 to 10 days. Oral tapers of prednisone usually are instituted for 3-week periods. Severity of symptoms at presentation dictates the length of the steroid course; optic neuritis and spinal cord involvement require 1 full week of treatment. Because of the paucity of pediatric cases available, randomized controlled trials are difficult to perform, and treatment recommendations are based mostly on case reports and case series [36,37,46,51–53]. In the larger case series of 84 patients [36], all patients received supportive care that included symptomatic antiepileptic therapy if required (35%) and acyclovir (69%) for possible HSV infection until laboratory studies were negative. Nearly half (43%) required ICU care, and 16% required mechanical ventilation. In this cohort, 80 children (95%) were treated with high-dose corticosteroids, including 43 patients receiving 1 mg/kg/d of dexamethasone for 10 days and 21 patients receiving intravenous methylprednisolone at a dose of 30 mg/kg/d (for children weighing <30 kg) and 1 g/day (for children weighing >30 kg) for 3 to 5 days followed by 10 days of oral prednisolone. The remaining patients received oral steroid preparations, including 10 patients who received oral prednisolone (2 mg/kg/d) for 10 days and 6 who received oral deflazacort (3 mg/kg/d). All patients were treated with 4- to 6-week oral steroid tapers. In this case series, which followed patients 1 to 19 years (mean 6.6 years), 89% had normal neurologic examinations or had minor findings that did not result in disability. The investigators were unable to show an association with degree of abnormal radiologic involvement and degree of recovery. Residual deficits in this study included hemiparesis (7 children, 8%), partial epilepsy (6%), decreased visual acuity (6%), mild paraparesis (4%), and cognitive deficits (4%). A proposed algorithm for the evaluation of acute mental status changes in children is shown in Fig. 1.

Although ADEM is classically thought of as a monophasic illness, a few patients have one or more relapses. A relapse of ADEM sometimes can be distinguished from transition to MS by the absence of oligoclonal bands in the CSF [46,54–56]. The relapse rate in this series of 84 children was 10%, although because of differences in treatment regimens, this rate may reflect these differences partially. Relapses occurred 2 months to 8 years (mean 2.9 years) after the initial illness in this series. Anlar et al [35] found that relapse after corticosteroid therapy was associated with failure to taper the steroids gradually. Other case series have reported relapses of ADEM indicating that although the overall success rate of corticosteroid therapy is high, a few cases require alternative treatment modalities after corticosteroid failures.

Secondary treatments for relapsed or refractory ADEM include plasmapheresis and intravenous immunoglobulin (IVIG). The most compelling evidence for plasmapheresis was offered by Weinshenker et al [57], who conducted a randomized, sham-controlled, double-masked study of plasma exchange in refractory CNS inflammatory demyelinating disease (including MS, ADEM, acute transverse myelitis, Marburg's variant of MS, optic neuromyelitis, recurrent myelitis, and focal cerebral myelination). This study included a crossover treatment limb if no improvement was noted after the first phase. Overall, moderate to marked improvement based on functional impairment was noted in 5 of 11 patients randomized to plasmapheresis compared with only 1 of 11 patients who received sham treatment. An additional eight patients were treated with plasmapheresis in the crossover limb of the study, three of whom had marked improvement of symptoms. Functional improvement occurred in 8 of 19 (42%) patients who received plasmapheresis, as opposed to 1 of 17 (5.9%) receiving sham treatment. Although the study included some teenagers, average age of the patients receiving active treatment was 40.5 years, with a female-to-male predominance of 7:4, and most patients were treated for the diagnosis of MS (12 of 22). Earlier work by Weinshenker [58,59] summarizes the previous uses of plasmapheresis for CNS demyelinating disease. Specifically regarding the use of plasmapheresis and ADEM, two cases with improved neurologic status after plasmapheresis were reported by Lin et al in 2004 [60].

Literature support for the use of IVIG for the treatment of children who fail high-dose steroids consists entirely of case reports. Three children with ADEM, reported by Nishikawa et al [61], were given a dose of 400 mg/kg/d for 5 consecutive days because of difficulty distinguishing their presentation from acute infectious encephalitis. The first patient initially was given a diagnosis of viral encephalitis and was described as "semicomatose" before CSF and MRI findings that were consistent with a diagnosis of ADEM. Therapy with IVIG was initiated 10 days after presentation without first receiving corticosteroids, and the child was discharged on hospital day 21 without any residual sequelae. The second patient was diagnosed initially with meningitis and was treated with a courses of antibiotics 20 days before transfer to the accepting hospital on day 50 of symptoms. IVIG therapy was initiated, and 10 days after completing the course, all neurologic symptoms had resolved. The final patient was a 2-year-old with mumps diagnosed by parotid enlargement and serum serology. After typical MRI findings, the child was started on IVIG with an excellent neurologic outcome. Two additional case reports using IVIG for initial or recurrent ADEM were published by Hahn et al [62] and Kleiman and Brunquell [63].

Summary

The unique microenvironment and structure of the CNS preclude the CNS to a relative resistance to infection and inflammation and to selective vulnerability to specific pathogens. With CNS inflammation, there is a balance between wound healing and repair and injury propagation and further scar formation. Pediatric patients pose special challenges to the diagnosis and treatment of CNS diseases, especially when symptoms are vague and nonspecific. This challenge directly applies to neonates, in whom fever and other localizing signs may be absent. Given that the time to treatment with acyclovir in a neonate with HSV encephalitis correlates directly with morbidity and mortality, having a high index of suspicion for the treatable causes of altered mental status is imperative. Likewise, the presentations of ADEM can range from subtle to devastating; the prognosis is generally good when high-dose steroids are instituted early in the course of the disease. In a child with altered mental status, as with most medical differential diagnoses, having a framework or algorithm to guide the initial history, laboratory workup, and imaging evaluation is helpful in narrowing a long list of possible diagnoses. Treatment decisions that ultimately affect the patient's outcome can be made in a time-efficient manner.

Acknowledgments

Dr. Licht is a Pfizer Scholar and is funded in part by a grant from the W.W. Smith Charitable Trust. The authors thank Mr. David Silvestre and Mr. Erin O'Tool for their cooperation, critical comments, and technical assistance.

References

[1] Cserr HF, Knopf PM. Cervical lymphatics, the blood-brain barrier and the immunoreactivity of the brain: a new view. Immunol Today 1992;13:507–12.

[2] Wekerle H. Immune protection of the brain—efficient and delicate. J Infect Dis 2002; 186(Suppl 2):S140–4.

[3] Bradl M, Hohlfeld R. Molecular pathogenesis of neuroinflammation. J Neurol Neurosurg Psychiatry 2003;74:1364–70.

[4] Prat A, Biernacki K, Wosik K, Antel JP. Glial cell influence on the human blood-brain barrier. Glia 2001;36:145–55.

[5] Pachter JS, de Vries HE, Fabry Z. The blood-brain barrier and its role in immune privilege in the central nervous system. J Neuropathol Exp Neurol 2003;62:593–604.

[6] Hickey WF. Basic principles of immunological surveillance of the normal central nervous system. Glia 2001;36:118–24.

[7] Fuller GN, Goodman JC. Cells of the central nervous system. In: Fuller GN, Goodman JC, editors. Practical review of neuropathology. 1st edition. Philadelphia: Lippincott Williams & Wilkins; 2001. p. 7–73.

[8] DeGirolami U, Anthony DC, Frosch MP. The central nervous system. In: Cotran RS, Kuman V, Collins T, editors. Pathologic basis of disease. 6th edition. Philadelphia: WB Saunders; 1999. p. 1295–7.

[9] Tyor WR. Fundamentals of immunology. In: Rolak LA, Harati Y, editors. Neuro-immunology for the clinician. 1st edition. Newton: Butterworth-Heinemann; 1997. p. 24–5.

[10] Xiao BG, Link H. Immune regulation within the central nervous system. J Neurol Sci 1998;157: 1–12.

[11] Eddleston M, Mucke L. Molecular profile of reactive astrocytes—implications for their role in neurologic disease. Neuroscience 1993;54:15–36.

[12] Fierz W, Endler B, Reske K, Wekerle H, Fontana A. Astrocytes as antigen-presenting cells: I. induction of Ia antigen expression on astrocytes by T cells via immune interferon and its effect on antigen presentation. J Immunol 1985;134:3785–93.

[13] Fontana A, Fierz W, Wekerle H. Astrocytes present myelin basic protein to encephalitogenic T-cell lines. Nature 1984;307:273–6.

[14] Eng LF, Ghirnikar RS. GFAP and astrogliosis. Brain Pathol 1994;4:229–37.

[15] Dowling P, Shang G, Raval S, Menonna J, Cook S, Husar W. Involvement of the CD95 (APO-1/ Fas) receptor/ligand system in multiple sclerosis brain. J Exp Med 1996;184:1513–8.

[16] Pryce G, Male D, Campbell I, Greenwood J. Factors controlling T-cell migration across rat cerebral endothelium in vitro. J Neuroimmunol 1997;75:84–94.

[17] Merrill JE, Jonakait GM. Interactions of the nervous and immune systems in development, normal brain homeostasis, and disease. Faseb J 1995;9:611–8.

[18] Greenberg SB. Viral meningitis and encephalitis. In: Samuels MA, Feske S, editors. Office practice of neurology. 1st edition. New York: Churchill Livinstone Inc.; 1996. p. 401–4.

[19] Scheld W, Whitley RJ, Durack DT, editors. Infections of the central nervous system. 2nd edition. Philadelphia: Lippincott-Raven; 1997.

[20] Boossw J, Esiri MM. Viral encephalitis in humans, vol 1. Washington (DC): ASM Press; 2003.

[21] Whitley RJ, Lakeman F. Herpes simplex virus infections of the central nervous system: therapeutic and diagnostic considerations. Clin Infect Dis 1995;20:414–20.

[22] Aurelius E, Johansson B, Skoldenberg B, Staland A, Forsgren M. Rapid diagnosis of herpes simplex encephalitis by nested polymerase chain reaction assay of cerebrospinal fluid. Lancet 1991;337:189–92.

[23] Lakeman FD, Whitley RJ. Diagnosis of herpes simplex encephalitis: application of polymerase chain reaction to cerebrospinal fluid from brain-biopsied patients and correlation with disease. National Institute of Allergy and Infectious Diseases Collaborative Antiviral Study Group. J Infect Dis 1995;171:857–63.

[24] Kimberlin DW, Lin CY, Jacobs RF, et al. Natural history of neonatal herpes simplex virus infections in the acyclovir era. Pediatrics 2001;108:223–9.

[25] Whitley R, Arvin A, Prober C, et al. Predictors of morbidity and mortality in neonates with herpes simplex virus infections. The National Institute of Allergy and Infectious Diseases Collaborative Antiviral Study Group. N Engl J Med 1991;324:450–4.

[26] Whitley RJ, Corey L, Arvin A, et al. Changing presentation of herpes simplex virus infection in neonates. J Infect Dis 1988;158:109–16.

[27] Kimberlin DW. Advances in the treatment of neonatal herpes simplex infections. Rev Med Virol 2001;11:157–63.

[28] Kimberlin DW, Lin CY, Jacobs RF, et al. Safety and efficacy of high-dose intravenous acyclovir in the management of neonatal herpes simplex virus infections. Pediatrics 2001;108:230–8.

[29] Rotbart HA. Enteroviral infections of the central nervous system. Clin Infect Dis 1995;20: 971–81.

[30] Whitley RJ, Cobbs CG, Alford Jr CA, et al. Diseases that mimic herpes simplex encephalitis:

diagnosis, presentation, and outcome. NIAD Collaborative Antiviral Study Group. JAMA 1989; 262:234–9.

[31] Modlin JF, Dagan R, Berlin LE, Virshup DM, Yolken RH, Menegus M. Focal encephalitis with enterovirus infections. Pediatrics 1991;88:841–5.

[32] Rotbart HA, Webster AD. Treatment of potentially life-threatening enterovirus infections with pleconaril. Clin Infect Dis 2001;32:228–35.

[33] Chang CW, Bleck TP. Status epilepticus. Neurol Clin 1995;13:529–48.

[34] Leake JA, Albani S, Kao AS, et al. Acute disseminated encephalomyelitis in childhood: epidemiologic, clinical and laboratory features. Pediatr Infect Dis J 2004;23:756–64.

[35] Anlar B, Basaran C, Kose G, et al. Acute disseminated encephalomyelitis in children: outcome and prognosis. Neuropediatrics 2003;34:194–9.

[36] Tenembaum S, Chamoles N, Fejerman N. Acute disseminated encephalomyelitis: a long-term follow-up study of 84 pediatric patients. Neurology 2002;59:1224–31.

[37] Murthy SN, Faden HS, Cohen ME, Bakshi R. Acute disseminated encephalomyelitis in children. Pediatrics 2002;110(2 Pt 1):e21–7.

[38] Hart MN, Earle KM. Haemorrhagic and perivenous encephalitis: a clinical-pathological review of 38 cases. J Neurol Neurosurg Psychiatry 1975;38:585–91.

[39] Dun V, Bale Jr JF, Zimmerman RA, Perdue Z, Bell WE. MRI in children with postinfectious disseminated encephalomyelitis. Magn Reson Imaging 1986;4:25–32.

[40] Kuker W, Ruff J, Gaertner S, Mehnert F, Mader I, Nagele T. Modern MRI tools for the characterization of acute demyelinating lesions: value of chemical shift and diffusion-weighted imaging. Neuroradiology 2004;46:421–6.

[41] Kimura S, Nezu A, Ohtsuki N, Kobayashi T, Osaka H, Uehara S. Serial magnetic resonance imaging in children with postinfectious encephalitis. Brain Dev 1996;18:461–5.

[42] Khong PL, Ho HK, Cheng PW, Wong VC, Goh W, Chan FL. Childhood acute disseminated encephalomyelitis: the role of brain and spinal cord MRI. Pediatr Radiol 2002;32:59–66.

[43] Sakakibara R, Hattori T, Yasuda K, Yamanishi T. Micturitional disturbance in acute disseminated encephalomyelitis (ADEM). J Auton Nerv Syst 1996;60:200–5.

[44] Mader I, Wolff M, Niemann G, Kuker W. Acute haemorrhagic encephalomyelitis (AHEM): MRI findings. Neuropediatrics 2004;35:143–6.

[45] Gupte G, Stonehouse M, Wassmer E, Coad NA, Whitehouse WP. Acute disseminated encephalomyelitis: a review of 18 cases in childhood. J Paediatr Child Health 2003;39:336–42.

[46] Hynson JL, Kornberg AJ, Coleman LT, Shield L, Harvey AS, Kean MJ. Clinical and neuroradiologic features of acute disseminated encephalomyelitis in children. Neurology 2001;56:1308–12.

[47] Inglese M, Salvi F, Iannucci G, Mancardi GL, Mascalchi M, Filippi M. Magnetization transfer and diffusion tensor MR imaging of acute disseminated encephalomyelitis. AJNR Am J Neuroradiol 2002;23:267–72.

[48] Dousset V, Grossman RI, Ramer KN, et al. Experimental allergic encephalomyelitis and multiple sclerosis: lesion characterization with magnetization transfer imaging. Radiology 1992;182:483–91.

[49] Dale RC, Morovat A. Interleukin-6 and oligoclonal IgG synthesis in children with acute disseminated encephalomyelitis. Neuropediatrics 2003;34:141–5.

[50] Ichiyama T, Shoji H, Kato M, et al. Cerebrospinal fluid levels of cytokines and soluble tumour necrosis factor receptor in acute disseminated encephalomyelitis. Eur J Pediatr 2002;161:133–7.

[51] Jones CT. Childhood autoimmune neurologic diseases of the central nervous system. Neurol Clin 2003;21:745–64.

[52] Pasternak JF, De Vivo DC, Prensky AL. Steroid-responsive encephalomyelitis in childhood. Neurology 1980;30:481–6.

[53] Straub J, Chofflon M, Delavelle J. Early high-dose intravenous methylprednisolone in acute disseminated encephalomyelitis: a successful recovery. Neurology 1997;49:1145–7.

[54] Dale RC, de Sousa C, Chong WK, Cox TC, Harding B, Neville BG. Acute disseminated encephalomyelitis, multiphasic disseminated encephalomyelitis and multiple sclerosis in children. Brain 2000;123(Pt 12):2407–22.

[55] Rust RS. Multiple sclerosis, acute disseminated encephalomyelitis, and related conditions. Semin Pediatr Neurol 2000;7:66–90.

[56] Prabhakar S, Kurien E, Gupta RS, Zielinski S, Freedman MS. Heat shock protein immunoreactivity in CSF: correlation with oligoclonal banding and demyelinating disease. Neurology 1994;44:1644–8.

[57] Weinshenker BG, O'Brien PC, Petterson TM, et al. A randomized trial of plasma exchange in acute central nervous system inflammatory demyelinating disease. Ann Neurol 1999;46:878–86.

[58] Weinshenker BG. Plasma exchange for severe attacks of inflammatory demyelinating diseases of the central nervous system. J Clin Apheresis 2001;16:39–42.

[59] Weinshenker BG. Therapeutic plasma exchange for acute inflammatory demyelinating syndromes of the central nervous system. J Clin Apheresis 1999;14:144–8.

[60] Lin CH, Jeng JS, Yip PK. Plasmapheresis in acute disseminated encephalomyelitis. J Clin Apheresis 2004;19:154–9.

[61] Nishikawa M, Ichiyama T, Hayashi T, Ouchi K, Furukawa S. Intravenous immunoglobulin therapy in acute disseminated encephalomyelitis. Pediatr Neurol 1999;21:583–6.

[62] Hahn JS, Siegler DJ, Enzmann D. Intravenous gammaglobulin therapy in recurrent acute disseminated encephalomyelitis. Neurology 1996;46:1173–4.

[63] Kleiman M, Brunquell P. Acute disseminated encephalomyelitis: response to intravenous immunoglobulin. J Child Neurol 1995;10:481–3.

ELSEVIER
SAUNDERS

PEDIATRIC CLINICS
OF NORTH AMERICA

Pediatr Clin N Am 52 (2005) 1127–1146

Apparent Life-Threatening Event: A Review

Craig C. DeWolfe, MD

Department of Pediatrics, Pediatric Hospitalist Division, Children's National Medical Center,
George Washington University School of Medicine and Health Sciences, 111 Michigan Avenue NW,
Washington, DC 20010, USA

The term "apparent life-threatening event" (ALTE) refers to a complex of symptoms that presents unexpectedly in an infant and is of concern to the caregiver and often cannot be characterized easily by the health care provider. Although in most cases its natural history is benign, there is a risk for subsequent morbidity and mortality. Therefore, when caring for a patient who experiences an ALTE, the provider must stabilize the infant as needed, obtain key history, identify and address any underlying causes, educate the caregivers, and provide a safe disposition. This article summarizes the body about ALTE, with specific attention to the diagnosis and management of these cases.

In September 1986, the National Institutes of Health [1] convened an expert panel to review the literature of ALTE and discuss the relationship among infantile apnea, ALTE, and sudden infant death syndrome (SIDS). The consensus group described ALTE as "an episode that is frightening to the observer and that is characterized by some combination of apnea (central or occasionally obstructive), color change (usually cyanotic or pallid but occasionally erythematous or plethoric), a marked change in muscle tone (usually marked limpness), choking, or gagging" [1]. With this definition, the group standardized a previously inconsistent description and offered data on its incidence, pathogenesis, and causes, and provided recommendations regarding the evaluation, treatment, and outcome. They also suggested eliminating the terms "near-miss SIDS" and "aborted crib death" because no causal link could be established between ALTE and SIDS. Moreover, they were responsible for the first consensus recommendations on the use of monitors for the condition and proposed future research directions. In the nearly 20 years since this consensus statement, progress has

---

E-mail address: cdewolfe@cnmc.org

been made concerning ALTE and its management, but questions persist. This article summarizes the body about ALTE, with specific attention to the diagnosis and management of these cases.

Study of the apparent life-threatening event complex

The study of ALTE is particularly complex and difficult [2]. As a result, many authors and clinicians have felt uncomfortable classifying, managing, and providing anticipatory guidance for the condition [3,4].

There are concerns that the working definition consisting of apnea, change in color, change in tone, choking, and gagging may be too broad. Some practitioners have suggested that an ALTE should not include obvious cases of choking or gagging when they are associated with feeding or upper respiratory infections [5]. Others have suggested limiting the term to infants who have required vigorous stimulation for resuscitation [6] or to patients who have no obvious abnormalities on physical examination [7]. Still others, however, consider the current case definition too restrictive. Some researchers have explicitly included infants with altered mental status in their definition of ALTE [8]. In summary, the debate regarding the ALTE case definition and heterogeneity in selection criteria for various published reports makes it difficult to develop a coherent approach to the literature.

The investigation of ALTE also depends on the descriptions of an inexperienced or medically naïve caregiver involved in a frightening and often brief event. The examination of the patient after the episode also is typically normal. Therefore, practitioners and researchers depend heavily on historical cues rather than measurable data to define ALTE.

Study design also is complex. Some researchers use referral for subspecialty evaluation to enroll patients who have experienced an ALTE, but the resultant selection bias limits the generalizability of findings. Retrospective study methods are difficult in ALTE as well. A chart review is complicated by the fact that the "Disease Index" of the "International Classification of Diseases (ICD.9.CM)" does not list ALTE as a discharge diagnosis. Although dyspnea, respiratory abnormalities, and apnea often are included in retrospective studies, cyanosis, change in tone, and choking and gagging are not. Furthermore, in cases in which a cause is found for an ALTE, there may be no mention of apnea in the discharge coding.

Even basic assumptions regarding events such as "pathologic apnea," on which many studies have been based, have been called into question. A multicentered, prospectively designed study that monitored healthy children and those with a history of idiopathic ALTE has found no difference in the incidence of 20-second apneic spells. As a result, previous observational studies that characterize the type and frequency of similar apneic spells in preselected populations may prove to be irrelevant [9].

Definitions

Although the definitions of terms associated with ALTE are not always consistent, the following descriptions may provide a reference for future discussion. Apnea refers to a cessation of airflow and may result from central or obstructive causes. Central apnea is defined as the absence of respiratory effort caused by a lack of output from the central respiratory centers or by neuromuscular insufficiency. Chest wall movement will be absent and no breath sounds will be evident on auscultation of the chest. Obstructive apnea is defined as breaths associated with paradoxical inverse movements of the chest wall and abdomen with a corresponding decrease in oxygen saturation by 3%. Significant apnea has been defined as a cessation of air movement for at least 20 seconds. Shorter episodes also are included if they are associated with central cyanosis, bradycardia, pallor, or loss of muscle tone. Pathologic apnea is associated with physiologic compromise, whereas apneic events without these changes are considered normal.

When an unexplained pathologic apnea event occurs for the first time in an infant older than 37 weeks postconceptional age, it is called "apnea of infancy." It is distinct from "apnea of prematurity," which resolves by 37 weeks postconceptional age. In rare circumstances, apnea of prematurity may persist beyond term, particularly in infants born at less than 28 weeks of gestation.

Periodic breathing is defined as three or more respiratory pauses of greater than 3 seconds' duration, with less than 20 seconds of respiration between pauses. It is common and physiologic in preterm infants and may persist beyond term in other infants. Periodic breathing is considered pathologic if it is associated with cardiorespiratory instability. Clinically, the pattern may appear as short periods (eg, 5–10 seconds) of increased rate and rigor of breathing alternating with periods of shallow or undetectable breathing [1].

Central cyanosis represents the arterial circulation of desaturated blood and becomes clinically apparent at 5 g/dL of desaturated hemoglobin. It is best determined by a bluish discoloration of the oral mucus membranes, usually evident in the lips and tongue. Peripheral cyanosis occurs when there is an increased extraction of oxygen by peripheral tissues, as can be seen with sepsis, circulatory shock, hypovolemia, and vasoconstriction.

Acrocyanosis refers to a bluish discoloration of the hands and feet and is a common, normal phenomenon in newborns, believed to be caused by distal vasomotor instability or vasoconstriction from heat-retention efforts. Circumoral cyanosis is another benign entity that often is seen in fair-skinned infants and is characterized by a bluish mustache or circular blue or purple color in the perioral area. It is usually more pronounced with crying, straining, or other Valsalva-like maneuvers. It represents a prominence of the superficial perioral venous plexus. Acrocyanosis and circumoral cyanosis are not signs of a central cyanotic state, unless the overall clinical picture supports sepsis or another shock-like state [10].

Idiopathic ALTE is the term offered for an ALTE that occurs when an underlying cause cannot be found. SIDS is the unexpected death of an infant less than 1 year old that is unexplained by history and in which a thorough autopsy and death scene investigation fail to demonstrate an adequate explanation of the cause of death. No causal link has been made between these two entities.

Epidemiology

A longitudinal cohort study of monitored children suggests that 43% of healthy term infants have at least one 20-second apneic episode over a 3-month period [9]. Another study suggests that 5.3% of parents recall seeing such events [11]. The rates do not differ among healthy controls, patients with a history of idiopathic ALTE, or patients with a sibling who died of SIDS. Only preterm infants less than 34 weeks postconceptional age have significantly higher rates of apnea; however, these differences resolve when the premature infants reach 43 weeks postconceptional age. Thirty-second apnea occurs in 2.3% of healthy infants and 13.1% of patients with a history of idiopathic ALTE. Although a difference in percentage was found in the study, it did not reach statistical significance [9].

It is reported that 0.2% to 0.9% of infants will have apnea that leads to admission and that 0.05% of infants will have events that occur during sleep and require vigorous stimulation [11–13]. This is likely an underestimation of the ALTE admission rate because changes in color and tone, choking, and gagging exclusive of apnea were not included in the estimate. Moreover, discharge diagnoses may not reflect the true ALTE presentation if an alternative diagnosis was provided during the admission. In these studies of infants admitted for apnea, the researchers found maternal smoking and single-parent households to be risk factors for ALTE. The infants with ALTE had a median age at presentation of approximately 8 weeks and were equally likely to be male or female [11,12].

Presentation

A case series of 243 infants admitted to a tertiary care hospital has characterized the presentation of infants with ALTE [8]. The researchers found that nearly half of admitted patients had experienced more than one ALTE before being admitted to the hospital. The most common individual symptoms included, in order of frequency, apnea, cyanosis, hypotonia, unresponsiveness, labored breathing, and lethargy. Approximately 10% of these patients required supplemental oxygen or assisted ventilation by a caregiver or an emergency medical services provider.

Pathophysiology

The potential underlying abnormalities in ALTE are numerous, thus precluding any discussion of a unifying pathophysiology. Rather, the events common to an ALTE will be related to disease processes and their general pathophysiology. Therefore, the discussion begins with the sign most commonly associated with ALTE: apnea.

Central apnea results from a disruption in the generation of propagation of respiratory signals in the brainstem and descending neuromuscular pathways. Causes include prematurity, head trauma, or even the rare condition of congenital central hypoventilation syndrome (Ondine's curse). These conditions may disturb the respiratory generators, alter the pulmonary vasomotor tone, and disrupt reflexes arising from and around the pulmonary vascular bed that match perfusion to ventilation in the lungs [14]. In apnea of prematurity, studies have demonstrated a delayed and diminished central response to increasing carbon dioxide levels [15]. It is hypothesized that with decreasing respiratory effort, the Hering-Breuer inflation reflex may be disrupted. Normally, activation of these stretch receptors in this reflex terminates the inspiratory effort. During hypopnea or apnea, lung volumes fall, and the afferent input decreases. At this point, the Hering-Breuer reflex is down-regulated, resulting in increased efferent signal to terminate inspiratory effort at low levels of stretch. This causes further compromise of the breathing pattern. When positive-pressure ventilation is provided, it resets the stretch reflex, which helps to normalize breathing. The autonomic nervous system also has been implicated in syndromes associated with central apnea, and it contributes to the heart rate and blood pressure variability [16]. These mechanisms are believed to be manifest in Ondine's curse [17].

Obstructive apnea results from breathing through an occluded airway despite neuromuscular respiratory efforts. It may result from several pathophysiologic mechanisms. The obstruction may be caused by masses that occlude the airway, as seen in infants with Pierre Robin syndrome, in which the poorly anchored tongue is displaced posteriorly when the person is in the supine position. Another common cause is adenotonsillar hypertrophy, in which snoring and apnea are associated with sleep. An aspirated foreign body also can be a barrier to air movement. Functional or dynamic obstruction occurs when the airway collapses due to positive pressure inspiration. This can be seen in infants with laryngomalacia or intraluminal cysts. Finally, vocal cord paralysis, as seen in central compression of the abductor vocal cord nerves from hydrocephalus or Chiari type II malformations, may produce stridor and obstructive apnea [18].

Mixed apnea has features of both central and obstructive apnea. It may result from an underlying obstructive condition (eg, adenotonsillar hypertrophy) with a superimposed insult (eg, preoperative sedation). Conversely, children with an underlying condition of central apnea (eg, premature infants) with an acquired obstructive burden (nasal congestion from a viral respiratory illness) also may develop a mixed picture. Alternatively, single conditions may present with features of both entities, as seen in gastroesophageal reflux (GER) or infection with respiratory syncytial virus (RSV); in the former, suspected mechanisms of apnea include choking on regurgitated gastric contents, bronchospasm, and laryngeal chemoreceptor reflex central apnea [19]. With RSV infection, the virus has been believed to alter the sensitivity of laryngeal chemoreceptors to regurgitated gastric contents, resulting in reflex central apnea [20,21], and to cause inflammation of the airway that leads to obstructive apnea.

Decreased oxygenation or differential blood flow to a portion of the body may cause cyanosis, erythema, plethora, and pallor. Cyanosis may manifest centrally or peripherally. It is a consequence of hemoglobin desaturation and can result from impaired oxygen exchange or distribution. The former may occur during periods of apnea, whereas the latter may result from conditions such as sepsis. The presence of 5 g/dL desaturated hemoglobin will manifest as cyanosis. Normally, 2 g/dL desaturated hemoglobin is present in the venules, so an additional 3 g/dL reduced hemoglobin in the arterial blood produces clinical cyanosis [52]. A polycythemic infant with a hemoglobin concentration of 20 g/dL will appear cyanotic when oxygen saturations reaches 85% (ie, [20 g/dL − 3 g/dL]/ 20 g/dL). An anemic infant with a hemoglobin concentration of 6 g/dL will appear cyanotic only at 50% desaturation ([6g/dL − 3g/dL]/6 g/dL).

Transient plethora may result from hyperemia and localized vasodilation (often venous), whereas pallor may result from vasoconstriction. Both conditions tend to be mediated by autonomic activity. The practitioner should recognize that pathologic and physiologic states may be difficult for lay people to differentiate. It has been suggested that as many as two of 150 patients presenting on referral after mouth-to-mouth resuscitation had physiologic pallor with normal oxygenation [22].

Altered muscle tone may appear as limpness, hypertonia, and rhythmic movements of the extremities. The source of the defect may originate in the nervous system, as seen in hydrocephalus. However, the defect may result secondary to a systemic process such as crying in a vasovagally mediated breath-holding spell. Other more general neurologic triggers of ALTE may include central or autonomic nervous system disorders.

Choking, coughing, and gagging are normal protective responses to stimulation of the posterior nasopharynx, hypopharynx, larynx, and lower airway. These reflexes result in the temporary interruption of ventilation by two key processes. Mechanical obstruction can occur from the foreign material present or from the reflexive occlusion of soft tissue designed to prevent passage of the material. Also, the forceful effort to expel the offending material prevents effective ventilation. These forceful efforts may cause plethora and erythema of the face and head because the increased intrathoracic pressures that are generated cause increased blood flow and venous congestion superiorly. Sustained efforts may result in hypoxia or limpness caused by the vagal stimulation, but typically, the coughing, gagging, and retching responses are self-limited when the offending stimulus is removed. These responses have been associated with digestive, neurologic, vasovagal, and acute airway obstruction abnormalities [2].

Differential diagnosis

Because ALTE is a description rather than a diagnosis, the hospitalist must consider the broad range of possible underlying causes. Table 1 [23–35] provides a suggested grouping of causes and their relative percentages from a systematic review of the literature that has examined patients on their first presentation to

Table 1
Differential diagnosis of ALTE

Gastrointestinal (33%)[a]	Cardiovascular (1%)
Gastroesophageal reflux [19]	Congenital heart disease
Gastroenteritis	Cardiomyopathy
Esophageal dysfunction	Cardiac arrhythmia/*prolonged QTc* [30]
Colic	*Myocarditis*
Surgical abdomen	Metabolic/endocrine
Dysphagia[b]	Electrolyte disturbance
Neurologic (15%)	Hypoglycemia
Seizure [23]	Inborn error of metabolism [31]
Central apnea/hypoventilation syndromes	Other infections
(apnea of prematurity, Ondine's curse)	*Sepsis*
Head injury (intraventricular hemorrhage,	Urinary tract infections
subarachnoid hemorrhage)	*Child maltreatment syndrome*
Meningitis/encephalitis	*Shaken baby syndrome* [40]
Hydrocephalus	*Intentional suffocation* [22]
Brain Tumor	*Munchausen-by-proxy syndrome* [22]
Neuromuscular disorders	Other diagnoses
Vasovagal reaction [24]	Physiologic event (periodic breathing,
Congenital malformation of the brainstem [18]	*acrocyanosis*)
Respiratory (11%)	Breath-holding spell [14]
Respiratory syncytial virus [25]	Choking
Pertussis [26,27]	Drug or *toxin reaction* [32]
Aspiration pneumonia	*Unintentional smothering* [33]
Other lower or upper respiratory tract infection	*Anemia* [34]
Reactive airway disease	*Hypothermia* [35]
Foreign body	Idiopathic/apnea of infancy (23%)
Otolaryngologic (4%)	ALTE
Laryngomalacia [28]	
Subglottal and/or laryngeal stenosis [28]	
Obstructive sleep apnea [29]	

McGovern and Smith [36] described the relative frequency of specific diagnoses (%)[a] across all patients in studies reviewed by them. Using the same methods and studies, these figures are shown with respect to broader diagnostic groupings (eg, gastrointestinal rather than gastroesophageal reflux). The table includes broad categories and potential diagnoses (*italics*)[b] not considered by McGovern and Smith based on their inclusion criteria. Thus, the reader is provided a wider range of diagnostic possibilities to consider, with references to additional studies.

a medical system [36]. The data were extrapolated from a large number of case series with varying selection criteria and ALTE definitions, but it provides useful estimates of the relative frequency of a wide range of causes. Diagnoses that were not identified in the study were added (in *italics*) to provide a more complete illustration of the differential diagnosis. "Idiopathic ALTE" is the term used when an underlying cause could not be identified.

Special consideration is given to GER because it may be a coexistent but not necessarily a causative entity. A case series [37] involving a standard battery of tests on all patients presenting with ALTE has found that 89% of a subpopulation of screened infants had radioisotope-labeled milk scan evidence of GER. More than half of these cases also had an alternative diagnosis that the authors considered more likely than GER as the cause of the ALTE (eg, seizures, pertussis, or urinary tract infection). With the extremely high prevalence of GER in young infants, practitioners should be wary of assigning this condition as the cause for ALTE because it may be detected in most children presenting for ALTE evaluation.

History

A history is the single most important component in the evaluation of infants with ALTE. In many cases, a history may determine the diagnosis and thereby abrogate the need for further diagnostic testing. In other cases, it may suggest a particular diagnosis or diagnoses that direct the work-up. The practitioner, however, may find it difficult to gather or interpret the data from a sudden and irreproducible event in a child who otherwise appears to be well [4]. Some caregivers may not be familiar with the physiologic nature of periodic breathing or acrocyanosis. Others, by contrast, may minimize more serious pathologic events. The entire event may not have been witnessed, and caregivers commonly overlook or distort features during the unexpected and distressing event. Despite these shortcomings, the practitioner should make every attempt to obtain a history of the event from all observers. Important features of the history are included in Box 1.

The chief complaint often clearly illustrates the element of most concern to the parent. It also will allow the practitioner to focus on the same element when explaining potential mechanisms of action in relation to the evaluation and diagnosis or when providing anticipatory guidance and reassurance.

Another important aspect of the history is differentiating between true apnea and central or obstructive symptoms. Sometimes it is difficult to distinguish true apnea from shallow respiratory efforts that are undetectable to the observer. Lighting conditions, proximity to the patient, and the amount of clothes or bedding present may influence the ability to detect breathing motions.

Central apnea will appear as an effortless pause, whereas obstructive apnea in an awake or awakened infant presents as a sudden onset of choking, gasping, coughing, or gagging, with or without an appearance of distress. The appearance of gastric contents (milk, mucus, or gastric secretions) may proceed, accompany, or follow the event and may be a causative or an associated phenomenon. The caregiver should be asked about events leading up to the spell, milk or mucus coming from the nose or mouth, a history of spitting up, relationship to feedings, or any possibility of a foreign body aspiration. Obstructive sleep apnea often is associated with stridor, snoring, or other evidence of partial airway obstruction along with repeated episodes of self-limited apnea. The cause of an obstructive event may be suggested by the recent or past medical history, for example in recent symptoms of upper respiratory tract infection or a past history of endotracheal intubation. Attention to more long-standing symptoms and more recent superimposed symptoms may be key when a mixed apnea picture presents [10].

Box 1. Focused history

Chief complaint
Presence of apnea with attention to obstructive or central
   symptoms
Type of color change and distribution
Any change in tone, rhythmic shaking, and its distribution
Choking, gagging, coughing, vomiting
Duration
Relationship to feedings
Feeding difficulties such as aversion, choking, fatigue,
   diaphoresis, sloppiness
Eye deviation
Loss of consciousness
Coryza
Fever
History of trauma: intentional or unintentional
State of alertness prior to ALTE
Location of the infant at the time of the ALTE
Sleep position
Witness to the ALTE
Type of resuscitation needed and who performed it
Review of the prehospital (emergency medical service) record,
   if available
Current condition of the child in the caretaker's opinion or the
   amount of time to reach baseline
Presence of a monitor
Medicines taken by the child or by the mother who is breast
   feeding him/her
History of ALTE in the past and type of evaluation
Medical history, including pregnancy, birth, delivery, diet, and
   development
Family history of ALTE, SIDS, or unexpected sudden death

Although GER should be considered in the child who has events around the time of feedings, the astute practitioner also will consider any difficulties with feedings. Swallowing difficulty, inability to complete a feeding without respite, diaphoresis, or respiratory distress with feedings may suggest oromotor difficulties, cardiac dysfunction, or an aerodigestive fistula.

A history of fever or hypothermia may be an important harbinger of infection. However, apnea alone may be a presenting sign of serious infections in an infant who appears to be ill with meningitis or sepsis. It also may be the initial symptom of an RSV infection.

Finally, the practitioner should have a low threshold for consideration of nonaccidental trauma. The American Academy of Pediatrics Committee on Child Abuse and Neglect [38] has suggested that certain circumstances should alert the practitioner to the possibility of abuse, including recurrent ALTE or previous infant death while in the care of the same person, especially if the child and the caregiver are unrelated; previous unexplained deaths or simultaneous symptoms in siblings; or discovery of blood in the infant's mouth or nose in association with ALTE [38,39]. Studies have demonstrated that intentional suffocation, shaken-baby syndrome, and Munchausen-by-proxy may manifest with nonspecific symptoms and few, if any, clinical signs [22,40]. Moreover, these children are at continuing risk if they are returned to an unsafe environment. In one prospective study [8], two of three infants presenting with an ALTE who ultimately died presented secondary to child abuse. Another study [22] has documented deliberate suffocation in over 10% of patients evaluated after active resuscitation. Finally, 3% to 5% of SIDS cases are believed to be a result of infanticide [38].

Examination

Although the event of concern has resolved typically by the time the patient presents for medical evaluation, there are important features on which to focus the physical examination. Aside from residual findings of the event (eg, post-ictal somnolence and dried formula at the nares), the practitioner is looking for any

---

Box 2. Areas of focus for the physical examination of an ALTE

General condition: arousal, irritability, somnolence
Vital signs, including the pulse oximetry
Growth curves, including head circumference
Examination of the:
Head for evidence of trauma or fontanelle size and fullness
Tympanic membrane for hemotympanum
Eyes for pupil reactivity and conjunctival and retinal hemorrhages
Nasopharynx for congestion or presence of milk or formula
Lungs for work of breathing and stridor, wheeze, crackles, rhonchi, or transmitted upper airway sounds
Heart for rate and rhythm, murmur, and capillary refill
Abdomen for signs of an acute abdomen
Musculoskeletal system for range of motion or signs of trauma
Skin for bruising or other signs of trauma or rash
Neurologic examination for tone, movement, head control, and reflexes
Features suggestive of a genetic or metabolic syndrome

---

evidence of an underlying process that might have caused or contributed to the ALTE (eg, rhinorrhea or micrognathia). Box 2 details some of these important aspects.

Other areas and methods of observation may be informative. Interactions between the caregiver and the child may reveal areas of concern. Observing a feeding may allow the practitioner to confirm or detect previously unrecognized difficulties. Cardiovascular monitoring during the entire intake process would allow detection of subclinical cardiorespiratory events as well as provide valuable data, if an event recurs.

Evaluation

The medical evaluation of an ALTE is directed at uncovering any underlying cause, determining the severity, frequency, and nature of the events, and detecting any progression of symptoms or clinical deterioration. Immediate medical evaluation and referral for cardiorespiratory monitoring may be warranted in many cases and often is accomplished best initially in an emergency department.

The initial assessment includes determining and establishing cardiorespiratory stability. Once this has been achieved, taking the history and performing a physical examination can proceed with cardiorespiratory monitoring and pulse oximetry in place.

The extent and direction of further evaluation will depend on the initial assessment and the clinician's clinical judgment. No medical protocol has ever been tested for ALTE, therefore the practitioner should not be confined to a minimum or maximum number of tests. The enormous number of tests available to the practitioner makes it challenging to embark on an appropriate work-up. Aside from the discomfort, inconvenience, risk, and cost of the various tests, the sheer number performed may affect the reliability of the results. The more tests that are performed, the more likely an abnormality (real or spurious) will be detected, whether related to the ALTE event or not.

An organized approach is helpful, and a flow sheet is provided that is useful as a general guide (Fig. 1). As indicated in this guide, in some cases the history, physical examination, and initial period of cardiorespiratory monitoring may be sufficiently reassuring to preclude the need for further work-up. This is especially true if the event was promptly reversible, short lived, and self-limited. Some examples might include an unintentional brief smothering event leading to external airway obstruction (eg, from a pillow or stuffed animal over the face); infrequent, isolated choking episodes either during feeding or with vomiting; hypothermia caused by unintentional, unexpected exposure to cold, such as after bathing; or a frank breath-holding spell. Each of these situations mandates counseling, anticipatory guidance, and education to avoid or manage repeat events and to prevent unintentional behaviors that portend subsequent risk.

If the clinical presentation is consistent with central apnea, and the health care provider is unable to elicit any diagnostic clues on initial assessment, a set of screening tests may be warranted. These tests may include a complete blood

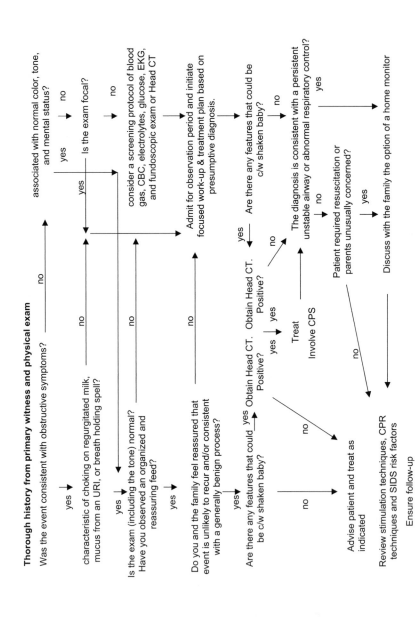

Fig. 1. An untested approach to the evaluation of an ALTE.

count, a basic serum metabolic panel, and a venous blood gas or lactate level. Acidosis with or without an elevated serum lactate level would prompt a more thorough investigation of metabolic disorders and could provide clues about the extent of respiratory compromise. Other electrolyte abnormalities such as hypo- or hypernatremia, hypo- or hypercalcemia, and hypoglycemia in neonates may suggest metabolic disorders manifesting as seizures or lethargy. An elevated white blood count would suggest infection, leading to other microbiologic studies and possibly empiric therapy. Anemia may be, in and of itself, an explanation for an apneic event, or it may be a clue to an underlying hematologic disorder. A screening CT scan of the head is recommended by some experts, especially when the practitioner has any concern for abuse. Studies suggest that the scan may be more sensitive for abuse, with fewer false-positive results than a dilated fundoscopic examination and could detect nontraumatic causes of ALTE such as hydrocephalus [41]. Performing a scan on a patient who is unsedated would likely be more accessible and arguably safer than administering mydriatic and cycloplegic drugs to a patient who requires serial neurologic examinations. If seizure activity or a focal neurologic deficit is suggested by the history or physical examination, electroencephalography should be considered in addition to brain imaging.

If a sudden event with poor perfusion or seizure suggested a possible rhythm disturbance, then an electrocardiogram should be performed, looking for a prolonged QTc interval. If, however, long-standing feeding issues, a failure to thrive, or diaphoresis with feedings accompanies the presentation, a chest radiograph, four-extremity blood pressure measurements, and pre- and postductal oxygen saturation measurements should be included, along with a consultation with cardiology.

If the oxygen saturation was abnormal, arterial blood gas evaluation and chest radiography would be indicated. If oxygen saturation cannot be corrected with the inspiration of 100% oxygen supplementation, a right-to-left vascular shunt becomes another important consideration.

When a patient presents with a history consistent with an obstructive event or physical examination findings reveal features that predispose to such an event, the work-up should be directed at localizing a lesion. The recent onset of upper respiratory tract symptoms with nasal congestion, a barky cough, or hoarseness could reassure the clinician or lead to testing of the nasal secretions for common viral respiratory pathogens. A history of long-standing stridor or hoarseness may direct anatomic or functional assessment of the airway, including radiographs of the neck with or without airway fluoroscopy, chest radiography, contrast esophagram, nasopharyngolaryngoscopy, or occasionally, bronchoscopy. A visible hemangioma, especially in the beard distribution, should raise the concern for airway involvement. Circumstances of concern for foreign body aspiration might lead the clinician to obtain neck and chest radiographs and bilateral decubitus films.

If an event occurred during feeding, it would be prudent to observe another feeding and to refer a child with suspected dysfunction for a modified barium swallow evaluation with a speech, occupational, or feeding specialist. If the infant's neurologic examination and feeding technique are normal but aspiration (especially chronic) is still a consideration, then evaluation by endoscopy or contrast radiography for the detection of a tracheoesophageal fistula might be prudent. If clinical evidence of GER disease is present (eg, emesis with discomfort or apnea, food aversion, or documented esophagitis) and no other diagnosis seems likely, an evaluation may be pursued, but many clinicians start with a trial of empiric therapy. Finally, in patients who do not have classic symptoms of GERD but do have a history that suggests central apnea in the absence of other pathology, an isotope-labeled milk scan or a pH probe could help identify subtle laryngochemoreceptor reflex apnea. In an infant who presents while on a home cardiorespiratory monitor or because of frequent alarms, an expedited monitor download should be conducted to determine if and to what extent true apnea or bradycardia occurred.

Sleep studies may be indicated in the case of a history suggestive of apnea of infancy or prematurity, when the practitioner wishes to further characterize hospital cardiorespiratory (CR) monitor or home apnea monitor alarms, or when no physiologic mechanism can be found to explain repeated ALTE during sleep. The sleep study can record and characterize the extent of desaturation, the breathing pattern, and changes in heart rate. It also can differentiate between central apnea and obstructive apnea by means of a nasal thermistor and sensors that detect chest wall movement. Additionally, sleep studies may identify seizures and cardiac arrhythmias. In special circumstances, a sleep study can be performed with an esophageal pH probe to characterize the role of GER. Despite these impressive capabilities, there are significant limitations to the sleep study. If an event occurs when the patient is not on a monitor, the event will not be recorded, which may give a false sense that the event has resolved, especially if it has not been witnessed. The hope is that the sleep study detects an event that is similar to the presentation, but a normal test does not rule out future ALTE. Moreover, the sleep study is time and labor intensive, with results that often take days to process. It may be best to reserve the sleep study for events that are consistently and repeatedly found during sleep, after a period of observation in the hospital on a CR monitor or when a home monitor suggests concern.

Treatment and discharge planning

Although hospitalization is not required for all infants who present with an ALTE, there are several benefits to this approach. Prolonged cardiovascular monitoring will allow further evaluation of any recurrences and possibly provide information regarding severity, progression, sequelae, or cause. During this time, diagnostic testing can be more judiciously and expeditiously performed, and subspecialty consultation can be enlisted. Hospitalization also allows for the reassurance and education of caregivers regarding the events, and it allows them to receive specific training in cardiopulmonary resuscitation and modifiable SIDS risk factors.

Practitioners and researchers have advocated observation periods of 23 to 72 hours [4,6,42]. In a case series of 65 infants admitted for a 72-hour period of monitoring after an ALTE, only four patients had a subsequent event. Three of these infants had apnea within the first 24 hours, and the fourth patient manifested the subsequent event by 48 hours [43]. The authors made no mention of the severity of the episodes or the intervention provided during the hospitalization for these four patients, but they did state that all 65 patients were followed for 1 year and experienced no further ALTE or deaths.

Treatment is directed at the underlying pathology that is amenable to therapy, whether it consists of simple techniques that the caregivers can institute at home (eg, upright positioning for GER or suctioning for RSV infection), medical therapy (eg, the use of antacids with or without prokinetic agents for GER disease), or surgical intervention (eg, a tracheostomy for critical subglottal stenosis).

Patients with apnea of prematurity or infancy may benefit from treatment with methylxanthine therapy that is coordinated with a pulmonologist. The best choice is caffeine, which has the best safety-efficacy profile of this group of agents but also exacerbates reflux symptoms.

Infants who demonstrate cardiorespiratory instability during hospitalization need to complete the necessary intervention and demonstrate subsequent stability before discharge. Appropriate home environment and medical support must be established. Communication with the primary care clinician and any subspecialists needs to be ensured to create a safe transition to the home and for outpatient follow-up.

Ultimately, parents should be counseled on appropriate resuscitation techniques in the event of a future ALTE. Specifically, they should be instructed on appropriate stimulation techniques (reinforcing the fact that an infant should never be shaken) and provided with cardiopulmonary resuscitation (CPR) instruction. Moreover, they should be counseled on ways to minimize the risk of SIDS, including the proper supine sleep position, use of a firm crib mattress while avoiding excessive blankets, and avoidance of exposure to environmental tobacco smoke.

Natural history and relationship to sudden infant death syndrome

Although the literature on the natural history of infants who present with ALTE is incomplete, most infants will never experience another event and will develop normally. A study of 65 infants presenting to an emergency room with an ALTE found that none of the infants less than 2 months of age with a normal clinical examination and a lactate level less than 2 mmol/L had experienced a subsequent ALTE or were diagnosed with an underlying disorder. Moreover, none of the larger population of patients died within 3 years after presentation, although eight infants were readmitted and were diagnosed ultimately with a "significant underlying disorder." Any delay in diagnosis did not have a lasting impact on the natural history of the underlying disease [37].

The relationship between ALTE and SIDS also is unknown. Studies have reported a mortality rate of 0% to 6% in infants who presented with ALTE and a 13% mortality rate in subpopulations of infants who presented with idiopathic apnea discovered during sleep that required mouth-to-mouth resuscitation [9,44–47]. These studies had significant methodological differences and were not designed to illustrate causation, but they do illustrate the major concern for families and practitioners.

By contrast, there are striking epidemiologic and clinical differences between ALTE and SIDS. First, the incidence of SIDS peaks at 3 to 5 months of life, whereas ALTE peaks 1 to 3 months earlier [12]. Second, only 4% to 13% of SIDS cases had a history of apnea, a percentage only slightly higher than healthy controls [11,13,48]. Moreover, there is no statistical difference between parental reports of apneic episodes in the 2 weeks preceding a SIDS episode and the frequency reported in healthy controls. Finally, after extensive research, most researchers believe that apnea of prematurity is not a risk factor for SIDS [9,48].

The CR monitor, an intervention designed to target at-risk infants, has not affected significantly the rate of SIDS. Instead, the "Back to Sleep" campaign has been the most important factor in the 30% to 50% decline in the SIDS rate, since its inception [39]. During this same period of time, admissions for ALTE have not significantly changed. Furthermore, beyond maternal smoking, which is a shared risk factor for SIDS and ALTE, environmental factors for SIDS such as prone sleeping position and co-sleeping have not been found to be statistically associated with ALTE.

Apnea monitors

The role of home CR monitors designed to detect central apnea and bradycardia in patients with ALTE remains an area of debate in the medical literature and among practitioners. The original 1986 National Institutes of Health consensus statement [1], in the absence of definitive literature, has suggested that monitors are indicated in cases of ALTE that require vigorous stimulation or resuscitation. A subsequent policy statement offered in 2003 by the Committee on the Fetus and Newborn of the American Academy of Pediatrics [49] offered more specific indications. The committee suggested that monitors might be used to alert the family of a patient with a known unstable airway, abnormal respiratory control, or symptomatic and technologically dependent chronic lung disease [49]. Although the committee did not differentiate the source of ALTE, one might suggest that if it were a result of the above criteria, a monitor may be justified.

The provider should be aware that obstructive apnea often is not identified by conventional monitors because chest wall motion is maintained despite a lack of airflow [9]. These monitors have devices to detect only chest wall motion and heart rate. Without a device that detects ribcage and abdominal movements, nasal airflow or oxygen saturation, the only detectable abnormality of an obstructive event would be bradycardia if the event were sufficiently severe or prolonged.

Moreover, the parents should be counseled that monitoring has not been shown to prevent SIDS. A multicenter study conducted by the Collaborative Home Infant Monitoring Evaluation (CHIME) Study Group [9] has suggested that apneic events are common to both normal infants and those who are diagnosed with idiopathic ALTE who had previously required CPR or vigorous stimulation. Moreover, the number of extreme apneic events (lasting 30 seconds or more) did not significantly differ between the groups (although the sample size may not have been large enough to detect a difference) [9].

Practitioners must also be familiar with the possible adverse effects of the monitor technology. First, monitors often cannot differentiate between true cardiorespiratory events and disrupted connections, with resultant frequent false alarms. Second, monitors generally increase caregiver anxiety, depression, and hostility, especially during the first few months of use, compared with matched controls [50]. Finally, and perhaps most debatably, infants who were monitored over the course of a year may have worse developmental consequences, and some authors speculate that increased parental stress levels and perceptions of infant vulnerability may be to blame [51].

In appropriate situations, the parents should be empowered to participate in the decision regarding the use of a monitor. Some parents will feel more comfortable with an alarm, whereas others will find it intrusive or potentially more worrisome. Because false alarms are a clinical reality, the parents should be counseled to use the assessment techniques that they have learned in the event of an alarm and should have ready access to medical personnel who can answer immediate questions and refer for follow-up.

If it is prescribed, the CR monitor should have an event recorder and be set with age-appropriate physiologic parameters (Table 2). Most experts agree that the CR monitoring may be discontinued once it is clear of apnea for 2 consecutive months. Furthermore, no subsequent sleep study may be needed if an event recorder is used and sufficient data is gathered.

A home monitor with an oxygen event recorder has been studied and used in rare circumstances. These monitors record the date, time, oxygen saturation, plethysmographic waveforms, partial pressure of oxygen of the skin, breathing

Table 2
Suggested age-appropriate cardiorespiratory monitor settings

Premature infants		Full-term infants	
Age (PCA in weeks)	Bradycardia threshold (beats per minute)	Age (months)	Bradycardia threshold (beats per minute)
≤40	100	≤1	80
40–44	80	1–3	70
≥44	Use corrected age in months with full-term limits	3–12	60
		≥12	50

Apnea, 15 seconds for preterm infants; 20 seconds for term infants.
Abbreviation: PCA, postconceptional age.

movements, and electrocardiograms. With these additional features, researchers have been able to assess features of altered skin perfusion, suffocation, and fabricated illness [22].

Future directions

Because of its prevalence, its potential to consume significant medical resources, and its unpredictable natural history, further research interest and funding are needed to clarify ALTE. The following study designs and objectives suggest immediate research strategies in the field but are not intended to be exhaustive.

First, prospective observational cohort studies are needed to describe the epidemiology and risk factors for ALTE in the United States population. Other epidemiologic studies should follow up on the evidence that 20- or 30-second apneic episodes may be common events in the lives of infants and help to identify which patients may be at risk for adverse outcomes. Second, bench and translational research protocols should continue to describe the pathophysiology of apnea and other neurocardiorespiratory events to describe potential causative mechanisms. Finally, trials are needed to compare the natural history of patients who present with an ALTE based on an intervention such as a diagnostic algorithm, GER treatment, or monitor use. Ultimately, the intention of future study should be to predict and intervene before an ALTE occurs, while limiting the morbidity and mortality associated with it.

Summary

ALTE is a common, nonspecific, and primarily benign disorder that also may be potentially serious. A firm understanding of the definition and differential diagnosis is crucial to allow the practitioner to swiftly differentiate between events that may require minimal intervention and those that demand immediate investigation and therapy. Providing education and anticipatory guidance to concerned parents and caregivers also is critical to the effective management and discharge planning for these infants.

References

[1] National Institutes of Health Consensus Development Conference on Infantile apnea and home monitoring. Pediatrics 1987;79:292–9.
[2] Kahn A, Rebuffat E, Franco P, et al. Apparent life-threatening events and apnea of infancy. In: Hunt C, Brouillette R, editors. Respiratory control disorders. Baltimore: Baltimore Press; 1991. p. 178.
[3] Gray C, Davies F, Molyneux E. Apparent life-threatening events presenting to a pediatric emergency department. Pediatr Emerg Care 1999;15:195–9.

[4] Rosenberg NM, Cruz MN, Chamberlain JM, et al. The least expensive diagnostic tool. Pediatr Emerg Care 1995;11:389–91.

[5] Stratton SJ, Taves A, Lewis RJ, et al. Apparent life-threatening events in infants: high risk in the out-of-hospital environment. Ann Emerg Med 2004;43:711–7.

[6] Wennergren G, Milerad J, Westphall I, et al. Consensus statement on clinical management. Acta Paediatr Suppl 1993;82(Suppl 389):S114–6.

[7] Maffei FA, Powers KS, van der Jagt EW. Apparent life-threatening events as an indicator of occult abuse. Arch Pediatr Adolesc Med 2004;158:402 [author reply, p. 402].

[8] Altman RL, Brand DA, Forman S, et al. Abusive head injury as a cause of apparent life-threatening events in infancy. Arch Pediatr Adolesc Med 2003;157:1011–5.

[9] Ramanathan R, Corwin MJ, Hunt CE, et al. Cardiorespiratory events recorded on home monitors: comparison of healthy infants with those at increased risk for SIDS. JAMA 2001;285: 2199–207.

[10] Park MK. Pediatric cardiology for practitioners. 4th edition. St Louis: Mosby; 2002. p. 11.

[11] Mitchell EA, Thompson JM. Parental reported apnoea, admissions to hospital and sudden infant death syndrome. Acta Paediatr 2001;90:417–22.

[12] Kiechl-Kohlendorfer U, Hof D, Peglow UP, et al. Epidemiology of apparent life threatening events. Arch Dis Child 2005;90:297–300.

[13] Wennergren G, Milerad J, Lagercrantz H, et al. The epidemiology of sudden infant death syndrome and attacks of lifelessness in Sweden. Acta Paediatr Scand 1987;76:898–906.

[14] Southall DP, Samuels MP, Talbert DG. Recurrent cyanotic episodes with severe arterial hypoxaemia and intrapulmonary shunting: a mechanism for sudden death. Arch Dis Child 1990; 65:953–61.

[15] Katz-Salamon M. Delayed chemoreceptor responses in infants with apnoea. Arch Dis Child 2004;89:261–6.

[16] Kahn A, Groswasser J, Sottiaux M, et al. Clinical problems in relation to apparent life-threatening events in infants. Acta Paediatr Suppl 1993;82(Suppl 389):S107–10.

[17] Chen ML, Keens TG. Congenital central hypoventilation syndrome: not just another rare disorder. Paediatr Respir Rev 2004;5:182–9.

[18] Ruff ME, Oakes WJ, Fisher SR, et al. Sleep apnea and vocal cord paralysis secondary to type I Chiari malformation. Pediatrics 1987;80:231–4.

[19] Veereman-Wauters G, Bochner A, Van Caillie-Bertrand M. Gastroesophageal reflux in infants with a history of near-miss sudden infant death. J Pediatr Gastroenterol Nutr 1991;12:319–23.

[20] Lindgren C, Jing L, Graham B, et al. Respiratory syncytial virus infection reinforces reflex apnea in young lambs. Pediatr Res 1992;31:381–5.

[21] Lindgren C, Lin J, Graham BS, et al. Respiratory syncytial virus infection enhances the response to laryngeal chemostimulation and inhibits arousal from sleep in young lambs. Acta Paediatr 1996;85:789–97.

[22] Samuels MP, Poets CF, Noyes JP, et al. Diagnosis and management after life threatening events in infants and young children who received cardiopulmonary resuscitation. BMJ 1993;306: 489–92.

[23] Hewertson J, Poets CF, Samuels MP, et al. Epileptic seizure-induced hypoxemia in infants with apparent life-threatening events. Pediatrics 1994;94:148–56.

[24] Kahn A, Montauk L, Blum D. Diagnostic categories in infants referred for an acute event suggesting near-miss SIDS. Eur J Pediatr 1987;146:458–60.

[25] Rayyan M, Naulaers G, Daniels H, et al. Characteristics of respiratory syncytial virus-related apnoea in three infants. Acta Paediatr 2004;93:847–9.

[26] Heininger U, Kleemann WJ, Cherry JD. A controlled study of the relationship between Bordetella pertussis infections and sudden unexpected deaths among German infants. Pediatrics 2004;114:e9–15.

[27] Southall DP, Thomas MG, Lambert HP. Severe hypoxaemia in pertussis. Arch Dis Child 1988;63:598–605.

[28] McMurray JS, Holinger LD. Otolaryngic manifestations in children presenting with apparent life-threatening events. Otolaryngol Head Neck Surg 1997;116:575–9.

[29] Harrington C, Kirjavainen T, Teng A, et al. Altered autonomic function and reduced arousability in apparent life-threatening event infants with obstructive sleep apnea. Am J Respir Crit Care Med 2002;165:1048–54.

[30] Schwartz PJ, Stramba-Badiale M, Segantini A, et al. Prolongation of the QT interval and the sudden infant death syndrome. N Engl J Med 1998;338:1709–14.

[31] Arens R, Gozal D, Williams JC, et al. Recurrent apparent life-threatening events during infancy: a manifestation of inborn errors of metabolism. J Pediatr 1993;123:415–8.

[32] Hickson GB, Altemeier WA, Martin ED, et al. Parental administration of chemical agents: a cause of apparent life-threatening events. Pediatrics 1989;83:772–6.

[33] Byard RW, Burnell RH. Apparent life threatening events and infant holding practices. Arch Dis Child 1995;73:502–4.

[34] Poets CF, Samuels MP, Wardrop CA, et al. Reduced haemoglobin levels in infants presenting with apparent life-threatening events–a retrospective investigation. Acta Paediatr 1992;81: 319–22.

[35] Dunne KP, Matthews TG. Hypothermia and sudden infant death syndrome. Arch Dis Child 1988;63:438–40.

[36] McGovern MC, Smith MB. Causes of apparent life threatening events in infants: a systematic review. Arch Dis Child 2004;89:1043–8.

[37] Davies F, Gupta R. Apparent life threatening events in infants presenting to an emergency department. Emerg Med J 2002;19:11–6.

[38] Committee on Child Abuse and Neglect of the American Academy of Pediatrics. Distinguishing sudden infant death syndrome from child abuse fatalities. Pediatrics 1994;94:124–6.

[39] Farrell PA, Weiner GM, Lemons JA. SIDS, ALTE, apnea, and the use of home monitors. Pediatr Rev 2002;23:3–9.

[40] Pitetti RD, Maffei F, Chang K, et al. Prevalence of retinal hemorrhages and child abuse in children who present with an apparent life-threatening event. Pediatrics 2002;110:557–62.

[41] Sezen F. Retinal haemorrhages in newborn infants. Br J Ophthalmol 1971;55:248–53.

[42] Kahn A. Recommended clinical evaluation of infants with an apparent life-threatening event: consensus document of the European Society for the Study and Prevention of Infant Death, 2003. Eur J Pediatr 2004;163:108–15.

[43] Tal Y, Tirosh E, Even L, et al. A comparison of the yield of a 24 h versus 72 h hospital evaluation in infants with apparent life-threatening events. Eur J Pediatr 1999;158:954.

[44] US Department of Health and Human Services. Infantile apnea and home monitoring: report of a consensus development conference. NIH Publication no. 87-2905; 1987.

[45] Ariagno RL, Guilleminault C, Korobkin R, et al. "Near-miss" for sudden infant death syndrome infants: a clinical problem. Pediatrics 1983;71:726–30.

[46] Duffty P, Bryan MH. Home apnea monitoring in "near-miss" sudden infant death syndrome (SIDS) and in siblings of SIDS victims. Pediatrics 1982;70:69–74.

[47] Oren J, Kelly D, Shannon DC. Identification of a high-risk group for sudden infant death syndrome among infants who were resuscitated for sleep apnea. Pediatrics 1986;77:495–9.

[48] Hoffman HJ, Damus K, Hillman L, et al. Risk factors for SIDS: results of the National Institute of Child Health and Human Development SIDS Cooperative Epidemiological Study. Ann N Y Acad Sci 1988;533:13–30.

[49] American Academy of Pediatrics Committee on Fetus and Newborn. Apnea: sudden infant death syndrome, and home monitoring. Pediatrics 2003;111:914–7.

[50] Abendroth D, Moser DK, Dracup K, et al. Do apnea monitors decrease emotional distress in parents of infants at high risk for cardiopulmonary arrest? J Pediatr Health Care 1999;13:50–7.

[51] Baroni MA. Apparent life-threatening events during infancy: a follow-up study of subsequent growth and development. J Dev Behav Pediatr 1991;12:154–61.

[52] Pasterkamp K. The history and physical exam. In: Chernick V, Boat TF, editors. Kendig's disorders of the respiratory tract in children. 6th edition. Philadelphia: WB Saunders; 1998. p. 101–2.

ELSEVIER
SAUNDERS

PEDIATRIC CLINICS
OF NORTH AMERICA

Pediatr Clin N Am 52 (2005) 1147–1163

Diabetic Ketoacidosis in Children

Michael S.D. Agus, MD[a,b], Joseph I. Wolfsdorf, MB, BCh[a,b],*

[a]*Division of Endocrinology, Children's Hospital Boston, 300 Longwood Avenue,
Boston, MA 02115, USA*
[b]*Department of Pediatrics, Harvard Medical School, 25 Shattuck Street,
Boston, MA 02115-6092, USA*

Severe diabetic ketoacidosis (DKA) is a life-threatening complication of diabetes mellitus. Approximately 15% to 67% of patients with newly diagnosed type 1 diabetes in Europe and North America present with DKA, and it accounts for 65% of all hospital admissions of patients with diabetes mellitus who are younger than 19 years old [1,2]. The frequency of DKA at onset of diabetes correlates inversely with the regional incidence of type 1 diabetes and is more common in young children, children without a first-degree relative with type 1 diabetes, and individuals whose families are of lower socioeconomic status [3,4]. The mortality rate for DKA in children is 0.15% to 0.31% [5,6]. Despite the more apparent issues of hypovolemia and acidosis, clinically significant cerebral edema, which occurs in 1% of cases, is the most serious risk to children [7,8].

In Canada and Europe, rates of hospitalization for DKA in established and new patients with type 1 diabetes have remained stable at approximately 10 per 100,000 children over the past 20 years. The risk of DKA in patients with established type 1 diabetes is 1% to 10% per patient per year [9,10]. Risk is increased in children with poor metabolic control or previous episodes of DKA, peripubertal and adolescent girls, children with psychiatric disorders, including individuals with eating disorders, and children with difficult family circumstances, including lower socioeconomic status and lack of health insurance [10]. Interruption of insulin delivery, regardless of the reason, is an important cause of DKA in patients who use continuous subcutaneous insulin infusion (insulin pump) therapy. Children rarely have DKA when insulin administration is closely

---

* Corresponding author. Division of Endocrinology, Children's Hospital Boston, 300 Longwood Avenue, Boston, MA 02115.
E-mail address: joseph.wolfsdorf@childrens.harvard.edu (J.I. Wolfsdorf).

0031-3955/05/$ – see front matter © 2005 Elsevier Inc. All rights reserved.
doi:10.1016/j.pcl.2005.03.006
pediatric.theclinics.com

Box 1. Clinical manifestations of diabetic ketoacidosis

- Dehydration
- Rapid, deep, sighing (Kussmaul) respiration
- Nausea, vomiting, and abdominal pain that may mimic an acute abdomen
- Increased leukocyte count with left shift
- Nonspecific elevation of serum amylase
- Fever when infection is present
- Progressive obtundation and loss of consciousness

---

supervised or performed by a responsible adult. In established patients, most instances of DKA are probably associated with insulin omission or treatment error, whereas the rest of the instances are caused by inadequate insulin therapy during intercurrent illness.

The biochemical criteria for the diagnosis of DKA include hyperglycemia (blood glucose >11 mmol/L (approximately 200 mg/dL) with acidosis (venous blood pH < 7.3 or serum bicarbonate ≤ 15 mmol/L), ketonemia with total serum ketones (β-hydroxybutyrate and acetoacetate) >3 mmol/L, and ketonuria. DKA usually is categorized by the severity of the acidosis: from mild (venous pH < 7.30, bicarbonate < 15 mmol/L), to moderate (pH < 7.2, bicarbonate < 10 mmol/L), to severe (pH < 7.1, bicarbonate < 5 mmol/L) [11]. Clinical symptoms also may vary from mild to severe (Box 1) [12].

Pathophysiology

DKA is the result of absolute or relative deficiency of circulating insulin and the combined effects of increased levels of the counterregulatory hormones, catecholamines, glucagon, cortisol, and growth hormone. Absolute insulin deficiency occurs in previously undiagnosed type 1 diabetes and when patients on treatment deliberately or inadvertently do not take insulin. Relative insulin deficiency occurs when the concentrations of counterregulatory hormones increase in response to stress in conditions such as sepsis, trauma, or gastrointestinal illness with diarrhea and vomiting.

Low serum levels of insulin and high concentrations of the counterregulatory hormones result in an accelerated catabolic state whose effects include increased glucose production by the liver and kidney (via glycogenolysis and gluconeogenesis), impaired peripheral glucose use that results in hyperglycemia and hyperosmolality, and increased lipolysis and ketogenesis, which cause ketonemia and metabolic acidosis. Hyperglycemia that exceeds the renal threshold of approximately 180 mg/dL and hyperketonemia cause osmotic diuresis, dehydration, and obligatory loss of electrolytes, which often is aggravated by vomiting. These

Table 1
Usual losses of fluids and electrolytes in diabetic ketoacidosis and normal maintenance requirements

	Average losses per kg (range)	Maintenance requirements per meter^2
Water	70 mL (30–100)	1500 mL
Sodium	6 mmol (5–13)	45 mmol
Potassium	5 mmol (3–6)	35 mmol
Chloride	4 mmol (3–9)	30 mmol
Phosphate	(0.5–2.5) mmol	10 mmol

These data are from measurements in only a few children and adolescents.

changes stimulate further catecholamine and stress hormone production, which induces more severe insulin resistance and worsening hyperglycemia and hyperketonemia. If uninterrupted with exogenous insulin, fluid, and electrolyte therapy, this cycle progresses to fatal dehydration and metabolic acidosis. Ketoacidosis may be aggravated by lactic acidosis from poor tissue perfusion or sepsis.

DKA is characterized by severe depletion of water and electrolytes from the intra- and extracellular fluid compartments; the range of losses is shown in Table 1. Despite their dehydration, patients continue to have considerable urine output until renal blood flow and glomerular filtration are critically decreased as a result of extreme volume depletion. The magnitude of specific deficits in an individual patient at the time of presentation varies depending on the duration of illness, the extent to which the patient was able to maintain intake of fluid and electrolytes, and the content of food and fluids consumed before presentation.

Intracellular potassium is depleted because of transcellular shifts of this ion caused by hypertonicity (ie, increased plasma osmolality causes solvent drag in which water and potassium are pulled out of cells), and glycogenolysis and proteolysis secondary to insulin deficiency cause potassium efflux from cells. Potassium is lost from the body through vomiting and as a consequence of osmotic diuresis. Volume depletion causes secondary hyperaldosteronism, which promotes urinary potassium excretion. Total body depletion of potassium occurs, although at the time of presentation, the plasma potassium concentration may not reflect the deficit [13].

Management of diabetic ketoacidosis

During the initial evaluation, the clinician should take the following steps:

- Perform a clinical evaluation to establish the diagnosis and determine its cause (while carefully looking for evidence of infection). Weigh the patient and measure height or length. Determine body surface area. Assess the patient's degree of dehydration.

- Determine the blood glucose concentration with a glucose meter and the blood or urine ketone concentration.
- Obtain a blood sample for laboratory measurement of serum glucose, electrolytes and total carbon dioxide (TCO_2), blood urea nitrogen, creatinine, serum osmolality, venous (or arterial in critically ill patients) pH, partial pressure of carbon dioxide (pCO_2), partial pressure of oxygen (pO_2), hemoglobin, hematocrit, total and differential white blood cell count, calcium, phosphorus and magnesium concentrations.
- Perform a urinalysis and obtain appropriate specimens for culture (eg, blood, urine, throat).
- Perform an electrocardiogram for baseline evaluation of potassium status.

In the management of DKA, several supportive measures should be undertaken:

- Secure the airway and empty the stomach by continuous nasogastric suction to prevent pulmonary aspiration in the unconscious or severely obtunded patient.
- Give antibiotics to febrile patients after obtaining appropriate cultures of body fluids.
- Provide supplementary oxygen to patients with severe circulatory impairment or shock.
- Catheterize the bladder if a child is unconscious or unable to void on demand (eg, infants and ill young children).
- A heparin-locked peripheral intravenous catheter should be placed for convenient and painless repetitive blood sampling.
- A cardiac monitor should be used for continuous electrocardiographic monitoring.
- Use a flow chart to record a patient's clinical and laboratory data, including vital signs (eg, heart rate, respiratory rate, blood pressure, level of consciousness [Glasgow coma scale]), details of fluid and electrolyte therapy, amount of administered insulin, and urine output. A key to successful management of DKA is meticulous monitoring of a patient's clinical and biochemical response to treatment so that timely adjustments in the treatment regimen can be made when indicated by a patient's clinical or laboratory data. Frequent re-examination of laboratory parameters is required to prevent serious electrolyte imbalance and administration of either insufficient or excessive fluid.

A child with DKA should be cared for in a unit that has experienced nursing staff trained in monitoring and management, clear written guidelines, and access to a laboratory that can provide frequent and timely measurements of relevant biochemical variables. A pediatrician with training and expertise in the management of DKA should supervise inpatient management of these children. Children with signs of severe DKA, including compromised circulation or depressed level of consciousness, and children who are at increased risk for cerebral edema

(<5 years of age, new onset) should be considered for treatment in a pediatric intensive care unit or in a pediatric ward that specializes in diabetes care that has equivalent resources and supervision [11].

Fluid and electrolyte therapy

Sodium and water

All patients with DKA are dehydrated and suffer total body depletion of sodium, potassium, chloride, phosphate, and magnesium (Table 1). The high effective osmolality of the extracellular fluid compartment and restriction of glucose to the extracellular space result in a shift of water from the intracellular fluid compartment to the extracellular fluid compartment, which causes a decrease in the measured serum sodium concentration. A commonly used correction factor is 1.6 mmol/L decrease in serum sodium concentration per 5.6 mmol/L (100 mg/dL) increase in blood glucose concentration above normal [14]. Experimental evaluation of its accuracy is lacking, and based on acute experimental observations, other researchers have suggested a correction factor of 2.4 mmol/L decrease in serum sodium concentration per 5.6 mmol/L (100 mg/dL) increase in blood glucose concentration above normal [15]. The presence of hyperlipidemia also may lower the measured serum sodium concentration (depending on the methodology used to measure serum sodium concentration). The serum sodium concentration may give a misleading estimate of the degree of sodium loss. The effective osmolality (see formula in following section) at the time of presentation is frequently in the range of 300 to 350 mOsm/L. Increased serum urea nitrogen and hematocrit are useful markers of severe extracellular fluid contraction [16,17]. At the time of presentation, patients are extracellular fluid contracted, and clinical estimates of the deficit in patients with severe DKA, although notoriously inaccurate, are usually in the range of 5% to 10% [18,19]. In cases of mild to moderately severe DKA, fluid deficits are more modest—in the range 30 to 50 mL/kg. Shock with hemodynamic compromise is rare in childhood.

The onset of dehydration is associated with a reduction in glomerular filtration rate, which results in decreased glucose and ketone clearance. Intravenous fluid administration expands the intravascular volume and increases glomerular filtration, which increases renal excretion of glucose and ketoanions, and results in a prompt decrease in blood glucose concentration in the first 2 to 4 hours after rehydration is initiated [20,21].

The goals of fluid and salt replacement therapy in DKA are restoration of circulating volume, replacement of sodium and the extracellular fluid and intracellular fluid water deficit, and restoration of glomerular filtration rate with enhanced clearance of glucose and ketones from the blood and avoidance of cerebral edema (Box 2). In animals and humans, intracranial pressure rises as intravenous fluids are given [22,23]. Although no compelling evidence shows superiority of any fluid regimen over another, some data suggest that rapid

---

Box 2. Goals of therapy

- Correct dehydration
- Restore blood glucose to near normal levels
- Correct acidosis and reverse ketosis
- Avoid complications of treatment
- Identify and treat the precipitating event

---

fluid replacement with hypotonic fluid is associated with an increased risk of cerebral edema, and slower fluid deficit correction with isotonic or near-isotonic solutions results in earlier reversal of acidosis [11,24,25]. Large amounts of 0.9% saline also have been associated with the development of hyperchloremic metabolic acidosis.

Initial intravenous fluid administration and, when necessary, volume expansion should begin immediately with an isotonic solution (0.9% saline or balanced salt solution such as Ringer's lactate). The volume and rate of administration depend on a patient's circulatory status. When volume expansion is clinically indicated, 10 to 20 mL/kg is given over 1 to 2 hours and may be repeated if necessary. The goal of this initial fluid therapy is to re-establish adequate perfusion of end organs, not restoration of euvolemia. Success in achieving this goal may be judged best by monitoring mental status, capillary refill, and presence of urine output.

Subsequent fluid management should be with a solution that has a tonicity of 0.45% saline or more (0.9% saline or balanced salt solution [Ringer's lactate] or 0.45% saline with added potassium). The rate of intravenous fluid administration should be calculated to rehydrate a patient at an even rate over 48 hours. Because the severity of dehydration may be difficult to determine and is often overestimated, the daily volume of fluid usually should not exceed 1.5 to 2 times the usual daily requirement based on age, weight, or body surface area (Table 1). Urinary losses should not be added to the calculation of replacement fluids. The development of hyponatremia or failure to observe a progressive rise in serum sodium concentration with a concomitant decrease of blood glucose concentration during treatment is a risk factor for cerebral edema [7,26]. The composition of the hydrating fluid should be changed appropriately to increase the serum sodium concentration.

When the blood glucose concentration reaches approximately 17 mmol/L (300 mg/dL), 5% dextrose is added to the infusion fluid. It is often necessary to use 10% or even 12.5% dextrose to prevent hypoglycemia while continuing to infuse insulin to correct the metabolic acidosis. Administration of intravenous fluids should be continued until acidosis is corrected and a patient can tolerate fluids and food. Inadequate fluid administration should be evident from examination of the cumulative fluid balance and persistent tachycardia in the absence of a fever.

Insulin and glucose

Insulin is essential for restoring blood glucose to normal and suppressing lipolysis and ketogenesis. Rehydration alone decreases the blood glucose concentration but does not reverse ketoacidosis. Several routes (ie, subcutaneous, intramuscular, and intravenous) of insulin administration and doses have been used and are effective in managing DKA [27–29]; however, "low dose" intravenous insulin administration is the current standard of care [11,27,28]. A loading dose of insulin is not required to initiate insulin therapy [30]. At a continuous dose of 0.1 U/kg/h, intravenous regular (soluble) insulin achieves steady state serum insulin levels of 50 to 200 μU/mL within 60 minutes. These serum insulin levels are adequate to offset the insulin resistance characteristic of DKA. They suppress glucose production, significantly increase peripheral glucose uptake, and inhibit lipolysis and ketogenesis. The dose of insulin should remain at 0.1 U/kg/h until resolution of ketoacidosis (pH > 7.30 and bicarbonate >15 mmol/L or closure of the anion gap). It should be noted, however, that resolution of ketoacidemia takes longer than restoration of blood glucose concentrations to normal. Intravenous insulin therapy must not be discontinued until ketoacidosis has resolved, even if the blood glucose concentration is normal or near to normal. To prevent an unduly rapid fall in blood glucose concentration and development of hypoglycemia, dextrose should be added to the intravenous fluid when the plasma glucose has fallen to approximately17 mmol/L (300 mg/dL), as noted previously.

The amount of dextrose in the intravenous infusion should be increased in stepwise fashion up to a maximum concentration of 12.5% to maintain the blood glucose between 100 and 200 mg/dL. If the blood glucose continues to drop, the rate of intravenous fluid administration should be increased to twice the maintenance rate. If the blood glucose still cannot be maintained and the serum bicarbonate is approaching normal, the insulin infusion rate may be decreased by decrements of 0.02 U/kg/h.

Continuous intravenous insulin should be administered via an infusion pump. Regular insulin is diluted in normal saline (50 U regular insulin in 50 mL saline) and is given at a rate of 0.1 U/kg/h. An intravenous priming dose of 0.1 U/kg is not necessary but may be used at the start of insulin therapy, particularly if insulin treatment has been delayed. This rate of insulin infusion is sufficient to reverse ketoacidosis in most patients. If the response is inadequate (especially if blood glucose level is falling but acidosis is not improving; ie, the anion gap is not decreasing) because of severe insulin resistance, the rate of insulin infusion should be increased until a satisfactory response is achieved. There are rare patients with severe insulin resistance who do not respond satisfactorily to low-dose insulin infusion and require two or three times the usual dose. It is essential to monitor the response to insulin therapy in terms of blood glucose and degree of acidosis (ie, venous or arterial pH, anion gap, or end-tidal CO_2, as detailed later). One also should consider other possible explanations for failure to respond to insulin, especially an error in insulin preparation. When intravenous administration is not possible, the intramuscular or subcutaneous route of insulin administration may be used, and rapid-acting insulin (lispro or aspart) may be preferable to regular insulin in these circumstances. Treatment of adult patients who have uncomplicated DKA with subcutaneous insulin lispro every hour in a nonintensive care setting has been shown to be safe and more cost effective than treatment with intravenous regular insulin in the intensive care unit [29]. Poor tissue perfusion in a severely dehydrated patient may impair absorption of insulin from subcutaneous tissue, and insulin initially should be given intramuscularly.

The serum half-life of insulin is 5 minutes, so if the insulin infusion is stopped, the serum insulin concentration decreases rapidly. If the infusion were to infiltrate and was not recognized promptly, inadequate serum insulin levels would ensue rapidly. Low-dose intravenous insulin therapy must be supervised carefully.

When ketoacidosis has resolved and the change to subcutaneous insulin is planned, the first subcutaneous injection should be given at an appropriate interval before stopping the insulin infusion to allow sufficient time for the subcutaneously injected insulin to begin to be absorbed. The onset of action of rapid-acting insulin (lispro or aspart) is approximately 15 minutes, whereas that of regular insulin is 30 to 60 minutes. At the authors' institution, the starting dose of subcutaneous insulin in new-onset patients after recovery from DKA initially is based on a total daily dose (TDD) of insulin of 0.75 U/kg/d in prepubertal children and 1 U/kg/d in pubertal patients. Two thirds of the TDD is given before breakfast (one third as rapid-acting insulin and two thirds as intermediate-acting insulin; in young children, one fourth is given as rapid-acting insulin and three fourths are given as intermediate-acting insulin). One third of the remainder of the TDD is given before dinner as rapid-acting insulin, and two thirds of the remainder of the TDD is given as intermediate-acting insulin at bedtime. Likewise, in young children, the proportion of rapid-acting insulin given before dinner usually is decreased to one fourth of the remainder of the TDD. For example, if a 10-year-old prepubertal child weighs 30 kg, the starting dose would be 5 U rapid-acting insulin and 10 U intermediate-acting insulin before breakfast, 2 to 3 U rapid-acting insulin before dinner, and 5 U intermediate-acting insulin at bedtime. Supplemental rapid-acting insulin is given at approximately 4-hour intervals to correct blood glucose levels that exceed 200 mg/dL. Alternatively, one half of the estimated TDD may be given as basal insulin using insulin glargine, and the remaining one half of the estimated TDD is given as rapid-acting insulin, with the dose before each meal comprising approximately 15% to 20% of the TDD. In the hypothetical case cited previously, a child would receive a single dose of 11 to 12 U of insulin glargine either at dinnertime or bedtime and 3 to 4 U of rapid-acting insulin before each meal.

Potassium

Serum potassium concentrations at the time of presentation may be normal, increased or, infrequently, decreased. Hypokalemia at presentation may be related to prolonged duration of disease and persistent vomiting, whereas hyperkalemia primarily results from impaired renal function [13]. Adults with DKA have total body potassium deficits of the order of 4 to 6 mmol/kg and, although data in children are sparse, similar deficits have been described in a few carefully studied cases [31–35]. After treatment is started, insulin promotes cellular uptake of glucose and potassium, and correction of acidosis promotes the return of potassium to the intracellular compartment. The serum potassium concentration may decrease abruptly, which predisposes a patient to cardiac arrhythmias. Potassium replacement should be started immediately if a patient is hypokalemic. Otherwise, it should be started concurrent with commencing insulin therapy. If a patient presents with hyperkalemia, potassium administration should be deferred until urine output has been documented.

The amount of potassium administered should be sufficient to maintain serum potassium levels in the normal range. The usual starting potassium concentration in the infusate should be 40 mmol/L, and potassium administration should continue throughout the period of intravenous fluid therapy. Careful monitoring of the serum level and provision of adequate potassium are essential to prevent hypokalemia and life-threatening arrhythmias. An electrocardiogram can be used as a guide to therapy and is especially valuable while waiting for the serum potassium concentration to be measured. Flattening of the T wave, widening of the QT interval, and the appearance of U waves indicate hypokalemia. Tall, peaked, symmetrical T waves and shortening of the QT interval are signs of hyperkalemia. The plasma potassium concentration should be rechecked every 1 to 2 hours if the plasma concentration is outside the normal range. Potassium may be given as chloride, acetate, or phosphate salt. Use of potassium acetate and potassium phosphate reduces the total amount of chloride administered and partially corrects the phosphate deficit.

Phosphate

Depletion of intracellular phosphate occurs in DKA and phosphate is lost as a result of osmotic diuresis. In adults, deficits are in the range of 0.5 to 2.5 mmol/kg, but comparable data in children are sparse. After starting therapy, plasma phosphate levels rapidly decrease because of urinary excretion and because insulin causes phosphate to re-enter cells. Low serum phosphate levels have been associated with various metabolic disturbances; however, the effects of hypophosphatemia on 2,3-diphosphoglycerate concentrations and on tissue oxygenation are especially relevant to DKA management. Although phosphate depletion persists for several days after resolution of DKA, prospective studies have failed to show any significant clinical benefit from phosphate replacement [36–41]. Serum phosphate levels should be monitored, and severe hypophosphatemia should be treated with potassium phosphate while carefully monitoring serum calcium concentrations to avoid phosphate-induced hypocalcemia. This occurrence generally can be avoided if potassium phosphate concentration in the intravenous fluid does not exceed 20 mEq/L.

Acidosis and bicarbonate

Even severe acidosis is reversible by fluid and insulin replacement. Insulin stops further synthesis of ketoacids and promotes ketone use. The metabolism of ketoanions results in the regeneration of bicarbonate and correction of acidemia. Treatment of hypovolemia improves tissue perfusion and restores renal function, which increases the excretion of organic acids and reverses any lactic acidosis, which may account for up to 25% of the acidemia.

In DKA, the anion gap is increased primarily because of a marked increase in the concentrations of the major ketoanions, β-hydroxybutyrate and aceto-acetate. Acetone is formed by spontaneous decarboxylation of acetoacetate. Acetoacetate and acetone, but not β-hydroxybutyrate, are measured by the commonly used clinical reagent strip or tablet methods that use the sodium nitroprusside reaction. At initial presentation with DKA, the concentration of β- hydroxybutyrate is four to ten times higher than that of acetoacetic acid. With insulin therapy and correction of the acidosis, the β- hydroxybutyrate is reoxidized to acetoacetate, which is eventually metabolized. Blood ketone meters only measure β-hydroxybutyrate.

The indications for bicarbonate therapy in DKA are unclear. Controlled trials of sodium bicarbonate in children and adults have been unable to show clinical benefit or any important difference in the rate of rise in the plasma bicarbonate concentration [42–44]. There are physiologic reasons not to use bicarbonate. Its use may cause paradoxic central nervous system acidosis. Bicarbonate combines with H+ and then dissociates to CO_2 and H_2O. Bicarbonate diffuses poorly across the blood-brain barrier, whereas CO_2 diffuses freely into the cerebrospinal fluid. The use of bicarbonate may worsen acidosis within the central nervous system while serum acidosis improves [45]. Rapid correction of acidosis causes hypokalemia, may aggravate sodium load, and contributes to serum hypertonicity. It also may impair tissue oxygenation by increasing the affinity of hemoglobin for oxygen (ie, shift the hemoglobin-oxygen dissociation curve to the left). Alkali therapy may increase hepatic ketone production and slow the rate of recovery from ketosis [46]. The use of bicarbonate in children with DKA is associated with an increased risk of cerebral edema (Box 3) [7].

Box 3. Complications of therapy

- Inadequate rehydration
- Hypoglycemia
- Hypokalemia
- Hyperchloremic acidosis
- Cerebral edema

Selected patients may benefit from cautious alkali therapy, including patients with severe acidemia (arterial pH<6.9), in whom decreased cardiac contractility and peripheral vasodilatation can further impair tissue perfusion, and patients with life-threatening hyperkalemia. Administration of bicarbonate is indicated when acidosis is severe (arterial pH$\leq$6.9) and when there is hypotension, shock, or an arrhythmia. In these circumstances, 1 to 2 mmol/kg or 40 to 80 mmol/m^2 of sodium bicarbonate is infused over 2 hours and the plasma bicarbonate level is rechecked. Bicarbonate should not be given as a bolus because this may precipitate an acute cardiac arrhythmia.

Clinical and biochemical monitoring

Initially, plasma glucose should be measured hourly. Thereafter, plasma glucose, serum electrolytes (and calculated sodium), pH, pCO$_2$, TCO$_2$, anion gap, calcium and phosphorus levels should be measured every 2 to 4 hours for the first 8 hours and then every 4 hours until they are normal. The data must be recorded carefully on a flow sheet.

In all patients, continuous cardiovascular and respiratory monitoring should be performed. The end-tidal CO$_2$ has been shown to correlate well with degree of acidosis in DKA, and noninvasive capnography may be used continuously to monitor the degree of metabolic acidosis [47–49]. The end-tidal CO$_2$ can be expected to rise steadily toward normal (35–45 mm Hg) in the successfully treated patient. If the end-tidal CO$_2$ begins to trend downward, immediate investigation must be undertaken of the insulin infusion and a patient's neurologic status. Conversely, an upward trend in end-tidal CO$_2$ in an increasingly somnolent patient may be a sign of hypoventilation and evolving cerebral edema.

Investigating the cause of ketoacidosis

The management of DKA is not complete until its cause has been identified and treated. Leukocytosis is common but most likely reflects the severity of DKA rather than the presence of infection; most children with DKA have no evidence of infection [50]. An intercurrent infection is not the usual cause when a patient is properly educated in diabetes management, is receiving regular follow-up care by a competent physician, and has access to a diabetes treatment team [51,52]. In previously diagnosed patients on treatment with insulin, omission of insulin— either inadvertently or deliberately—is the most common cause [52,53]. There is often an important psychosocial reason for insulin omission, including an attempt by an adolescent girl with an eating disorder to lose weight, a means of escaping an intolerable or abusive home situation, clinical depression, or the inability of a patient to manage his or her own diabetes unassisted [11]. A psychiatric social worker or clinical psychologist should be consulted to help to identify the psychosocial reasons underlying the development of DKA.

The following calculations are useful for managing DKA [54]:

Effective osmolality $2[Na^+ + K^+] + glucose\ (mg/dL)/18$

Corrected sodium $= [Na^+]$
$$+ (1.6 \times [plasma\ glucose\ mmol/L - 5.6] \div 5.6])$$

Anion gap $= [Na^+] - [Cl^- + HCO_3^-]$
Evaluation for pure metabolic acidosis:

$pCO_2 =$ last two numbers of the pH
$pCO_2 = 1.5\ [serum\ HCO_3^-] + 8 \pm 2$

Effective serum osmolality correlates with mental status abnormalities. Blood or serum urea nitrogen freely diffuses into cells and does not contribute to effective osmolality. Corrected serum sodium assists in estimation of free water deficits. A decreasing anion gap indicates successful therapy of metabolic acidosis. A lower than predicted pCO_2 indicates respiratory alkalosis and may be a clue to sepsis.

Morbidity and mortality from diabetic ketoacidosis in children

Reported mortality rates from DKA in national population-based studies are reasonably constant in the range of 0.15% to 0.31% [11]. In areas with sparse medical facilities, the risk of dying from DKA is greater, and children may succumb before receiving treatment. Cerebral edema accounts for 57% to 87% of all deaths from DKA. The incidence of cerebral edema has been fairly consistent between national population-based studies: 0.46% in Canada to 0.87% in the United States. Mortality rates from cerebral edema in population-based studies are 21% to 25%. Significant morbidity is evident in 10% to 26% of survivors. Other causes of DKA-related morbidity and mortality include hypokalemia, hyperkalemia, hypoglycemia, sepsis, venous thrombosis [55], and other central nervous system complications, such as cerebrovascular thrombosis with brain infarction [56].

Cerebral edema

Clinically significant cerebral edema may develop at any time during the first 24 hours of therapy. It is more common in children with severe DKA, new-onset type 1 diabetes, younger age, and longer duration of symptoms [7,8]. The cause(s) of CE remains poorly understood. It occurs to some extent (subclinical) in all patients with DKA [57]. Patients who require treatment are the subset of patients who have clinical symptoms or signs. The onset of symptoms typically occurs 4 to 12 hours after commencement of treatment but can occur before treatment has begun or at any time during treatment. Symptoms and signs vary and are shown in Box 4 [58]. Children who develop significant CE during DKA usually exhibit definable signs and symptoms of neurologic collapse early enough to allow intervention to prevent brain damage. Initial cranial CT scans may be reported as normal. The diagnosis of this complication must be based on clinical criteria at the bedside.

Based on data generated in animal models, researchers have thought that because of the presence of a chronic hyperosmolar state associated with hyperglycemia, the cerebral cells compete with the osmotic force of the serum by

---

Box 4. Bedside evaluation of neurologic state of children with diabetic ketoacidosis

Diagnostic criteria

- Abnormal motor or verbal response to pain
- Decorticate or decerebrate postures
- Cranial nerve palsy (especially III, IV, and VI)
- Abnormal neurogenic respiratory pattern (eg, grunting, tachypnea, Cheyne-Stokes respiration, apneusis)

Major criteria

- Altered mentation/fluctuating level of consciousness
- Sustained heart rate deceleration (decrease >20 beats/min) not attributable to improved intravascular volume or sleep state
- Age-inappropriate incontinence

Minor criteria

- Vomiting
- Headache
- Lethargic or not easily arousable
- Diastolic blood pressure more than 90 mm Hg
- Age younger than 5 years

One diagnostic criterion, two major criteria, or one major and two minor criteria have a sensitivity rate of 92% and a false-positive rate of 4% [58].

storing intracellular osmoles (primarily taurine). It has been thought that with therapy plasma glucose concentrations decline over several hours and the cytosolic osmolality becomes disproportionately high; water is attracted by osmosis, and cellular swelling occurs. This longstanding theory was challenged recently when MRI with diffusion-weighted analysis demonstrated that among 12 subjects with DKA, none demonstrated significant cellular edema [59]. The edema in this series of patients was vasogenic, or extracellular. Because none of the patients studied had severe cerebral edema, the possibility that cellular edema complicates vasogenic edema only in those patients who develop clinical symptomatology has not been ruled out.

Treatment of cerebral edema

Treatment of cerebral edema should be initiated as soon as the condition is suspected. The rate of fluid administration should be reduced. Intravenous mannitol (0.25–1 g/kg) should be given over 20 minutes and can be repeated, if necessary, in 2 hours if there is no initial response. Hypertonic saline (3%), 5 to 10 mL/kg over 30 minutes, may be an alternative to mannitol [60]. Intubation may be necessary for a patient with impending respiratory failure, but aggressive hyperventilation (to a $pCO_2 < 22$ mm Hg) has been associated with poor outcome and is not recommended [61].

Summary

Although DKA should, theoretically, be largely preventable in patients with established diabetes, a recent report from the Barbara David Center for Childhood Diabetes in Denver, Colorado showed that children with type 1 diabetes remain at high risk for DKA, with an incidence of 8 per 100 patient-years [10]. Children who are uninsured or underinsured, have psychiatric disorders, have poorly controlled diabetes, and live in dysfunctional families are most vulnerable. The efficacy and cost effectiveness of strategies to reduce the incidence of DKA, before diagnosis and in patients with established diabetes, are important issues for future investigation.

References

[1] Levy-Marchal C, Papoz L, de Beaufort C, et al. Clinical and laboratory features of type 1 diabetic children at the time of diagnosis. Diabet Med 1992;9:279–84.
[2] Komulainen J, Lounamaa R, Knip M, et al. Ketoacidosis at the diagnosis of type 1 (insulin dependent) diabetes mellitus is related to poor residual beta cell function: Childhood Diabetes in Finland study group. Arch Dis Child 1996;75:410–5.
[3] Komulainen J, Kulmala P, Savola K, et al. Clinical, autoimmune, and genetic characteristics of very young children with type 1 diabetes: Childhood Diabetes in Finland (DiMe) study group. Diabetes Care 1999;22:1950–5.

[4] Pinkey JH, Bingley PJ, Sawtell PA, et al. Presentation and progress of childhood diabetes mellitus: a prospective population-based study: The Bart's-Oxford study group. Diabetologia 1994;37:70–4.

[5] Curtis JR, To T, Muirhead S, et al. Recent trends in hospitalization for diabetic ketoacidosis in Ontario children. Diabetes Care 2002;25:1591–6.

[6] Edge JA, Ford-Adams ME, Dunger DB. Causes of death in children with insulin dependent diabetes 1990–96. Arch Dis Child 1999;81:318–23.

[7] Glaser N, Barnett P, McCaslin I, et al. Risk factors for cerebral edema in children with diabetic ketoacidosis: the Pediatric Emergency Medicine Collaborative Research Committee of the American Academy of Pediatrics [see comment]. N Engl J Med 2001;344:264–9.

[8] Edge JA, Hawkins MM, Winter DL, et al. The risk and outcome of cerebral oedema developing during diabetic ketoacidosis. Arch Dis Child 2001;85:16–22.

[9] Smith CP, Firth D, Bennett S, et al. Ketoacidosis occurring in newly diagnosed and established diabetic children. Acta Paediatr 1998;87:537–41.

[10] Rewers A, Chase HP, Mackenzie T, et al. Predictors of acute complications in children with type 1 diabetes. JAMA 2002;287:2511–8.

[11] Dunger DB, Sperling MA, Acerini CL, et al. European Society for Paediatric Endocrinology/ Lawson Wilkins Pediatric Endocrine Society consensus statement on diabetic ketoacidosis in children and adolescents. Pediatrics 2004;113:e133–40.

[12] Klekamp J, Churchwell KB. Diabetic ketoacidosis in children: initial clinical assessment and treatment. Pediatr Ann 1996;25:387–93.

[13] Adrogue HJ, Lederer ED, Suki WN, et al. Determinants of plasma potassium levels in diabetic ketoacidosis. Medicine 1986;65:163–72.

[14] Katz MA. Hyperglycemia-induced hyponatremia: calculation of expected serum sodium depression. N Engl J Med 1973;289:843–4.

[15] Hillier TA, Abbott RD, Barrett EJ. Hyponatremia: evaluating the correction factor for hyperglycemia [see comment]. Am J Med 1999;106:399–403.

[16] Harris GD, Fiordalisi I. Physiologic management of diabetic ketoacidemia: a 5-year prospective pediatric experience in 231 episodes. Arch Pediatr Adolesc Med 1994;148:1046–52.

[17] Linares MY, Schunk JE, Lindsay R. Laboratory presentation in diabetic ketoacidosis and duration of therapy. Pediatr Emerg Care 1996;12:347–51.

[18] Mackenzie A, Barnes G, Shann F. Clinical signs of dehydration in children [see comment]. Lancet 1989;2:605–7.

[19] Koves IH, Neutze J, Donath S, et al. The accuracy of clinical assessment of dehydration during diabetic ketoacidosis in childhood. Diabetes Care 2004;27:2485–7.

[20] Owen OE, Licht JH, Sapir DG. Renal function and effects of partial rehydration during diabetic ketoacidosis. Diabetes 1981;30:510–8.

[21] Waldhausl W, Kleinberger G, Korn A, et al. Severe hyperglycemia: effects of rehydration on endocrine derangements and blood glucose concentration. Diabetes 1979;28:577–84.

[22] Harris GD, Fiordalisi I, Yu C. Maintaining normal intracranial pressure in a rabbit model during treatment of severe diabetic ketoacidemia. Life Sci 1996;59:1695–702.

[23] Clements Jr RS, Blumenthal SA, Morrison AD, et al. Increased cerebrospinal-fluid pressure during treatment of diabetic ketosis. Lancet 1971;2:671–5.

[24] Felner EI, White PC. Improving management of diabetic ketoacidosis in children. Pediatrics 2001;108:735–40.

[25] Adrogue HJ, Barrero J, Eknoyan G. Salutary effects of modest fluid replacement in the treatment of adults with diabetic ketoacidosis: use in patients without extreme volume deficit. JAMA 1989;262:2108–13.

[26] Harris GD, Fiordalisi I, Harris WL, et al. Minimizing the risk of brain herniation during treatment of diabetic ketoacidemia: a retrospective and prospective study [see comment]. J Pediatr 1990;117:22–31 [erratum appears in J Pediatr 1991;118(1):166–7].

[27] Burghen GA, Etteldorf JN, Fisher JN, et al. Comparison of high-dose and low-dose insulin by continuous intravenous infusion in the treatment of diabetic ketoacidosis in children. Diabetes Care 1980;3:15–20.

[28] Butkiewicz EK, Leibson CL, O'Brien PC, et al. Insulin therapy for diabetic ketoacidosis: bolus insulin injection versus continuous insulin infusion. Diabetes Care 1995;18:1187–90.

[29] Umpierrez GE, Latif K, Stoever J, et al. Efficacy of subcutaneous insulin lispro versus continuous intravenous regular insulin for the treatment of patients with diabetic ketoacidosis [see comment]. Am J Med 2004;117:291–6.

[30] Lindsay R, Bolte RG. The use of an insulin bolus in low-dose insulin infusion for pediatric diabetic ketoacidosis. Pediatr Emerg Care 1989;5:77–9.

[31] Atchley D, Loeb R, Richards D. On diabetic acidosis: a detailed study of electrolyte balances following withdrawal and reestablishment of therapy. J Clin Invest 1933;12:297–326.

[32] Nabarro JDN, Spencer AG, Stowers JM. Metabolic studies in severe diabetic ketosis. Q J Med 1952;82:225–48.

[33] Danowski T, Peters J. Studies in diabetic acidosis and coma, with particular emphasis on the retention of administered potassium. J Clin Invest 1949;28:1–9.

[34] Butler A, Talbot N. Metabolic studies in diabetic coma. Trans Assoc Am Physicians 1947;60: 102–9.

[35] Darrow DC, Pratt EL. Retention of water and electrolyte during recovery in a patient with diabetic acidosis. J Pediatr 1952;41:688–96.

[36] Gibby OM, Veale KE, Hayes TM, et al. Oxygen availability from the blood and the effect of phosphate replacement on erythrocyte 2,3-diphosphoglycerate and haemoglobin-oxygen affinity in diabetic ketoacidosis. Diabetologia 1978;15:381–5.

[37] Keller U, Berger W. Prevention of hypophosphatemia by phosphate infusion during treatment of diabetic ketoacidosis and hyperosmolar coma. Diabetes 1980;29:87–95.

[38] Wilson HK, Keuer SP, Lea AS, et al. Phosphate therapy in diabetic ketoacidosis. Arch Intern Med 1982;142:517–20.

[39] Becker DJ, Brown DR, Steranka BH, et al. Phosphate replacement during treatment of diabetic ketosis: effects on calcium and phosphorus homeostasis. Am J Dis Child 1983;137:241–6.

[40] Fisher JN, Kitabchi AE. A randomized study of phosphate therapy in the treatment of diabetic ketoacidosis. J Clin Endocrinol Metab 1983;57:177–80.

[41] Clerbaux T, Reynaert M, Willems E, et al. Effect of phosphate on oxygen-hemoglobin affinity, diphosphoglycerate and blood gases during recovery from diabetic ketoacidosis. Intensive Care Med 1989;15:495–8.

[42] Hale PJ, Crase J, Nattrass M. Metabolic effects of bicarbonate in the treatment of diabetic ketoacidosis. Br Med J (Clin Res Ed) 1984;289:1035–8.

[43] Morris LR, Murphy MB, Kitabchi AE. Bicarbonate therapy in severe diabetic ketoacidosis. Ann Intern Med 1986;105:836–40.

[44] Green SM, Rothrock SG, Ho JD, et al. Failure of adjunctive bicarbonate to improve outcome in severe pediatric diabetic ketoacidosis. Ann Emerg Med 1998;31:41–8.

[45] Assal JP, Aoki TT, Manzano FM, et al. Metabolic effects of sodium bicarbonate in management of diabetic ketoacidosis. Diabetes 1974;23:405–11.

[46] Okuda Y, Adrogue HJ, Field JB, et al. Counterproductive effects of sodium bicarbonate in diabetic ketoacidosis. J Clin Endocrinol Metab 1996;81:314–20.

[47] Agus MS, Alexander JA, Mantell P. Continuous non-invasive CO2 monitoring in pediatric inpatients with diabetic ketoacidosis. Diabetes 2004;53:A67.

[48] Fearon DM, Steele DW. End-tidal carbon dioxide predicts the presence and severity of acidosis in children with diabetes. Acad Emerg Med 2002;9:1373–8.

[49] Garcia E, Abramo TJ, Okada P, et al. Capnometry for noninvasive continuous monitoring of metabolic status in pediatric diabetic ketoacidosis [see comment]. Crit Care Med 2003;31: 2539–43.

[50] Flood RG, Chiang VW. Rate and prediction of infection in children with diabetic ketoacidosis. Am J Emerg Med 2001;19:270–3.

[51] Jacobson AM, Hauser ST, Willett J, et al. Consequences of irregular versus continuous medical follow-up in children and adolescents with insulin-dependent diabetes mellitus. J Pediatr 1997; 131:727–33.

[52] Thompson CJ, Cummings F, Chalmers J, et al. Abnormal insulin treatment behaviour: a major cause of ketoacidosis in the young adult. Diabet Med 1995;12:429–32.

[53] Morris AD, Boyle DI, McMahon AD, et al. Adherence to insulin treatment, glycaemic control, and ketoacidosis in insulin-dependent diabetes mellitus: the DARTS/MEMO Collaboration. Diabetes Audit and Research in Tayside, Scotland. Medicines Monitoring Unit [see comment]. Lancet 1997;350:1505–10.

[54] Fleckman AM. Diabetic ketoacidosis. Endocrinol Metab Clin North Am 1993;22:181–207.

[55] Gutierrez JA, Bagatell R, Samson MP, et al. Femoral central venous catheter-associated deep venous thrombosis in children with diabetic ketoacidosis. Crit Care Med 2003;31:80–3.

[56] Roe TF, Crawford TO, Huff KR, et al. Brain infarction in children with diabetic ketoacidosis. J Diabetes Complications 1996;10:100–8.

[57] Krane EJ, Rockoff MA, Wallman JK, et al. Subclinical brain swelling in children during treatment of diabetic ketoacidosis. N Engl J Med 1985;312:1147–51.

[58] Muir AB, Quisling RG, Yang MC, et al. Cerebral edema in childhood diabetic ketoacidosis: natural history, radiographic findings, and early identification. Diabetes Care 2004;27:1541–6.

[59] Glaser NS, Wootton-Gorges SL, Marcin JP, et al. Mechanism of cerebral edema in children with diabetic ketoacidosis [see comment]. J Pediatr 2004;145:164–71.

[60] Kamat P, Vats A, Gross M, et al. Use of hypertonic saline for the treatment of altered mental status associated with diabetic ketoacidosis. Pediatr Crit Care Med 2003;4:239–42.

[61] Marcin JP, Glaser N, Barnett P, et al. Factors associated with adverse outcomes in children with diabetic ketoacidosis-related cerebral edema [see comment]. J Pediatr 2002;141:793–7.

ELSEVIER
SAUNDERS

PEDIATRIC CLINICS
OF NORTH AMERICA

Pediatr Clin N Am 52 (2005) 1165–1187

Hospitalist Care of the Medically Complex Child

Rajendu Srivastava, MD, FRCP(C), MPH[a,b,*],
Bryan L. Stone, MD[a], Nancy A. Murphy, MD[a]

[a]Department of Pediatrics, University of Utah School of Medicine, 100 North Medical Drive,
Salt Lake City, UT 84132, USA
[b]Institute for Health Care Delivery Research, Intermountain Health Care, 36 South State Street,
21st Floor, Salt Lake City, UT 84111, USA

The nature of inpatient pediatrics is changing. Over the past decade, several factors have converged to influence the kinds of children currently being hospitalized. Managed care organizations have been under increasing pressure to control costs and reduce unnecessary prolonged hospital stays. Many emergency departments are using observational units to avoid hospitalizations while reserving inpatient wards for higher acuity and complex patients [1]. There has been a shift in the perception in the minds of clinicians as to what constitutes an appropriate hospital stay and what may be treated on an outpatient basis. Therapies such as home oxygen for certain pediatric conditions (eg, bronchiolitis) and home intravenous therapy for fluids and medications are being used increasingly. These developments have produced a shift in the relative proportion of otherwise healthy children with simple, self-limited acute illness being hospitalized to children with chronic illnesses presenting with acute exacerbations or consequences of their underlying illnesses being cared for in the hospital [2]. This article focuses on hospitalist care of these medically complex children (MCC) and provides an overview on (1) the challenges in defining this population, (2) the unique issues surrounding their inpatient care (using a family-centered care approach that includes coordinated care, minimizing secondary complications, nutritional needs, functional limitations, transdisciplinary collaboration, and pri-

---

* Corresponding author. Department of Pediatrics, University of Utah School of Medicine, 100 North Medical Drive, Salt Lake City, UT 84132.
E-mail address: raj.srivastava@hsc.utah.edu (R. Srivastava).

0031-3955/05/$ – see front matter © 2005 Elsevier Inc. All rights reserved.
doi:10.1016/j.pcl.2005.03.007

pediatric.theclinics.com

mary care issues), (3) technology devices commonly found, and (4) a proposal for a research agenda regarding MCC.

Defining the medically complex child

Defining this population has been challenging for health services researchers and clinicians. Several recent initiatives have shaped the current conceptual model. In 2001, the Institute of Medicine recommended that the Agency for Health care Research and Quality identify "15 priority conditions, taking into account frequency of occurrence, health burden, and resource use" [3]. The Institute of Medicine identified children with special health care needs (CSHCN) as a priority population [3,4]. Researchers and experts in this field have published the following definition: "Children with special health care needs are those who have or are at increased risk for a chronic physical, developmental, behavioral, or emotional condition and who also require health and related services of a type or amount beyond that required by children generally" [5]. Although CSHCN comprise between 13% and 18% of all children [6], they account for more than 80% of the cost of health care for children in the United States [5]. CSHCN are two to three times more likely than other children to have unmet health care needs that ultimately lead to belated, dramatic, and expensive interventions [7]. Children with chronic health conditions are three times more likely to have an unscheduled intensive care unit admission than healthy children, and 32% of these admissions are judged to be potentially preventable [8]. Of the potentially preventable events, 64% are related to health care system deficiencies, such as inadequate care coordination. Medical errors are an especially important example of preventable events, and errors in care for CSHCN are likely to be higher than for other children because of the complexity of their care [9,10]. Because these children are approximately four times as likely as children without disabilities to be hospitalized and, once hospitalized spend eight times as many days in the hospital, the total impact of health care system deficiencies in CSHCN is substantial [11].

The importance of understanding and improving care for CSHCN is widely recognized, but research to date has done little to improve measurably the quality of care that these children receive. A major reason for this deficiency is that CSHCN comprise a heterogeneous group with a multitude of conditions and diagnoses, each of which affects a relatively small group of children [12]. Single-center studies focused on children with a particular diagnosis suffer from small sample sizes, and results are rarely generalizable. Researchers recently moved toward a consequence-based definition for CSHCN in an attempt to capitalize on the similarities among diagnoses and allow for more robust statistical studies with greater clinical relevance [13–20]. Development of operational, valid, and easily administered methods of identifying CSHCN is challenging. To identify these children, several studies have used various survey-based tools, categorical lists that use codes as defined in the International Classification of Diseases

(ICD-9 CM), or methods that use administrative databases to predict children who are high resource users (as measured by cost or length of stay). Each approach has its own limitations; survey tools are generally laborious (with the exception of the CSHCN screener designed and validated in the outpatient setting by the Foundation for Accountability) [21,22], and the categorical lists or predictors of high resource use may be performed only after a patient is discharged from the hospital and the data are abstracted from administrative data.

What is urgently needed is a method to identify prospectively the subset of CSHCN who are medically complex. These children share several similar features that may be understood best by examining an example (Box 1).

Prospective, feasible identification would allow hospitalists to maximize the effectiveness of the hospital stay of these patients. For example, imagine a child with neurologic impairments who is repeatedly hospitalized for acute illnesses or elective surgical procedures who presents to the inpatient service. Patients such as these typically require an enormous amount of resources and services that ideally would be engaged at admission, such as social work to see how the family is coping and to review the current financial situation and need for assistance; pharmacy to review medications, look for interactions, and recheck dosing at home compared with directions written upon admission; physical and occupational therapy to assess how a patient is functioning and how best to maximize function and prevent the patient from developing any secondary complications (eg, decubitus ulcer or another aspiration episode). Typically these health care professionals would assess and treat the patient only once the hospitalist wrote the orders. A prospective identification method could be used to activate services

---

Box 1. Prototypic example of a medically complex child: the child with neurologic impairments

Diversity of conditions (eg, brain tumors, intraventricular hemorrhage, traumatic brain injury, tuberous sclerosis, congenital brain anomalies, cerebral palsy with global developmental delay)
Multisystemic disease (eg, respiratory, neurologic, gastrointestinal)
Multiple medications (eg, bronchodilators, anti-sialagogues, anti-convulsants, gastric motility agents)
Multiple specialists (eg, pulmonologist for recurrent aspiration pneumonia, otolaryngologist for salivary gland management, neurologist for seizures, gastroenterologist and surgeon for the management of gastroesophageal reflux disease)
Important subsets (eg, children who depend on technology)
Frequent admissions (eg, for recurrent aspiration pneumonia, seizures, antireflux surgeries)
Critical need for optimal coordination of their care in the inpatient and the outpatient settings

to care for these patients, however, and help the hospitalist coordinate inpatient care and ultimate discharge to the primary care provider.

Several definitions commonly are used in the literature to describe other subgroups of children with chronic medical conditions, such as technology-dependent children and medically fragile children. This terminology history was reviewed by Newacheck et al [5] in 1998. Although a formal definition is lacking, we prefer the term "medically complex children"(MCC) to capture the principles as outlined previously. Throughout this article we use the term "medically complex children" to be concise; however, we are more correctly referring to children with complex medical care needs.

Unique issues of inpatient care

A comprehensive approach by pediatric hospitalists is essential for delivering effective, efficient, coordinated, and family-centered care that best meets the multifaceted needs of these children and their families. Twenty-two percent of recurrent hospital admissions for children with chronic illness are related to medical controversy regarding the most appropriate treatment strategy, and approximately 33% are associated with medical dependency [23]. In general, parents of children with disabilities are less satisfied with medical care when compared with children with other medical conditions [24]. Increased patient and family satisfaction with in-hospital care may promote adherence with post-discharge care plans, minimize readmissions, and ultimately improve the health and well-being of MCC. When approaching MCC, hospitalists are encouraged to treat the "whole child" in the context of function rather than diagnosis-specific or organ-based categories [25–27]. In facilitating the coordination of care, pediatric hospitalists can ensure that the focus remains on the child and his or her function at the level of the individual, the family, and the community.

The American Academy of Pediatrics defined the medical home in 1992 [28] and further developed the concepts that focus on CSHCN. The medical home is characterized by care that is accessible, family centered, continuous, comprehensive, coordinated, compassionate, and culturally effective [29,30]. Although these principles apply primarily to ambulatory care, we believe that this model of care is a valuable way to view key elements of the inpatient care of children with complex medical conditions. For some of these children, hospitalists may find themselves as the inpatient medical home physician (especially for children without a primary care physician).

Family-centered care

Parents of MCC with associated complex medical regimens have responsibilities that differ from those of typical parents. They are responsible not only for the physical care of their children but also for dealing with medical, educational, and other service providers while balancing competing family needs

[31]. Parents of children with cerebral palsy have more chronic physical ailments, including back pain, migraine headaches, and stomach/intestinal ulcers, and higher overall distress when compared with other parents [32]. Caregivers of technology-dependent children experience more anxiety, anger, guilt, frustration, sorrow, social isolation, sleep deprivation, and depression when compared with parents of able-bodied children [33]. Thirty percent of all recurrent hospitalizations for children with chronic illnesses are related to a lack of respite services and community support, and 26% are related to psychological or medical issues that affect other family members [23]. There is an association between the health and well-being of MCC and that of their parents. Given the vital role that families play in providing care to MCC, it is critically important that hospitalists acknowledge parents as caregivers and position them centrally on inpatient treatment teams for their children.

In family-centered systems of care, parents are well informed, supported, and afforded ultimate control over decisions regarding the care of their child. Such care is associated with improvements in parents' emotional well-being, satisfaction with services, and the burden experienced [34]. The concept of family-centered care as described by the American Academy of Pediatrics includes physician recognition of key family members and their values and shared decision making between medical providers and families [35]. Pediatric hospitalists can promote family-centered care by regarding parents as the experts in their child's condition and including them in all facets of inpatient care.

Coordinated care

In inpatient settings, care coordination involves managing treatment planning and outcomes monitoring, coordinating input from subspecialists, organizing care to avoid duplication of services, sharing information among health care professionals and family members, managing discharge planning, and family training [36,37]. Hospitalists can lead transdisciplinary team meetings as a forum for care coordination through the establishment of common goals for hospitalization, the development and revision of care plans, and the defining of discharge criteria [38]. Up-to-date care plans that clearly include a problem list, key elements of a child's history, and therapeutic interventions can serve as an efficient and effective means of communication and care coordination [110]. Care plans should be accessible to the family and all members of the transdisciplinary treatment team [39]. Care coordination offers the additional advantage of minimizing hospital-reported medical errors, which occur more often with MCC [9,10].

Discharge planning is a key element of care coordination. The arrangement of home care services for skilled nurses, allied care providers, and durable medical equipment (eg, ventilators, suction machines, and feeding pumps) requires time and effort [40]. Early anticipation of discharge needs smoothes transitions from hospitals to homes for MCC and their families. Before discharge, the inpatient team should ensure the safety and accessibility of a child's home and the availability of uninterrupted phone, electrical, and transportation services for children who depend on medical technology [39,41]. In cooperation with parents, discharge planners can facilitate the scheduling of numerous recommended follow-up appointments. Hospitalists should communicate a timely summary of the hospitalization and recommendations for follow-up to the primary care physician to further ease the transition of MCC to their medical home. Novel approaches to maximize this transfer of the complexity of information between settings are urgently needed for this population, because the number and types of errors caused by the transitions of care are likely to be dramatic. One novel approach that focused on shared care plans and clinical care specialists in Whatcom County, Washington, was highlighted at the 2004 Institute for Health Improvement's annual forum, and a series of videos is being prepared to be released for television in 2006 [42].

Minimizing secondary complications

Although an acute illness prompts hospitalization for MCC, there are always concomitant comorbid conditions. Hospitalists must remain alert to the potential for exacerbation of these underlying conditions caused by the interdependent nature of organ systems and not focus solely on resolution of the acute illness. A complete medical history should include details of daily schedules, medications, diet, patterns of sleep, typical stool output, functional status, and usual behaviors and activities. This depth of information allows unfamiliar health care providers to identify and address promptly any secondary complications that may prolong hospitalization and increase stress for families. Most MCC require many medications for various standard and "off-label" indications on a long-term basis, which renders them at increased risk for drug interactions and medical errors [9]. Hospitalists should review with parents the dose, route, frequency, and indication of each medication, including homeopathic and over-the-counter medications. For example, valproic acid may be prescribed for aggressive outbursts and gabapentin may be prescribed for neuropathic pain syndromes. The assumption that either of these medications is administered to treat seizures would be an error. During the usual review of food and drug allergies, the hospitalist should explore each child's history of latex reactions, especially when caring for children who have had multiple reactions. A review of the home medication schedule reveals meaningful information, such as administration of phenytoin with meals rather than nonadherence as an explanation for subtherapeutic blood levels.

Nutritional needs

The nutritional needs of children with chronic conditions warrant special consideration during hospitalizations. Upon admission, hospitalists should discuss with families the details of their child's feeding program including route (eg, oral, tube feedings), content (eg, altered texture, preferred foods), and mealtime schedule. When children are fed at home with adapted cups, spoons, nipples, oral stimulation techniques, or positioning strategies, similar feeding approaches should be providing during the hospitalization. Nutritional assessments and periodic reassessments are indicated during every hospitalization. In addition to plotting heights and weights on standard growth curves, for certain populations (eg, children with Down syndrome) growth parameters can be plotted on specialized growth curves. The intake of calories and fluids should be monitored regularly. Intervention with enteral feedings or hyperalimentation is started when nutritional intake or status is deemed inadequate, particularly for children with dysphagia and a decreased likelihood of regaining weight lost during acute illness.

Functional limitations

Many children with chronic conditions also experience functional limitations and benefit from adaptive equipment, including standers, wheelchairs, and orthotics, during hospitalization to promote independence and mobility. Children should participate in their usual activities as much as possible to minimize complications of immobility (eg, constipation, atelectasis, joint contractures, muscle deconditioning). Hospitalists can consult with physical, occupational, and speech therapists to ensure that the necessary equipment and support are available for each child.

Transdisciplinary coordination

Hospitalization can be stressful and disruptive for MCC and their families. Pediatric hospitalists can collaborate with child life specialists, chaplains, social workers, and other treatment team members to address their emotional needs. Efforts to minimize disruption of schoolwork are encouraged, and schoolwork should continue when possible. Strategies for return to school after discharge should be developed. Educational consultants should guide parents in negotiating the school services best suited to their child's unique needs, including special educational programming through an individualized educational plan. For children unable to return to school in the short term, homebound education can be prescribed for a period of time.

Primary care issues

CSHCN have more unmet medical needs than typically developing children [43]. Because hospitalists and specialists provide most of their care, well-child care issues may be overlooked. Hospitalists should provide missed immunizations or prophylaxis against influenza, respiratory syncytial virus, or pneumococcal infections as needed. Hospitalization may be a time to consider programs of early intervention, discuss eligibility for social security, or explore community-based services for recreation and socialization.

Application of the concepts

Because the scope of diagnoses involved when considering children who are "medically complex" or "technology-dependent" or have "special health care needs" is broad, we chose children with cerebral palsy as the model of MCC. Children with cerebral palsy present a heterogeneous group of disabilities that range from mild motor impairments to complex developmental and functional limitations. The breadth of experience of children with cerebral palsy and their families is expected to generalize to various developmental disabilities [44].

Consider a child with quadriplegic cerebral palsy. She has global developmental delays, spasticity, gastrointestinal dysmotility, dysphagia with gastrostomy tube dependency, failure to thrive, epilepsy, neuromuscular scoliosis, and functional limitations. Let us assume that she is hospitalized with acute respiratory distress secondary to interstitial viral pneumonia. Because of her tachypnea, feedings are held for 3 days, after which she improves with a regimen of chest physical therapy, postural drainage, and supportive care. She then experiences a generalized tonic clonic seizure, however, which is associated with vomiting and significant aspiration pneumonitis. Was this an avoidable event? On careful review, it is noted that when gastrostomy tube feedings were resumed, formula was delivered continuously rather than in periodic boluses. Although she had stable epilepsy with therapeutic phenytoin levels upon admission, a random serum phenytoin level at the time of her seizure was grossly subtherapeutic. In hindsight, it is evident that her parents provided intermittent gastrostomy tube feedings at home and gave her phenytoin at least 1 hour before or 2 hours after meals to ensure adequate absorption [45,46]. Familiarity with all details of her care should alert the hospitalist to potential food and drug interactions in this child.

After recovering from the seizure and aspiration pneumonitis, the girl with quadriplegic cerebral palsy is clinically improving and discharge is anticipated in 1 to 2 days. She then develops recurrent emesis with feeding intolerance. On physical examination, her abdomen is moderately distended but nontender. Radiographs confirm fecal impaction with obstipation, which is not surprising in a child with gastrointestinal dysmotility exacerbated by immobilization, interrupted enteral feedings, and analgesic medications. Constipation in children with cerebral palsy can present as anorexia, abdominal pain, sleep disturbances, irritability, urinary retention, nausea, and vomiting. Because these nonspecific symptoms could suggest several illnesses, a standardized comprehensive care process for MCC is a primary strategy to the anticipation, prevention, and early recognition of common complications of hospitalization such as this.

Finally, the patient is ready for discharge. When her parents are dressing her in anticipation of going home, they are upset to find a decubitus overlying her left ischium. Pressures sores can develop quickly in children with compromised nutrition, depleted fat stores, and bed rest [47]. A standardized care process approach would anticipate and reduce the increased risk during hospitalization of this preventable complication.

Technologic devices for medically complex children

Hospitalists should be familiar with enterostomy tubes, tracheostomy, indwelling central venous catheters, noninvasive ventilatory support, and ventricular shunts in terms of indications, complications, and the hospital-based evaluation of these devices.

Enterostomy tubes

Children who depend on feeding technologies have a long-term gastrostomy, gastrojejunostomy (GJ), or jejunostomy tube. Indications for enterostomy tubes include oral motor feeding problems, mechanical esophagopharyngeal occlusion/stricture/atresia for any reason, inadequate oral caloric intake for growth, altered adsorption or metabolism that requires constant infusion nutrition, unpalatable diets as disease treatment, excess unpalatable medications (such as in HIV), and conditions requiring venting of the stomach for obstruction. GJ or jejunostomy tubes are used for patients with severe gastroesophageal reflux and individuals at high risk for aspiration. Neurologically impaired children comprise the largest category of patients who depend on enterostomy tube feedings, with failure to thrive and risk of aspiration being two primary indications [48].

Tubes are placed surgically with laparotomy or laparoscopy or are placed percutaneously with endoscopic or radiologic guidance. Surgical placement is usually accomplished with another primary surgery, such as fundoplication for gastroesophageal reflux. GJ tubes simply add guided placement of a tube into the jejunum.

Complications of gastrostomy are divided into "early or late," and "major or minor." Early major complications are more common with surgical placement (19.9%) than percutaneous endoscopic gastrostomy (9.4%) or percutaneous radiologic gastrostomy (5.9%), which offers the least risk [49]. Minor and late complications are independent of the approach. Overall, complications that lead to gastrostomy tube revisions occur in 6% of children [50]. Tube design and location can influence risk of late complications; GJ tubes have higher risk [51,52]. Major complications include procedure-related aspiration pneumonia [53], dislodgement before tract maturation, gastrointestinal bleeding, peritonitis, severe wound/abdominal wall infection, intussusception, gastrocolocutaneous fistula, sepsis, and death. Major complications are heralded by typical signs and symptoms that may be more difficult to recognize in the neurologically impaired enterostomy population. Pneumoperitoneum is common with tube placement, may be a complication in very small infants [54], and can obscure the diagnosis of some major early complications in all children. Worsening of gastroesophageal reflux is reported in some studies, particularly in neurologically impaired children, but not all studies support this finding [55]. Careful consideration of the need for fundoplication surgery should precede enterostomy.

Minor complications include tube dislodgement after tract maturation, tube blockage, migration, leakage, gastrostomy tube site infection, granulation tissue formation and "buried bumper syndrome." Recognition of minor complications can be straightforward for tube dislodgement and blockage, whereas other presentations may be obscure. Vomiting with a gastrostomy tube may indicate migration with blockage of the duodenum by the balloon or malposition; with GJ tubes, it may indicate leakage in the gastric coil, back-migration or malposition into the stomach, and intussusception. Diarrhea "like formula" or aspiration of fecal material may indicate a gastrocolocutaneous fistula. Redness at the site may be caused by tape sensitivity, leakage, granulation tissue, or infection. Tube leakage should be distinguished from gastric contents leakage around the tube. Excess mobility of the tube may enlarge the tract and lead to gastric leakage, which can be difficult to treat. For gastric contents leakage, air drying, barrier agents, and sucralfate powder may help. Using an acid-reducing agent, placing a temporary GJ tube, ordering no oral intake for the child with gastrostomy tube suction, and removing the tube for hours or days to allow the tract to heal and shrink may be necessary. Granulation tissue tends to be friable and bleed easily. If present, it can be treated with warm saline compresses and may need cautery with silver nitrate. Buried bumper syndrome occurs when excess traction leads to the internal bumper eroding through the stomach wall, with re-epithelialization covering or burying the bumper. Symptoms may include abdominal pain with feedings, resistance to flow through the tube, and inability to rotate the tube. Treatment requires tube removal and replacement.

Approximately 20% of patients experience infection; it is usually local but may progress to cellulitis and, rarely, necrotizing fasciitis [49]. Local infection can be treated with cleaning and use of local antibacterial agents and oral antibiotics. Cellulitis requires systemic antibiotics, and necrotizing fasciitis is a surgical/infectious emergency.

Tube blockage is best treated by prevention. Treatment of blockage includes using water, pancreatic enzymes, and carbonated drinks. Tube dislodgement before 4 weeks is a major complication because tract maturation occurs between 4 weeks and 3 months. It likely requires a repeat procedure, with peritonitis being a potential complication caused by separation of the stomach wall from the inner abdominal wall. A mature stoma still may close within hours to days if the tube is dislodged. Parents may be taught to insert gently a temporary Foley catheter, with the balloon deflated, until its location can be determined radiologically if it occurs within 8 weeks of placement. After that, a correct sized Foley catheter or a spare gastrostomy tube can be reinserted gently followed by balloon inflation. If gastric contents are aspirated and air injection verifies the correct position, feedings can be reinstituted until proper replacement. Many gastrostomy tubes are currently replaced by a low-profile "button" within 2 to 4 months. Removal and replacement of a button requires special expertise and equipment that may necessitate consultation with the service that placed the gastrostomy tube. A dislodged button still necessitates placement of a Foley catheter to maintain patency of the ostomy until the button can be replaced.

Jejunal tubes have unique potential complications. Because of the size of the small bowel, a smaller internal bumper is needed, which leads to difficulties anchoring the tube and incurs higher risk of dislodgement. Gastrointestinal complaints are also higher, including abdominal distention, pain, tenderness, and diarrhea. Small intestinal ischemia and necrosis can develop as a consequence of direct small bowel feeding, particularly in hemodynamically unstable patients. An ostomy care nurse can be invaluable in troubleshooting enterostomy tube problems for the pediatric hospitalist who cares for such patients.

Tracheostomy

Tracheostomy tubes are indicated in cases of upper airway obstruction, for children who cannot protect their airway, and for patients with long-term mechanical ventilation. Children usually remain hospitalized until the first tube change, which allows some maturation of the stoma. Optimal tracheostomy care starts with the proper tube of appropriate size and shape to fit the airway without exerting pressure on the tracheal mucosa. It also must fit well enough to prevent aspiration (if that is its primary purpose) or loosely enough to allow translaryngeal air escape for vocalization and mucous clearance. It must have an adequate inside diameter to prevent airflow restriction. This should be tailored to each child's specific circumstances.

Standards of care in the hospital should include 24-hour 1:1 care from a provider trained in acute troubleshooting of tracheostomy complications. Frequent respiratory therapist care and input, attention to clearing of secretions, humidification, and ready availability of a replacement tracheostomy tube that matches the patient's tube—and one size smaller—are also essential. Most pediatric tracheostomy tubes are not cuffed; if a cuffed tube is used, that fact should be apparent to all caregivers who might provide emergency management. One should notify the otolaryngology or general surgery services of the patient's admission and the potential for emergency airway management needs.

Complications include accidental decannulation, creating of a false passage, obstruction, infection, hemorrhage, pneumothorax, pneumomediastinum, peritracheal cellulitis, and lower airway infection. Although accidental decannulation and obstruction are the most common overall complications, they are rarely encountered in the inpatient setting. Because of their acuity, they are rapidly addressed by bedside caregivers and rarely impact the hospitalist directly. Peritracheal infection usually can be treated with oral antibiotics and local wound care, but it can lead to mediastinitis if not addressed. Lower respiratory tract infections are common. Children with tracheostomies are colonized with multiple pathogens, including *Staphylococcus aureus*, *Pseudomonas aeruginosa*, and *Candida albicans*. Empiric antibiotic therapy should reflect this. A rare (1%–2%), life-threatening complication is erosion into the innominate artery, which leads to massive hemorrhage. Extensive hemorrhage in the postoperative period or significant hemorrhage after the first 48 hours should prompt evaluation for this critical complication.

Perhaps the single most important preparation for safe home tracheostomy management is good training of at least two adult caregivers. Although the mortality rate of children with tracheostomy is 11% to 40%, death from a tracheostomy complication is rare. In January 2000, the Pediatric Assembly of the American Thoracic Society published a consensus statement to serve as a standard of pediatric tracheostomy care that provides detailed guidelines and the evidence supporting it [56].

Long-term intravenous access catheters

Many patients currently require extended or long-term intermittent intravenous medication, frequent blood draws, or parenteral hyperalimentation. There are three general categories of central venous catheters (CVCs): (1) external partially implanted (Broviac, Hickman, Groshong), (2) totally implanted with a subcutaneous port (Portacath, Mediport, Infusaport), and (3) percutaneously inserted (PICC line). Whereas the first two CVCs are inserted for long-term access, with reported durations of 12 to 32 months [57,58], PICC lines are used for briefer periods, with reported average durations varying from 16.6 to 72.7 days [59,60]. Complications associated with CVCs include thrombosis, infection, malfunction (discussed later in detail), fractures or breaks, dislodgement, noninfectious phlebitis, and air embolism. Cardiac dysrhythmia, mediastinitis, cardiac tamponade, hemorrhage, and pneumothorax can occur more commonly as acute complications of line placement and must be considered in the first hours after placement. Factors associated with removal of a line are primarily completion of therapy but also include infection (eg, gram-negative bacilli and yeast), migration, use for obtaining blood samples rather than infusion alone, catheter material (polyurethane > silicone), and mechanical failure.

Thrombosis occurs with all CVCs. Symptomatic vascular thrombosis is less common, with reported rates of 4.6% to 9%, but is still the primary cause of thrombosis in children [61]. Thrombosis may involve only the catheter (obstruction) or the insertion vessel (subclavian vein) with ipsilateral limb venous outflow obstruction and associated symptoms, or it may extend centrally into the superior vena cava and lead to clinical signs and symptoms of superior vena cava syndrome. Pulmonary embolus is an underdiagnosed complication [62]. Asymptomatic pulmonary embolus was diagnosed indirectly by ECG or echocardiographic criteria in 12 of 21 (57%) children with a long-term CVC in one study [63]. The clinical relevance of asymptomatic pulmonary embolus remains unstudied, however.

Infections may involve the skin at the exit site, the subcutaneous tunnel, or systemic line sepsis. Reported rates of infection vary from 4% to 60%, with rates of line sepsis ranging from 4% to 9%. Factors associated with a higher risk of infection include frequency of accessing the line, the first month after placement or more than 24 months of use, and thrombosis/fibrin sheath formation [64–66]. The most common organisms are skin flora, but in immunocompromised children, gram-negative bacilli and yeast are recovered. Treatment initially involves empiric antibiotics and then proceeds to appropriate antibiotics based on culture results. Most gram-positive bacteremias/sepsis can be treated successfully without CVC removal. If bacteremia recurs after treatment, the CVC can be sterilized successfully with an "antibiotic lock," usually with vancomycin and a thrombolytic agent, such as urokinase. A prospective, randomized, double-blind trial compared prophylactic "antibiotic lock" with vancomycin and heparin for 1 hour every 2 days to heparin lock alone. The hub colonization and bacteremia rates were 15.8% and 7% with heparin, 0% for both with treatment [67]. Gram-negative line sepsis and yeast line sepsis generally require line removal as part of treatment, but there is recent evidence of successful line salvage with antibiotics and a thrombolytic agent together [65,68,69]. A Cochrane review of dressings used to cover CVC exit site and infection risk found no risk difference among dressings and recommended that dressings reflect patient preference [70]. A 1-year prospective study that monitored the difference in infection rate with or without an inline filter found no difference [71]. Little information exists to document the infectious risks from PICC lines, which are low overall because of shorter duration of use, although a sepsis rate of 25.7% (7/25 catheters) was reported in one study of patients with solid tumors [72]. Minor exit site infections, including yeast infections, have been reported.

Malfunction of CVCs is common and presents as total occlusion, lines that infuse but do not withdraw blood, and lines that are intermittently nonfunctional. Malfunction can be evaluated by Trendelenburg positioning, raising the ipsilateral arm over the head, or hydrating the patient. If these approaches result in a normally functioning line, one should obtain a radiograph to check tip location. Inability to withdraw blood may be caused by a one-way valve-like thrombus on the tip. Complete occlusion is usually the result of thrombus. Treatment with thrombolytic agents, such as urokinase, 2500 to 5000 U for 30 minutes, or tissue plasminogen activator (tPA), 0.5 to 1 mL, left to rest in the line for 2 hours before attempting aspiration can restore function [73]. A study that evaluated the efficacy of tPA in clearing CVCs showed 86% success with a first dose and 95% with two attempts [74]. Other line-associated complications are less frequent and include air embolism at the time of placement, which was shown to be less frequent in well-sedated patients, and complications associated with general anesthesia [75], which also occur rarely with home infusion mistakes [76]. Catheter breaks and leaks occur; each manufacturer has catheter-specific repair kits that can be used to repair them. Accidental dislodgement usually requires replacement of the catheter; a radiograph should be obtained to check for migration of the tip. PICC lines sometimes can be replaced over a wire. Complications with PICC lines are reported to range from 0 to 40.7%, with occlusion and infection being the most frequently reported. Complications more common with PICC lines include external breaks, shoulder pain, phlebitis without infection, exit site irritation, dislodgement, and occlusion. A study that compared PICC line function with non–central tip location versus central tip location showed comparable results and complication rates, with the exception that non-central PICC lines failed sooner (11.4 days versus 16.6 days), and fewer patients completed their course of therapy (69% versus 73%) [60].

Noninvasive positive pressure ventilatory assistance

Noninvasive positive airway pressure (NiPAP) assisted ventilation can be continuous (CPAP), bi-level, or automatically adjusted (auto-CPAP). NiPAP is indicated in obstructive sleep apnea, chronic neuromuscular disease, apnea of prematurity, syndromes with facial/pharyngeal malformation and dysfunction, acute chest syndrome in sickle cell disease [77], poorly controlled epilepsy with concurrent obstructive sleep apnea, bilateral diaphragm paralysis after surgery, and some instances of chronic and acute respiratory disease. Tracheostomy-delivered CPAP has been used to reduce the incidence of aspiration of saliva with its consequences in neurologically impaired children [78]. Bi-level positive airway pressure delivers two levels of positive pressure that vary by inspiration/expiration to improve comfort and tolerance.

NiPAP may be delivered by full face mask (covers mouth and nose), nasal route (nasal CPAP prongs, nasal mask), or tracheostomy. Automated CPAP is new to pediatrics and has been tested only in a monitored setting, but is likely to see more widespread use [79]. It essentially automatically titrates CPAP to an optimal pressure and adjusts for changes in sleep variables that affect frequency of apneas and hypopneas. Algorithms specific to pediatrics for recognizing apneas and hypopneas are yet to be validated. In all forms of NiPAP, intolerance of the intervention is the most common cause of failure. Mask fit is essential. When a patient on NiPAP is hospitalized, the successful continuation of their respiratory intervention is optimized with use of their home mask and delivery device. A process in place in the hospital to expedite this is useful. In some hospitals, the use of NiPAP ventilation assist necessitates admission to the pediatric intensive care unit. In many patients with chronic NiPAP ventilation, admission to the floor is allowed, but if home equipment is used, a caregiver (parent) trained on that equipment is asked to be available around the clock.

NiPAP ventilatory assistance has been shown to reduce hospital days by up to 85% in children with neuromuscular disease, with documented improvements in apnea/hypopnea index and transcutaneous PCO_2 level [80]. Three neurologically impaired children with tracheostomies and documented chronic saliva aspiration saw reduction in frequency of aspiration by radionuclide salivagram and only "rare hospitalization" after tracheostomy CPAP [78]. In children with obstructive sleep apnea who are successfully started on long-term NiPAP, approximately 96% can be expected to have measurable improvements [81]. There are no published guidelines for amount of pressure support by age or disease. Published studies do not show a consistent relation between degree of CPAP and clinical parameters. It is reasonable to institute therapy at 4 cm H_2O in infants and 6 cm H_2O in older children and titrate to response while monitoring for complications. In most patients cared for on the pediatric medical floor, NiPAP is at a preestablished level and no changes would be anticipated in the hospital. In acute illness, there may be a need for more support; generally this necessity should prompt a transfer to the pediatric intensive care unit. In children chronic disease, the measures of response to therapy include days hospitalized, frequency of pneumonia, measures of ventilatory function, daytime sleepiness scales, and measures of school performance, and the goal is the minimal long-term NiPAP that will maintain the clinical response. Titration of NiPAP is not indicated during an acute hospital stay.

Complications of NiPAP ventilation assist include pneumothorax, skin irritation and pressure injury, nasal drying, nasal pain, drying of the throat, claustrophobia, and nasal deformities in preterm infants. A high index of suspicion for pneumothorax, particularly with acute respiratory illness, attention to potential complications when hospital policy dictates use of standardized equipment while hospitalized, extra care by ancillary services in mask or nasal prong fitting, a protocol for early identification of pressure-induced skin injury with appropriate treatment, use of humidification, and acclimation to NiPAP use likely will reduce the risk of complications.

Cerebrospinal fluid shunts

Shunts are placed to treat increased intracranial pressure. Shunts are named based on their proximal and distal insertion locations. Most originate in the lateral ventricles; other locations include the third or fourth ventricles or an intracranial or spinal cyst. Most shunts terminate in the peritoneal cavity; other locations include the right atrium, pleural space, gall bladder, ureter, urinary bladder, bone marrow, mastoid, thoracic duct, and fallopian tube. Each shunt has three basic parts: (1) the proximal catheter, which exits the central nervous system through a bur hole, (2) a one-way valve that allows unidirectional flow when a specific pressure differential is exceeded, and (3) the distal catheter, which is tunneled under the skin to its destination, sometimes with extra length to allow for growth. Modern shunts also may incorporate reservoirs for cerebrospinal fluid sampling and drug instillation, antisiphon devices to prevent excessive run-off, and on-off valves. They also may be externally programmable. Shunts are placed by neurosurgical procedure, and the neurosurgical service should be consulted whenever a complication is suspected.

Complications include malfunction that leads to inadequate drainage and increased intracranial pressure, infection that may lead secondarily to malfunction, and overdrainage that may lead to the ventricle syndrome. Headache is a common long-term clinical challenge.

Malfunction eventually complicates 30% to 40% of all shunt procedures. Nearly half of all shunt revision procedures are for malfunction, and up to 71% of all patients experience a malfunction during their lifetime [73,82,83]. Symptoms of shunt malfunction are those of increased intracranial pressure, including headache, nausea, and vomiting, irritability, increased seizures, neck pain, back pain, blurred vision, lethargy, and "just not acting right" [84]. Fever is also seen in 22% of uninfected malfunctions [85] but actually may signal infected hardware despite negative cultures [86,87]. Signs include a bulging fontanelle, separating sutures, increased occipital-frontal circumference, papilledema, sun-setting eyes, redness and tenderness along the shunt tubing route, and altered mental status, although these signs may be subtle [88]. Sterile shunt malfunctions may be immunologically mediated and associated with cerebrospinal fluid eosinophilia [89–93]. Eighty-five percent of results of head CT scans are abnormal in shunt malfunction when compared with a baseline CT; more sensitive methods of comparison are being developed [94]. Approximately 15% of cases of malfunction are caused by discontinuity of shunt tubing or kinks and can be excluded by obtaining a plain radiographic "shunt series" [95]. A radionucleotide shunt function study can demonstrate patency of the proximal and distal tubing, but it involves accessing the shunt reservoir. Other evaluations include manipulation of the shunt reservoirs/valve and tapping the shunt to confirm or exclude obstruction of the proximal or distal catheters. These maneuvers are best performed by the consulting neurosurgeon. One should be aware that some patients have more than one shunt, which may or may not be connected. Symptoms can be vague and nonspecific. In one study, the average time between onset of symptoms and diagnosis of shunt malfunction was 11.5 days [73]. In another study, vomiting, lack of fever, and parental suspicion were the most sensitive clinical features. Parents have been shown to be as accurate as physicians in diagnosing shunt malfunction before diagnostic testing [73].

Infection complicates between 2% and 30% of shunt procedures, although the incidence has been declining over time [73,96]. Risk may be higher in infancy and in the recent postoperative period after a shunt procedure. Half of shunt infections occur in the first 2 weeks, 70% to 80% within 2 months, and 80% to 90% within 4 months [73,97]. Lumbar puncture, ventricular taps, cerebrospinal fluid withdrawal, and ventriculograms are not independently associated with an increased risk of shunt infection. Common pathogens in postoperative infection up to 6 to 9 months include coagulase-negative staphylococcal species, *Staphylococcus epidermidis,* and *S. aureus.* Gram-negative bacilli are isolated in 6% to 20% [97], and other pathogens commonly associated with meningitis have been isolated in late shunt infections (>6–9 months), such as pneumococcus and *Haemophilus influenzae* [98]. Symptoms can be vague and nonspecific but often include fever and may include irritability, feeding problems, nausea, vomiting, lethargy, headache, and change in sensorium. Symptoms of meningeal irritation are often absent. Signs include erythema, swelling, cellulitis, or wound infection overlying the shunt tract, fever, altered mental status, and—with a ventriculo-peritoneal shunt—abdominal pain, diarrhea, and clinical signs of peritonitis. Approximately 50% of infected shunts also malfunction. Evaluation includes a head CT scan and shunt series. Tapping the shunt to obtain a cerebrospinal fluid sample for laboratory evaluation and culture is essential, although there is controversy about the number of white blood cells and protein level that are "acceptable," particularly close to the time of a shunt procedure [89,99]. A Gram stain can be particularly helpful if the results are positive. Multiple studies have shown that use of systemic antibiotics and removal of the infected shunt hardware have a high probability of resolving the infection [100]; however, the ideal length of treatment is unknown [101]. Empiric therapy should begin with vancomy-cin and a third-generation cephalosporin [102]. Ventriculoatrial shunts may be associated with systemic sepsis symptoms when infected, and complications can include endocarditis, glomerulonephritis, hypocomplementemia, and throm-boembolic events.

Rare complications of ventriculoperitoneal shunts include development of an inguinal hernia (up to 16.8%), migration of the distal tip, and perforation of a wide variety of intra-abdominal organs, the incisions, and the diaphragm. An abdominal pseudocyst also can develop with symptoms that can be a diagnostic dilemma. Other rare complications attributed to shunts include intussusception, intractable hiccup, omental cyst torsion, and volvulus around the catheter.

Slit ventricles on head CT occur within 6.5 months in 21% of patients and 48% after 6 years, but symptomatic slit ventricle syndrome is uncommon [103]. One successful approach to treatment has included lumboperitoneal shunt-ing [104].

Future research agenda

Research on MCC as a subgroup of CSHCN is critical to study and improve the quality of care they currently receive. Challenges to studying this population include the enormous diversity of conditions and absolute small number of patients at a single hospital. One study that examined the impact of a pediatric hospitalist system for MCC (as defined by a positive response to the CSHCN screener, transfers from an intensive care unit or an All Payer Refined Diagnosis-Related Group of three or four [those of the highest severity of illness]) found that those children had proportionally lower length of stay and total costs, compared with the already lower length of stay and total costs of the cohort of all children who were cared for by hospitalists, as compared with the traditional academic attending model or community physicians [105]. Future research must determine, however, how to measure effectively the quality of care MCC receive (in terms of processes and outcomes of care). It is important to determine how a new inpatient system of care may best integrate the care of these children across the continuum of inpatient and outpatient care and across several disciplines and specialties.

For these children to receive the highest quality of care, three critical steps in research must occur to improve the current system of inpatient care. First, prospective methods of identifying MCC that are feasible, valid, and reproducible must be developed and allow for comparative studies across institutions. Recent novel studies are currently being undertaken to accomplish this goal [106,107,111].

Second, measures of inpatient processes of pediatric care must be defined, validated, and tested explicitly (disease-dependent and disease-independent). Process measures have been particularly challenging in inpatient pediatrics because few diseases have well-defined quality measures with strong evidence to link particular processes of care with improved outcomes. In particular, disease-dependent measures require the evidence base to be developed, tested, and refined and are largely lacking in pediatrics (with a notable exception of inpatient asthma care). The challenge is particularly great in assessing the quality of care of MCC who have few well-studied process measures. For example, children who are neurologically impaired have various conditions that may be responsible for their hospitalization, including seizures, aspiration pneumonia, and fever, but research in their care is sparse, at best. Disease-independent process measures are one method of addressing quality of care in the face of such a large range of infrequent conditions. MCC are an ideal group to study given their vulnerability that leads to repeated hospitalizations and allows researchers to understand better the aspects of their care. For example, when using parental expectations with care as an outcome measure, examining how parents of MCC rate their inpatient care compared with parents of children who are not medically complex allows for a more in-depth analysis of the system of inpatient care in the eyes of a frequent user, exemplifying aspects of poor- and high-quality care.

Third, pediatric hospitalists must be studied in their natural laboratory (ie, the hospital) to understand the mechanisms for the successful and unsuccessful models of translating research findings into clinical practice using quality improvement techniques. Various aspects of inpatient care can be studied, tested, and retested after changes in serial interventions using quasi-experimental study designs. For example, at Primary Children's Medical Center in Salt Lake City, we have undertaken a quality improvement study that evaluates the optimum method of improving written medication orders for newly admitted MCC. Pharmacists have been reviewing the initial orders, comparing them to home medication lists provided by parents, and contacting the outpatient pharmacies, the primary care physicians, and the hospital pharmacy database using the last hospital discharge as a comparison point. These medication reconciliations of new admissions from the emergency department and transfers from within the hospital provide insight into the system of care that allows for such errors to occur [108]. Hospitalists are often inpatient unit medical directors who work closely with hospital administration and are poised to see the implementation of and ongoing impact on outcomes of quality improvement and research findings translated into clinical inpatient practice.

As these three things occur, the care being delivered to hospitalized MCC will undergo a paradigm shift, because that care will be able to be measured, benchmarked against best performers, and improved on to deliver care that is effective, efficient, safe, patient centered, and timely [109].

References

[1] Daly S, Campbell DA, Cameron PA. Short-stay units and observation medicine: a systematic review. Med J Aust 2003;178(11):559–63.
[2] Wise PH. The transformation of child health in the United States. Health Aff 2004;23(5): 9–25.
[3] Institute of Medicine. Committee on Identifying Priority Areas for Quality Improvement. Priority actions for national action: transforming healthcare quality. Washington, DC: National Academy Press; 2003.
[4] Clancy CM, Andresen EM. Meeting the health care needs of persons with disabilities. Milbank Q 2002;80(2):381–91.
[5] Newacheck PW, Strickland B, Shonkoff JP, et al. An epidemiologic profile of children with special health care needs. Pediatrics 1998;102(1 Pt 1):117–23.
[6] Newacheck PW, Inkelas M, Kim SE. Health services use and health care expenditures for children with disabilities. Pediatrics 2004;114(1):79–85.
[7] Newacheck PW, Hung YY, Wong S, et al. The unmet health needs of America's children. Pediatrics 2000;105:989–97.
[8] Dosa NP, Boeing NM, Ms N, et al. Excess risk of severe acute illness in children with chronic health conditions. Pediatrics 2001;107(3):499–504.
[9] Sacchetti A, Sacchetti C, Carraccio C, et al. The potential for errors in children with special health care needs. Acad Emerg Med 2000;7(11):1330–3.
[10] Slonim AD, LaFleur BJ, Ahmed W, et al. Hospital-reported medical errors in children. Pediatrics 2003;111(3):617–21.
[11] Newacheck PW, Halfon N. Prevalence and impact of disabling chronic conditions in childhood. Am J Public Health 1998;88(4):610–7.
[12] Ireys HT, Grason HA, Guyer B. Assuring quality of care for children with special needs in managed care organizations: roles for pediatricians. Pediatrics 1996;98(2 Pt 1):178–85.
[13] Stein RE, Bauman LJ, Westbrook LE, et al. Framework for identifying children who have chronic conditions: the case for a new definition. J Pediatr 1993;122(3):342–7.
[14] Stein RE, Silver EJ. Operationalizing a conceptually based noncategorical definition: a first look at US children with chronic conditions. Arch Pediatr Adolesc Med 1999;153(1):68–74.
[15] Perrin EC, Newacheck P, Pless IB, et al. Issues involved in the definition and classification of chronic health conditions. Pediatrics 1993;91(4):787–93.
[16] McPherson M, Arango P, Fox H, et al. A new definition of children with special health care needs. Pediatrics 1998;102(1 Pt 1):137–40.
[17] Wagner EH, Austin BT, Von Korff M. Organizing care for patients with chronic illness. Milbank Q 1996;74(4):511–44.
[18] Bodenheimer T, Wagner EH, Grumbach K. Improving primary care for patients with chronic illness: the chronic care model, part 2. JAMA 2002;288(15):1909–14.
[19] Bodenheimer T, Wagner EH, Grumbach K. Improving primary care for patients with chronic illness. JAMA 2002;288(14):1775–9.
[20] Perrin JM. Health services research for children with disabilities. Milbank Q 2002;80(2): 303–24.

[21] Bethell CD, Read D, Neff J, et al. Comparison of the children with special health care needs screener to the questionnaire for identifying children with chronic conditions, revised. Ambul Pediatr 2002;2(1):49–57.

[22] Bethell CD, Read D, Stein RE, et al. Identifying children with special health care needs: development and evaluation of a short screening instrument. Ambul Pediatr 2002;2(1):38–48.

[23] Kelly AF, Hewson PH. Factors associated with recurrent hospitalization in chronically ill children and adolescents. J Paediatr Child Health 2000;36(1):13–8.

[24] Marchetti F, Bonati M, Marfisi RM, et al. Parental and primary care physicians' views on the management of chronic diseases: a study in Italy. The Italian Collaborative Group on Paediatric Chronic Diseases. Acta Paediatr 1995;84(10):1165–72.

[25] Rosenbaum P, Stewart D. The World Health Organization international classification of functioning, disability, and health: a model to guide clinical thinking, practice and research in the field of cerebral palsy. Semin Pediatr Neurol 2004;11(1):5–10.

[26] Baxter P. ICF: health vs disease. Dev Med Child Neurol 2004;46(5):291.

[27] Lansdown G. Implementing children's rights and health. Arch Dis Child 2000;83(4):286–8.

[28] American Academy of Pediatrics Ad Hoc Task Force. The medical home. Pediatrics 1992; 90(5):774.

[29] Anonymous. The medical home. Pediatrics 2002;110(1 Pt 1):184–6.

[30] Anonymous. Policy statement: organizational principles to guide and define the child health care system and/or improve the health of all children. Pediatrics 2004;113(5 Suppl):1545–7.

[31] Silver EJ, Westbrook LE, Stein RE. Relationship of parental psychological distress to consequences of chronic health conditions in children. J Pediatr Psychol 1998;23(1):5–15.

[32] Brehaut JC, Kohen DE, Raina P, et al. The health of primary caregivers of children with cerebral palsy: how does it compare with that of other Canadian caregivers? Pediatrics 2004; 114(2):e182–91.

[33] Wang KW, Barnard A. Technology-dependent children and their families: a review. J Adv Nurs 2004;45(1):36–46.

[34] King G, King S, Rosenbaum P, et al. Family-centered caregiving and well-being of parents of children with disabilities: linking process with outcome. J Pediatr Psychol 1999;24(1):41–53.

[35] Lindeke LL, Leonard BJ, Presler B, et al. Family-centered care coordination for children with special needs across multiple settings. J Pediatr Health Care 2002;16(6):290–7.

[36] Ziring PR, Brazdziunas D, Cooley WC, et al. American Academy of Pediatrics. Committee on children with disabilities. Care coordination: integrating health and related systems of care for children with special health care needs. Pediatrics 1999;104(4 Pt 1):978–81.

[37] American Academy of Pediatrics Committee on Hospital Care. Physician's role in coordinating care of hospitalized children. Pediatrics 1996;98(3 Pt 1):509–10.

[38] Percelay JM. Physicians' roles in coordinating care of hospitalized children. Pediatrics 2003; 111(3):707–9.

[39] American Academy of Pediatrics Committee on Pediatric Emergency Medicine. Emergency preparedness for children with special health care needs. Pediatrics 1999;104(4):e53.

[40] Bakewell-Sachs S, Carlino H, Ash L, et al. Home care considerations for chronic and vulnerable populations. Nurse Pract Forum 2000;11(1):65–72.

[41] National Task Force on Children with Special Health Care Needs. EMS for children: recommendations for coordinating care for children with special health care needs. Emergency Medical Services for Children. Ann Emerg Med 1997;30(3):274–80.

[42] Institute for Healthcare Improvement. Pursuing perfection in health care: navigating complex systems of care. Available at: http://www.ihi.org/IHI/Products/Video/NavigatingComplex SystemsofCare.htm. Accessed February 21, 2005.

[43] Mayer ML, Skinner AC, Slifkin RT. Unmet need for routine and specialty care: data from the National Survey of Children with Special Health Care Needs. Pediatrics 2004;113(2):e109–15.

[44] Raina P, O'Donnell M, Schwellnus H, et al. Caregiving process and caregiver burden: conceptual models to guide research and practice. BMC Pediatr 2004;4(1):1.

[45] Faraji B, Yu PP. Serum phenytoin levels of patients on gastrostomy tube feeding. J Neurosci Nurs 1998;30(1):55–9.

[46] Au Yeung SC, Ensom MH. Phenytoin and enteral feedings: does evidence support an interaction? Ann Pharmacother 2000;34(7–8):896–905.

[47] Curley MA, Quigley SM, Lin M. Pressure ulcers in pediatric intensive care: incidence and associated factors. Pediatr Crit Care Med 2003;4(3):284–90.

[48] Friedman JN, Ahmed S, Connolly B, et al. Complications associated with image-guided gastrostomy and gastrojejunostomy tubes in children. Pediatrics 2004;114(2):458–61.

[49] Friedman JN. Enterostomy tube feeding: the ins and outs. J Paediatr Child Health 2004; 9(10):695–9.

[50] Conlon SJ, Janik TA, Janik JS, et al. Gastrostomy revision: incidence and indications. J Pediatr Surg 2004;39(9):1390–5.

[51] Fortunato JE, Darbari A, Mitchell SE, et al. The limitations of gastro-jejunal (G-J) feeding tubes in children: a 9-year pediatric hospital database analysis. Am J Gastroenterol 2005; 100(1):186–9.

[52] Godbole P, Margabanthu G, Crabbe DC, et al. Limitations and uses of gastrojejunal feeding tubes. Arch Dis Child 2002;86(2):134–7.

[53] Siddique R, Neslusan CA, Crown WH, et al. A national inpatient cost estimate of percutaneous endoscopic gastrostomy (PEG)-associated aspiration pneumonia. Am J Manag Care 2000;6(4): 490–6.

[54] Wilson L, Oliva-Hemker M. Percutaneous endoscopic gastrostomy in small medically complex infants. Endoscopy 2001;33(5):433–6.

[55] Razeghi S, Lang T, Behrens R. Influence of percutaneous endoscopic gastrostomy on gastroesophageal reflux: a prospective study in 68 children. J Pediatr Gastroenterol Nutr 2002; 35(1):27–30.

[56] Sherman JM, Davis S, Albamonte-Petrick S, et al. Care of the child with a chronic tracheostomy. Am J Respir Crit Care Med 2000;161(1):297–308.

[57] Deerojanawong J, Sawyer SM, Fink AM, et al. Totally implantable venous access devices in children with cystic fibrosis: incidence and type of complications. Thorax 1998;53(4):285–9.

[58] Schwarz RE, Coit DG, Groeger JS. Transcutaneously tunneled central venous lines in cancer patients: an analysis of device-related morbidity factors based on prospective data collection. Ann Surg Oncol 2000;7(6):441–9.

[59] Cardella JF, Cardella K, Bacci N, et al. Cumulative experience with 1,273 peripherally inserted central catheters at a single institution. J Vasc Interv Radiol 1996;7(1):5–13.

[60] Thiagarajan RR, Bratton SL, Gettmann T, et al. Efficacy of peripherally inserted central venous catheters placed in noncentral veins. Arch Pediatr Adolesc Med 1998;152(5):436–9.

[61] Chan AK, Deveber G, Monagle P, et al. Venous thrombosis in children. J Thromb Haemost 2003;1(7):1443–55.

[62] Derish MT, Smith DW, Frankel LR. Venous catheter thrombus formation and pulmonary embolism in children. Pediatr Pulmonol 1995;20(6):349–54.

[63] Pollard AJ, Sreeram N, Wright JG, et al. ECG and echocardiographic diagnosis of pulmonary thromboembolism associated with central venous lines. Arch Dis Child 1995;73(2):147–50.

[64] McDonald LC, Banerjee SN, Jarvis WR. Line-associated bloodstream infections in pediatric intensive-care-unit patients associated with a needleless device and intermittent intravenous therapy. Infect Control Hosp Epidemiol 1998;19(10):772–7.

[65] Jones GR, Konsler GK, Dunaway RP, et al. Prospective analysis of urokinase in the treatment of catheter sepsis in pediatric hematology-oncology patients. J Pediatr Surg 1993;28(3):350–5 [discussion 355–7].

[66] McNelis J, Zarcone J, Marini C, et al. Outcome of subcutaneously implanted catheters in a teaching hospital. Am J Med Qual 2002;17(5):185–8.

[67] Carratala J, Niubo J, Fernandez-Sevilla A, et al. Randomized, double-blind trial of an antibiotic-lock technique for prevention of gram-positive central venous catheter-related infection in neutropenic patients with cancer. Antimicrob Agents Chemother 1999;43(9):2200–4.

[68] Hanna H, Afif C, Alakech B, Boktour M, et al. Central venous catheter-related bacteremia due to gram-negative bacilli: significance of catheter removal in preventing relapse. Infect Control Hosp Epidemiol 2004;25(8):646–9.

[69] De Sio L, Jenkner A, Milano GM, et al. Antibiotic lock with vancomycin and urokinase can successfully treat colonized central venous catheters in pediatric cancer patients. Pediatr Infect Dis J 2004;23(10):963–5.

[70] Gillies D, O'Riordan L, Carr D, et al. Gauze and tape and transparent polyurethane dressings for central venous catheters. Cochrane Database Syst Rev 2003;4:CD003827.

[71] Newall F, Ranson K, Robertson J. Use of in-line filters in pediatric intravenous therapy. J Intraven Nurs 1998;21(3):166–70.

[72] Cheong K, Perry D, Karapetis C, et al. High rate of complications associated with peripherally inserted central venous catheters in patients with solid tumours. Intern Med J 2004; 34(5):234–8.

[73] Teoh DL. Tricks of the trade: assessment of high-tech gear in special needs children. Clinical Pediatric Emergency Medicine 2002;3(1):62–75.

[74] Fisher AA, Deffenbaugh C, Poole RL, et al. The use of alteplase for restoring patency to occluded central venous access devices in infants and children. J Infus Nurs 2004;27(3):171–4.

[75] Morello FP, Donaldson JS, Saker MC, et al. Air embolism during tunneled central catheter placement performed without general anesthesia in children: a potentially serious complication. J Vasc Interv Radiol 1999;10(6):781–4.

[76] Laskey AL, Dyer C, Tobias JD. Venous air embolism during home infusion therapy. Pediatrics 2002;109(1):E15.

[77] Padman R, Henry M. The use of bilevel positive airway pressure for the treatment of acute chest syndrome of sickle cell disease. Del Med J 2004;76(5):199–203.

[78] Finder JD, Yellon R, Charron M. Successful management of tracheotomized patients with chronic saliva aspiration by use of constant positive airway pressure. Pediatrics 2001;107(6): 1343–5.

[79] Palombini L, Pelayo R, Guilleminault C. Efficacy of automated continuous positive airway pressure in children with sleep-related breathing disorders in an attended setting. Pediatrics 2004;113(5):e412–7.

[80] Katz S, Selvadurai H, Keilty K, et al. Outcome of non-invasive positive pressure ventilation in paediatric neuromuscular disease. Arch Dis Child 2004;89(2):121–4.

[81] Massa F, Gonsalez S, Laverty A, et al. The use of nasal continuous positive airway pressure to treat obstructive sleep apnoea. Arch Dis Child 2002;87(5):438–43.

[82] Vinchon M, Fichten A, Delestret I, et al. Shunt revision for asymptomatic failure: surgical and clinical results. Neurosurgery 2003;52(2):347–53 [discussion 353–6].

[83] Kestle J, Drake J, Milner R, et al. Long-term follow-up data from the shunt design trial. Pediatr Neurosurg 2000;33(5):230–6.

[84] Barnes NP, Jones SJ, Hayward RD, et al. Ventriculoperitoneal shunt block: what are the best predictive clinical indicators? Arch Dis Child 2002;87(3):198–201.

[85] Ashkenazi E, Umansky F, Constantini S, et al. Fever as the initial sign of malfunction in non infected ventriculoperitoneal shunts. Acta Neurochir (Wien) 1992;114(3–4):131–4.

[86] Steinbok P, Cochrane DD, Kestle JR. The significance of bacteriologically positive ventriculoperitoneal shunt components in the absence of other signs of shunt infection. J Neurosurg 1996;84(4):617–23.

[87] Vanaclocha V, Saiz-Sapena N, Leiva J. Shunt malfunction in relation to shunt infection. Acta Neurochir (Wien) 1996;138(7):829–34.

[88] Arnell K, Eriksson E, Olsen L. Asymptomatic shunt malfunction detected fortuitously by observation of papilloedema. Acta Neurochir (Wien) 2003;145(12):1093–6.

[89] McClinton D, Carraccio C, Englander R. Predictors of ventriculoperitoneal shunt pathology. Pediatr Infect Dis J 2001;20(6):593–7.

[90] Jimenez DF, Keating R, Goodrich JT. Silicone allergy in ventriculoperitoneal shunts. Childs Nerv Syst 1994;10(1):59–63.

[91] Pittman T, Williams D, Rathore M, et al. The role of ethylene oxide allergy in sterile shunt malfunctions. Br J Neurosurg 1994;8(1):41–5.

[92] Tanaka T, Ikeuchi S, Yoshino K, et al. A case of cerebrospinal fluid eosinophilia associated with shunt malfunction. Pediatr Neurosurg 1999;30(1):6–10.

[93] VandeVord PJ, Gupta N, Wilson RB, et al. Immune reactions associated with silicone-based ventriculo-peritoneal shunt malfunctions in children. Biomaterials 2004;25(17):3853–60.

[94] Sze RW, Ghioni V, Weinberger E, et al. Rapid computed tomography technique to measure ventricular volumes in the child with suspected ventriculoperitoneal shunt failure. II. Clinical application. J Comput Assist Tomogr 2003;27(5):668–73.

[95] Aldrich EF, Harmann P. Disconnection as a cause of ventriculoperitoneal shunt malfunction in multicomponent shunt systems. Pediatr Neurosurg 1990;16(6):309–11 [discussion 312].

[96] Kang JK, Lee IW. Long-term follow-up of shunting therapy. Childs Nerv Syst 1999; 15(11–12):711–7.

[97] Stamos JK, Kaufman BA, Yogev R. Ventriculoperitoneal shunt infections with gram-negative bacteria. Neurosurgery 1993;33(5):858–62.

[98] Baird C, O'Connor D, Pittman T. Late shunt infections. Pediatr Neurosurg 1999;31(5):269–73.

[99] Lan CC, Wong TT, Chen SJ, et al. Early diagnosis of ventriculoperitoneal shunt infections and malfunctions in children with hydrocephalus. J Microbiol Immunol Infect 2003;36(1): 47–50.

[100] Schreffler RT, Schreffler AJ, Wittler RR. Treatment of cerebrospinal fluid shunt infections: a decision analysis. Pediatr Infect Dis J 2002;21(7):632–6.

[101] Arthur AS, Whitehead WE, Kestle JR. Duration of antibiotic therapy for the treatment of shunt infection: a surgeon and patient survey. Pediatr Neurosurg 2002;36(5):256–9.

[102] Wang KW, Chang WN, Shih TY, et al. Infection of cerebrospinal fluid shunts: causative pathogens, clinical features, and outcomes. Jpn J Infect Dis 2004;57(2):44–8.

[103] Liniger P, Marchand S, Kaiser GL. Flow control versus antisiphon valves: late results concerning slit ventricles and slit-ventricle syndrome. Eur J Pediatr Surg 2003;13(Suppl 1):S3–6.

[104] Le H, Yamini B, Frim DM. Lumboperitoneal shunting as a treatment for slit ventricle syndrome. Pediatr Neurosurg 2002;36(4):178–82.

[105] Srivastava R, Muret-Wagstaff S, Young P, et al. Hospitalist care of medically complex children. Pediatr Res 2004;55(4):314–5A.

[106] Graham RJ, Dumas HM, O'Brien JE, et al. Congenital neurodevelopmental diagnoses and an intensive care unit: defining a population. Pediatr Crit Care Med 2004;5(4):321–8.

[107] Nicholson CE. Pediatric critical care for children with congenital neurodevelopmental diagnoses. Pediatr Crit Care Med 2004;5(4):407–8.

[108] Institute for Healthcare Improvement. Reconcile medications at all transition points. Available at: http://www.ihi.org/IHI/Topics/PatientSafety/MedicationSystems/Changes/ IndividualChanges/Reconcile+Medication+Orders+When+Patients+are+Transferred+to+ Other+Care+Units.htm. Accessed February 21, 2005.

[109] Institute of Medicine. Committee on Quality of Health Care in America. Crossing the quality chasm: a new health system for the 21st century. Washington, DC: National Academy Press; 2001.

[110] Committee of Pediatric Emergency Medicine. Emergency preparedness for children with special health care needs. Pediatrics 1999;104:e53.

[111] Srivastava R, Norlin C, Muret-Wagstaff S, et al. Identifying CSHCN in a pediatrics tertiary care hospital. Pediatr Research 2003;53:253A.

ELSEVIER
SAUNDERS

PEDIATRIC CLINICS
OF NORTH AMERICA

Pediatr Clin N Am 52 (2005) 1189–1208

Device-related Infections in Children

Samir S. Shah, MD[a,b,c,d,*], Michael J. Smith, MD[a],
Theoklis E. Zaoutis, MD, MSCE[a,c,d]

[a]Division of Infectious Diseases, The Children's Hospital of Philadelphia,
34th Street and Civic Center Boulevard, Philadelphia, PA 19104, USA
[b]Division of General Pediatrics, The Children's Hospital of Philadelphia,
34th Street and Civic Center Boulevard, Philadelphia, PA 19104, USA
[c]Center for Clinical Epidemiology and Biostatistics, University of Pennsylvania School of Medicine,
423 Guardian Drive, Philadelphia, PA 19104, USA
[d]Department of Pediatrics, University of Pennsylvania School of Medicine,
34th Street and Civic Center Boulevard, Philadelphia, PA 19104, USA

Medical devices such as central venous catheters (CVCs) and ventricular shunts are commonly used in children. Catheter-associated bloodstream infections (Ca-BSIs) are frequent complications of the use of long-term vascular access devices, with more than 200,000 cases occurring each year in the United States [1]. Local infections at insertion sites are another important catheter-associated complication. Insertion of a ventriculoperitoneal (VP) shunt is one of the most commonly performed operations in children [2]. These devices greatly increase the risk of infection by disrupting host defenses. This disruption provides a portal of entry for organisms to migrate from the skin and mucous membranes to sterile body sites. These devices also supply a site relatively sequestered from immune system surveillance, which allows bacteria to flourish unperturbed. Indwelling devices, such as catheters, can become seeded with bacteria as a result of bacteremia that arises at a distant site. This article discusses infectious complications of CVCs and ventricular shunts.

In the past, catheter-associated infections primarily were the purview of intensivists, oncologists, and gastroenterologists. The use of CVCs is increasing in the inpatient and outpatient settings. Consequently, previously healthy children

* Corresponding author. Division Infectious Diseases, Children's Hospital of Philadelphia, North Campus Room 1526, 34th Street and Civic Center Boulevard, Philadelphia, PA 19104.
  E-mail address: shahs@email.chop.edu (S.S. Shah).

0031-3955/05/$ – see front matter © 2005 Elsevier Inc. All rights reserved.
doi:10.1016/j.pcl.2005.05.003
pediatric.theclinics.com

with isolated infectious processes that require extended intravenous antibiotic therapy (eg, osteomyelitis, Lyme meningitis) often have these intravascular lines placed. Hospitalists are increasingly called on to assess patients for possible infectious complications as they appear in emergency departments or medical pediatric inpatient units or are referred through consultations from surgical or medical subspecialists. In many institutions, general pediatric hospitalist practice includes coverage of neonatal and pediatric intensive care units, in which central catheters commonly are used. Knowledge and expertise in assessing and managing catheter-associated infections become increasingly important in many settings.

The medical literature available to guide clinicians comes predominantly from adult studies, studies performed in pediatric or neonatal intensive care settings, and data collected from pediatric oncology patients. The generalizability of the information is yet to be determined, but until studies are performed in broader populations of pediatric patients, data from these more specialized patient populations will serve as the basis for our understanding of catheter-related infections.

Central venous catheter-related infections

Case presentation

A 5-year-old boy hospitalized with perforated appendicitis has an indwelling peripherally inserted CVC through which he is receiving one fourth of his daily fluid intake. Two days before anticipated hospital discharge, he develops a fever of 39°C (102.2°F). Physical examination reveals an ill-appearing boy with tachycardia and hypotension. There is mild induration and erythema at the catheter insertion site.

How should this child be evaluated for a catheter-related infection? Does he require central and peripheral blood cultures? What empiric antibiotics, if any, should he receive? Should the catheter be removed? How long are Ca-BSIs treated with antibiotics? The following information should address many of these concerns.

Epidemiology

BSIs are the most common health care–acquired infections experienced by hospitalized children, and they account for 21% to 34% of all nosocomial infections in pediatric intensive care unit patients. Most of these BSIs occur as a consequence of intravascular catheterization [3]. The attributable cost of these infections in patients in pediatric intensive care units is approximately $39,000 per episode [4] and is an increasingly common problem. In a prospective study of 49 hospitals, Wisplinghoff and colleagues [5] documented an increase in nosocomial BSIs. Some studies have attributed this increase to the more frequent use of CVCs.

Infection rates are affected by many factors, including patient location and comorbid illnesses. Most data on Ca-BSI are derived from hospitalized patients. Among patients in the pediatric intensive care unit studied by the National Nosocomial Infections Surveillance System between 2002 and 2004, the infection rate was 6.6 BSIs per 1000 catheter days. Among patients in the neonatal intensive care unit, the rates of infection ranged from 3.5 to 9.1 BSIs per 1000 catheter days [6]. A study to evaluate the infection rates in the home care setting found similar rates of Ca-BSI among pediatric oncology patients [7].

The rate of infection also varies by type of catheter. Table 1 provides a description of commonly used CVCs. Nontunneled catheters seem to have the highest rate of infection, whereas totally implanted venous access devices have the lowest rates of infection [8]. The following practices are associated with a reduced risk of catheter-associated infections: (1) use of maximal sterile barriers during catheter placement [9], (2) use of chlorhexidine/isopropyl alcohol solution to prepare the skin before placement or during routine care of the catheter, (3) prompt removal of catheters as soon as they are no longer required, (4) strict adherence to appropriate hand hygiene practices. In studies performed in adult intensive care units, antiseptic impregnated catheters have been associated with reduced rates of Ca-BSI [10].

Clinical manifestations and complications

A catheter-related infection may be local or systemic. In local infection, examination of the exit site may reveal erythema, induration, tenderness, fluctuance, and purulent or foul-smelling discharge. In a patient with a BSI in the context of a CVC, the catheter is often, but not always, the source of infection. The clinician should perform a detailed history and physical examination in an attempt to identify a primary source of infection. In Ca-BSI, fever is the most common presenting finding, and it occurs in 62% of children diagnosed with Ca-BSI after emergency department evaluation [11]. Most children with fever in

Table 1
Summary of commonly used central venous catheters

Catheter Type	Description
Peripherally inserted central catheter	Inserted via a peripheral vein (usually basilic, cephalic, or brachial) into superior vena cava
Nontunneled CVC	Inserted directly into a central vein (usually suvclavian, internal jugular, or femoral) through a skin incision
Tunneled CVC	Inserted through a subcutaneous tunnel on chest wall before entering the superior vena cava (eg, Broviac, Hickman, Groshong, or Quinton catheter); a dacron cuff located at the tunnel exit site contributes to long-term catheter stability by stimulating growth of tissue around the tunneled portion of the catheter
Totally implantable venous access device (port)	Subcutaneous port or reservoir with self-sealing septum that is accessed by a needle through intact skin; catheter tip located in subclavian or internal jugular vein

the context of a CVC do not have a Ca-BSI, however. Among cancer patients with fever with indwelling catheters, only 10% and 24% of all episodes of fever were associated with bacteremia in neutropenic and non-neutropenic patients, respectively [12].

Catheter malfunction also can be a manifestation of catheter-related infection. Thrombi and fibrin deposits on catheters impair blood flow through the catheter and serve as a nidus for microbial colonization and subsequent infection [13]. Potential complications of Ca-BSI include sepsis, disseminated infection with emboli in the retina, skin, bone, heart, and visceral organs (eg, lung, liver, spleen, and kidneys), and organ system function because of immune complex deposition (eg, nephritis).

Diagnosis

Types of catheter-related infections

Infections attributable to the CVC include exit, tunnel, and pocket infections and Ca-BSI (Table 2) [1]. A Ca-BSI is defined as bacteremia or fungemia in a patient with an intravascular catheter in which the catheter is the presumed source of infection. Identifying the catheter as the source is not always straight-forward. For example, a BSI in a patient with an indwelling catheter may originate from undocumented sources of infection (eg, postoperative incision infections, urinary tract infections) rather than from the catheter. In adult patients, only 15% to 20% of central catheters removed in the context of a BSI are

Table 2
Types of catheter-related infections

Infection	Clinical diagnosis
Exit site infection	Erythema or induration within 2 cm of catheter exit site
Tunnel infection	Tenderness, erythema, or induration along the subcutaneous tract of a tunneled catheter and more than 2 cm from catheter exit site
Pocket infection	Purulent fluid in the subcutaneous pocket of a totally implanted venous access device; may be accompanied by overlying tenderness, erythema, induration, visible drainage, and skin necrosis

Catheter-associated BSI	Positive simultaneous blood cultures from the CVC and peripheral vein yielding the same organism in the presence of at least one of the following:
	     Simultaneous quantitative blood cultures in which the number of CFUs isolated from blood drawn through the central catheter was at least fivefold more than the number isolated from blood drawn peripherally
	     Positive semiquantitative ($\geq$15 CFU/catheter segment) or quantitative ($\geq$100 CFU/catheter segment) catheter tip cultures
	     Simultaneous blood cultures in which the central blood culture grows $\geq$2 hours earlier than the peripheral blood culture

Abbreviation: CFU, colony-forming unit.

ultimately implicated as the infection source. Several methods have been proposed to improve our diagnosis of Ca-BSI, including quantitative cultures of blood obtained through the catheter and a peripheral vein, quantitative and semi-quantitative cultures of a catheter segment, and differential time to blood culture positivity (Table 2).

A diagnosis of Ca-BSI can be made by comparing quantitative differences between colony counts of a pathogen isolated from a blood culture obtained through the catheter and colony counts from a simultaneously obtained peripheral blood culture. A Ca-BSI is diagnosed when there is an incremental increase in the quantity of bacteria from blood obtained through the catheter compared with that obtained from peripheral venipuncture (Table 2). Because of the cost and relative unavailability of quantitative blood cultures, this technique has not been used widely. Until recently, the most commonly accepted methods of diagnosing a Ca-BSI have involved either quantitative or semi-quantitative cultures of the catheter tip. Removal of the catheter is necessary with this method. Quantitative culture of a catheter segment requires either flushing the segment with broth or vortexing it in broth, followed by culture of the broth on agar plates [14]. Semi-quantitative culture methods, also known as roll-plate methods, involve rolling a segment of the removed catheter across the surface of an agar plate; colony-forming units are counted after overnight incubation [15].

Differential time to positivity of blood cultures, which is defined as the difference in time necessary for the blood cultures taken by peripheral venipuncture and through the catheter to develop positive results using a continuous monitoring blood culture system, is the simplest of the three methods and does not require either specialized laboratory culture methods or catheter removal. This method is only accurate if the peripheral and central cultures are obtained at the same time and are of equal volume, because as discussed later, the volume of blood in the bottle contributes to time to positivity. Compared with quantitative and semi-quantitative methods, differential time to positivity of 2 or more hours had a sensitivity of 93% and a specificity of 75% for catheters in place for ≥30 days and a sensitivity of 81% and a specificity of 92% for catheters in place for <30 days [16]. Several smaller studies demonstrate similar results [17–19].

Timing of blood cultures

Few studies have evaluated the optimal timing of blood cultures. In clinical conditions with continuous bacteremia, such as endocarditis or septic thrombophlebitis, this issue is less relevant. In Ca-BSIs, the bacteremia is intermittent because the bacteria reside in the lumen of the catheters and are not continuously exposed to blood flow in the intravascular space. The traditional teaching suggests that bacteremia precedes the onset of fever and chills by 1 or more hours, which implies that blood cultures obtained at the time of fever onset may not detect intermittent bacteremia reliably. Anticipating fever and drawing blood samples for culture during a 1- or 2-hour time window before the fever is virtually impossible. Drawing multiple culture sets within a 24-hour period seems to detect intermittent bacteremia accurately, however [19], even if all the specimens were obtained at the same time [20]. In critically ill patients who are hemodynamically unstable, two blood culture sets should be drawn promptly before initiation of empiric antibiotic treatment. In less urgent cases, blood can be drawn at least twice within a 24-hour period. In patients who are already receiving antibiotics, samples obtained close to the time that antibiotic concentrations have reached trough levels (ie, just before next dose) theoretically improve blood culture yield [21]. This issue has not been studied and may not be clinically practical, however.

Volume of blood necessary for culture

Several important variables, including the magnitude of bacteremia and the sensitivity of the blood culture detection system, affect the volume of blood necessary for culture. The magnitude of bacteremia affects blood culture yield, especially when small blood volumes are used. The likelihood of growth was lower and the median time to detection was later when small volumes (≤ 0.5 mL) were used, particularly at ultralow concentrations of bacteria [22]. The volume of blood in the blood culture bottle is more important than the total number of blood cultures obtained, as indicated by a study that found that the pathogen recovery rate at 24 hours was 72% for a large volume (6 mL) single culture compared with a 47% combined yield of two smaller (2 mL) samples inoculated into separate culture bottles [23]. Similar results were found in studies in adult patients, in which standard adult volume cultures (mean, 8.7 mL) had a higher detection rate (92%) than low volume cultures (mean, 2.7 mL), which had a lower detection rate (69%) [24]. It is estimated that the yield of adult blood cultures increased approximately 3% per milliliter of blood cultured.

Although in pediatrics there is often difficulty in obtaining peripheral blood specimens, too much blood or too little blood can influence culture yield. Diluting the blood into the blood culture broth enhances recovery of pathogens, perhaps by diluting antimicrobial agents (if the patient is receiving antibiotic therapy) and blood components, such as phagocytes, antibodies, and complement factors, that are known to have bactericidal activity [25]. Too much blood in the bottle may dilute these factors insufficiently. Too little blood also affects the likelihood of bacterial growth in culture, because blood contains factors that enhance the growth of some bacteria (eg, *Haemophilus influenzae*). In such cases, too little blood volume leads to dilution of these factors by the blood culture bottle nutrient broth. The ideal blood/broth ratio depends on the blood culture system used, but a ratio between 1:5 and 1:10 is generally considered optimal [26]. For example, the PediBacT system, which is used at many institutions, contains 20 mL of broth. A 2-mL inoculum of blood provides a blood/broth ratio of 1:10 and a 4-mL inoculum provides a ratio of 1:5. Because many currently used blood culture systems supplement the broth with other materials that may help overcome cultures inoculated with suboptimal blood/broth ratios, slightly smaller blood volumes may be acceptable. If a single culture that contains 1 to 2 mL of blood is considered sufficient for detection of most clinically important bacteremias, a 0.5-mL blood sample, although not ideal, permits detection of some clinically important bacteremias.

Primary blood stream infection versus contaminated culture

Distinguishing between true BSIs and contaminated cultures poses a challenge when skin flora (eg, coagulase-negative staphylococci [CoNS], *Bacillus* species, micrococci) are isolated from blood culture. If multiple cultures are obtained before antibiotic administration, the situation becomes less ambiguous. Surveillance definitions provide a highly sensitive method for detecting primary BSIs. From a clinical perspective, however, these definitions may overestimate the incidence of BSI. Surveillance definitions have been developed through the combined efforts of the American Academy of Pediatrics and the Centers for Disease Control and Prevention [8]. Patients are considered to have a laboratory-confirmed primary BSI if they meet at least one of the following criteria:

1. The patient has a recognized pathogen (eg, *Staphylococcus aureus, Pseudomonas aeruginosa*) isolated from one or more blood cultures, and the pathogen cultured from the blood is not related to an infection at another site.
2. The patient has at least one sign or symptom of systemic infection, such as fever, chills, or hypotension, and at least one positive blood culture result for common skin flora in the context of a CVC and the physician institutes appropriate antimicrobial therapy.
3. A patient younger than 1 year has at least one sign or symptom of systemic infection, such as fever, chills, or hypotension, apnea, or bradycardia, and at least one positive blood culture result for common skin flora in the context of a CVC and the physician institutes appropriate antimicrobial therapy.

Cause of blood stream infection

Surveillance for nosocomial BSI is usually performed in high-risk patient areas, such as pediatric intensive care units, neonatal intensive care units, and oncology units. As a result, most data on the cause of nosocomial BSI is derived from patients in these units. We expect that the spectrum of organisms that cause nosocomial Ca-BSI in children hospitalized in non–intensive care unit settings will be similar, but at this point there is limited information. One study of outpatient parenteral antimicrobial therapy in children with osteoarticular infections found that the rate of infectious complications associated with the catheter was 6.3 per 1000 catheter days and occurred in approximately 10% of patients. The average time to development of infectious complications was 24.5 days [27]. Approximately 90% of nosocomial BSIs are associated with the presence of a CVC [3]. CoNS account for approximately 40% of the pathogens identified in children with nosocomial BSIs; in neonates, CoNS account for an even greater percentage of isolates (50%). Gram-negative aerobic bacilli account for approximately 25% of BSIs followed by enterococci (11%–15%) and *Candida* spp (6%) [3]. The most commonly encountered gram-negative bacilli include *Enterobacter* spp, *P aeruginosa*, *Klebsiella pneumoniae*, *Escherichia coli, Serratia marcescens, Acinetobacter* spp, and *Citrobacter* spp (Table 3) [3]. *Candida* spp are the fourth most common cause of nosocomial BSI in the United States [28]. Children with central catheters managed predominantly in home health care setting may be at higher risk for nonendogenous (eg, from water and other environmental sources) gram-negative pathogens, such as *Pseudomonas, Acinetobacter*, and *Agrobacterium* spp, particularly during summer months [7,29].

Interpretation of BSI rates and pathogens in children may be limited by the application of definitions developed for adults. For example, current National Nosocomial Infections Surveillance definitions for catheter-related BSI require the use of either a catheter tip culture or a central and peripheral blood culture [8]. There is often a reluctance to perform peripheral blood cultures in children because the procedure can be difficult and painful. Removal of a catheter for diagnostic purposes is avoided because of the difficulties inherent in placing CVCs and the limited venous access available in children.

Although CoNS are the most commonly reported isolate from children with nosocomial BSI, they are also common skin colonizers that frequently contaminate blood cultures. A study that used a mathematical model of blood cultures with positive results for CoNS in patients with a central venous line found that the positive predictive value of one positive culture (if only one culture was obtained) was 55%, 20% for one positive culture of two cultures performed, and only 5% for one positive result of three cultures performed. For two positive culture results of two cultures performed, the positive predictive value was 98% if both samples were obtained from a peripheral vein, 96% if one sample was obtained through a catheter and the other was obtained by through the vein, and only 50% if both samples were obtained through a catheter [30]. The distinction between pathogen and contaminant is affected by age and

Table 3
Distribution of most common pathogens identified from patients in pediatric intensive care units (NNIS 1992–1997)

Pathogen	Bloodstream infection % ($n=1887$)
Coagulase-negative staphylococci	37.8
Enterococcus	11.2
S aureus	9.3
Enterobacter spp	6.2
Candida albicans	5.5
P aeruginosa	4.9
Klebsiella *pneumoniae*	4.1
Escherichia coli	2.9

underlying condition of a child. CoNS as a true pathogen in neonates has been well described, but the issue remains controversial [31]. The identification of CoNS often results in clinical intervention with increased patient exposure to vancomycin. Overuse of vancomycin has implications for the continued increase of vancomycin resistance among gram-positive organisms [32–34].

Treatment

Limited data are available to guide the management of Ca-BSI in children, and most of the management recommendations are derived from adult populations. Even in adult populations, however, no randomized or controlled studies address the optimal management of Ca-BSI [1]. Empiric therapy in children with suspected Ca-BSI should include an antimicrobial agent with activity against gram-positive bacteria (eg, nafcillin, oxacillin, or vancomycin) and an agent effective against gram-negative bacteria, including *Pseudomonas* (eg, ceftazidime or cefipime with or without an aminoglycoside). The empiric use of an antipseudomonal beta-lactam agent and an aminoglycoside may be appropriate in severely ill patients or when infection with a resistant gram-negative organism is suspected. In institutions in which methicillin-resistant *S aureus* is common, the use of vancomycin is appropriate. Fluoroquinolones are commonly used in adults but have been approved for only limited indications in children.

One of the most commonly asked clinical questions in patients with Ca-BSI is whether the catheter should be removed (Table 4). In adult populations, it is recommended that most nontunneled CVCs should be removed in cases of Ca-BSI [1]. Removal of a catheter may not always be feasible in children because of potential complications associated with reinsertion and limited vascular

Table 4
Management of the catheter in patients with a central venous catheter–related infection

Type of infection	Catheter management
Exit site infection	Remove CVC if
	No longer required
	Alternate site exists
	Patient critically ill (eg, hypotension)
	Infection caused by *P aeruginosa* or fungi
Tunnel infection	Remove CVC
Pocket infection	Remove CVC
Catheter-related BSI	Remove CVC if
	No longer required
	Infection caused by *S aureus*, *Candida* spp, or mycobacteria
	Patient critically ill
	Failure to clear bacteremia in 48–72 hours
	Persistent symptoms of BSI beyond 48–72 hours
	Noninfectious valvular heart disease (increased risk of endocarditis)
	Endocarditis
	Metastatic infection
	Septic thrombophlebitis

access sites; treatment of Ca-BSI without removal of the catheter is often attempted. In patients with Ca-BSI associated with a tunneled catheter or implantable device, such as a port, the decision to remove the catheter is more complicated. Based on good evidence, it is strongly recommended that in patients with evidence of a tunnel infection or pocket infection (the subcutaneous pocket of an implanted device), the catheter should be removed [1]. Once culture data are available, treatment decisions can be tailored to specific organisms. Several studies have reported successful treatment of Ca-BSI without catheter removal [35–38], but treatment may depend on the pathogen identified.

Few data exist regarding the duration of antibiotic therapy for Ca-BSI. The duration of therapy depends in part on the pathogen, whether the catheter is removed, and whether infection is complicated by septic thrombosis, endocarditis, osteomyelitis, or other metastatic foci of bacteria. For complicated infections, the duration of therapy is based on the duration necessary to treat the complication. No data are available to determine the optimal duration of intravenous versus oral antibiotics for the treatment of Ca-BSI. Certain antibiotics with excellent oral bioavailability may be considered once a patient has cleared the bacteremia and has shown clinical improvement, the catheter has been removed, and compliance with therapy is ensured. Some pathogen-specific recommendations are provided later in this article.

Coagulase-negative staphylococci

CoNS are considered less virulent than other pathogens that cause Ca-BSI, and these infections usually present with fever alone or with inflammation of the catheter exit site. Patients rarely develop sepsis or have a poor outcome with this organism. CoNS Ca-BSI may resolve with just removal of the catheter without antibiotic therapy. Some experts recommend a short course of antibiotic therapy (ie, 3–5 days), even after removal of the catheter [39]. If the catheter remains in place, the recommended duration of treatment based on experience is 10 to 14 days after a negative blood culture result. In neonates with CoNS bacteremia, treatment without removal of the catheter can be attempted, but once a neonate has three positive blood culture results despite appropriate antimicrobial therapy, the catheter should be removed because of the risk for end-organ damage [40]. The relapse rate in adult patients with CoNS Ca-BSI is 20% if the catheter is not removed compared with 3% if the catheter is removed [41].

Staphylococcus aureus

Serious complications, including endocarditis and other deep-tissue infections, have been reported in association with S aureus–associated Ca-BSI [42]. Adult patients with S aureus bacteremia are at significant risk for endocarditis and often have echocardiography performed routinely as part of their management [43,44]. The frequency of infective endocarditis is low in children with S aureus bacteremia and structurally normal hearts, and echocardiography commonly is not performed [45]. Echocardiography should be considered in children with persistent bacteremia who are on appropriate antimicrobial therapy or in whom a new murmur is identified on physical examination. In a prospective study of 51 children with *S aureus* bacteremia, definite or possible endocarditis was diagnosed in 52% of patients with congenital heart disease but in only 3% of patients with structurally normal hearts [45]. Neonates may be more vulnerable to complications of *S aureus* BSI than older infants, however. Some researchers recommend catheter removal for neonates for a single positive blood culture for either *S aureus* or a gram-negative bacillus, because it significantly improves outcome [40]. Two weeks of appropriate antimicrobial therapy, chosen based on sensitivities, is recommended for uncomplicated *S aureus* Ca-BSI [1]. Longer durations of therapy may be necessary for patients with prolonged bacteremia (>3 days), persistent fever, or complicated infection [46].

Gram-negative bacilli

There is a paucity of data that addresses whether catheters should be removed in patients with Ca-BSI caused by the wide variety of gram-negative bacilli. Children with Ca-BSI caused by gram-negative bacilli have been treated successfully without catheter removal [1]. Catheter removal has been shown to be beneficial in the treatment of infections with specific gram-negative bacilli, such as *Pseudomonas* spp, *Burkholderia cepacia*, *Acinetobacter baumanni*, and *Stenotrophomonas* spp [1,42]. In a recent study of adult patients with Ca-BSI caused by gram-negative bacilli, catheter removal was associated with a reduced rate of relapse [47]. In general, antimicrobial therapy should be administered for 10 to 14 days after blood culture results become negative [1].

Fungemia

Treatment of fungemia without removal of the catheter has been associated with poor outcomes in children and adults [48–50]. Studies have not accounted for confounding effect of the severity of illness, however (eg, the sicker patients required catheter retention and were most likely to die) [51]. Failure to remove the catheter promptly may lead to prolonged candidemia, which in turn has been associated with higher rates of disseminated infection. Among 153 children with candidemia at our institution, the overall rate of disseminated candidiasis (ie, lung, liver, spleen, eye, brain, heart) was 17% [52]. Twenty-seven percent of children with candidemia were on a general pediatric or surgery ward at the time of infection. The crude mortality rate in children with candidemia was 26% [52]. The consensus opinion is that catheters should be removed in patients with candidemia whenever feasible [53]. Therapy with amphotericin B or fluconazole should be continued for 2 weeks. All patients with candidemia should have an ophthalmologic examination to evaluate for candidal endophthalmitis, preferably after the infection seems to be controlled and further disseminated disease is unlikely [53].

Ventriculoperitoneal shunts

Case presentation

A 6-month-old boy with a history of congenital hydrocephalus required a VP shunt placement at birth. The shunt required revision 4 weeks before the boy presented with fever, vomiting, and irritability. Physical examination reveals a febrile, inconsolable infant. How should this child be evaluated for a shunt-associated infection? Which, if any, antibiotics should be used for empiric treatment? Should the shunt be removed?

Introduction

The introduction of the VP shunt in the late 1960s revolutionized the treatment of hydrocephalus [54]. The VP shunt provided significant advantages over the previously used ventriculoatrial shunts and has become the mainstay of hydrocephalus management. Whereas VP shunts are associated with significantly less bacteremia then ventriculoatrial shunts, the shunts themselves frequently become infected, with a reported incidence of 2% to 30% [54]. This section summarizes the clinical manifestations, diagnosis, treatment, and prevention of shunt infections. Because ventriculoatrial shunts are rarely used currently, the main focus is on VP shunt-related infections.

Clinical presentation

A discussion of the clinical manifestations of shunt-associated infections requires making a distinction between the different locations along the track of the shunt that are prone to infection, including the lumen of the shunt itself, the

Table 5
Percent of patients with clinical finding of possible shunt infection

Presentation	Odio [58] $n = 59$	Ronan [57] $n = 49$	Kontny [56] $n = 28$	Mancao [55] $n = 29$	Total $n = 165$
Fever	87	72	96	62	77
Shunt malfunction	—	36	50	—	51 ($n = 57$)
Irritability	81	27	25	69[a]	49 ($n = 136$)
Vomiting	39	24	—		31 ($n = 108$)
Meningismus	—	20	21		18 ($n = 77$)
Cellulitis	19	15	—	24	18 ($n = 137$)
Abdominal pain	22	15	36	17[b]	21 ($n = 136$)
Lethargy	—	12	—	—	12 ($n = 49$)

[a] This percentage represents neurologic signs, which included vomiting, irritability, bulging fontanelle, and meningismus.
[b] This percentage represents patients with abdominal signs, which included abdominal pain, ileus, and diarrhea.

extraluminal ventricles, the cranial and distal surgical sites, and the peritoneal cavity. Given the multiple anatomic locations for potential shunt infections, the clinical manifestations of such infections can be varied. Table 5 summarizes the most common signs and symptoms. Most shunt infections occur within the first 6 months after shunt placement [55–57], with approximately one half occurring within the first 2 weeks [56,58].

Fever and shunt malfunction are commonly seen in shunt infections but are neither specific nor sensitive. Shunt malfunction usually presents clinical features of increased intracranial pressure, such as headache, vomiting, lethargy, or seizures. Distal shunt infection commonly presents with abdominal pain. A known complication of VP shunts is the formation of pseudocysts, which are pockets of cerebrospinal fluid (CSF) that collects at the distal end of the shunt, often related to decreased peritoneal absorption of CSF. Pseudocysts can be the direct consequence of a shunt infection or may develop in the absence of infection and become secondarily infected. If an infected pseudocyst leaks into the abdominal cavity, patients often present with frank peritonitis. If leakage does not occur, abdominal pain symptoms may be more indolent [59]. Patients with wound infections present with incisional erythema and purulence, with or without local collections of CSF.

Diagnosis

A commonly accepted definition of a shunt infection is isolation of a bacterial pathogen from ventricular fluid, lumbar CSF, or blood or pleocytosis more than 50 white blood cells/mm^3 and one or more of the following: fever, shunt malfunction, neurologic symptoms, or abdominal signs or symptoms [58]. Although cultures of blood and lumbar CSF can be helpful, sampling of the ventricular fluid is critical for making the diagnosis for three main reasons. First, positive blood cultures commonly are seen with ventriculoatrial shunting, in which infected CSF drains directly into the bloodstream [58]. Because VP shunting has become the standard of care, bacteremia is a relatively uncommon finding in shunt infections. Second, most patients who require CSF shunts often have an underlying impairment or absence of CSF reabsorption into the venous system, which would limit the passage of bacteria into the bloodstream. If the ventricles have little or no communication with the lumbar spinal fluid, it is possible to have a shunt-associated ventriculitis with a normal lumbar puncture. Finally, if a patient has more than one shunt, it is important to culture all of them, because they may be draining different collections of CSF that are not in communication.

CSF pleocytosis is a helpful marker; however, it alone does not diagnose infection. Many shunt infections occur shortly after placement, and it can be difficult to distinguish whether the CSF pleocytosis is caused by postoperative inflammation or infection. Shunt infections also can be caused by indolent organisms, which do not induce a vigorous immune response. This occurrence is exemplified by CoNS, the most common organisms cultured from infected shunts. These bacteria produce a biofilm that protects them from the host immune response and enhances adherence to the device. When taken in context with other clinical markers, however, the CSF white blood cell count can be useful. One recent study found that history of fever and ventricular fluid neutrophilia (>10%) had a specificity of 99% and positive and negative predictive values of 93% and 95%, respectively, for identifying or excluding shunt-related infection [60].

Etiology

Table 6 summarizes the organisms most commonly found in CSF shunt infections. *Staphylococcal* spp are by far the most common species identified, with CoNS being the most prevalent organism. Various gram-negative organisms have been implicated in shunt infections. Anaerobic bacteria—especially *Propionibacteria*—are also known to cause shunt infections [61]. Historically they have been implicated in culture-negative infections because they can be difficult to grow, especially when CSF is not sent for anaerobic culture. Fungi, predominantly *Candida* spp, rarely have been reported [62].

One study analyzed pathogens isolated from shunt infections by time to infection [58]. Eighty-five percent of infections that occurred within the first 15 days after surgery were caused by *Staphylococci*. Seventy-five percent of all *S aureus* infections also occurred in this period. In contrast, gram-negative infections generally occur further out from initial surgery, and researchers believe that they arise from ascending infection of enteric organisms that colonize the distal portion of the shunt [58]. Sixty-four percent of infections that occurred after 15 days were caused by gram-negative organisms. Another study found an association between shunt infections that occurred more than 30 weeks after shunt placement and *H influenzae* [57]. This study was conducted before routine vaccination against *H influenzae*. Finally, a recent review of 94 shunt infections found 8 that occurred more than 9 months after surgery, none of which were caused by *S aureus* [63]. These observations support the common belief that most shunt infections are caused by the introduction of skin organisms at the time of shunt placement [58,64,65]. Gram-negative infections tend to occur later and have been attributed to ascending infection of enteric organisms that have colonized the distal portion of the shunt.

Many studies have attempted to define factors that predispose children to shunt infections. Several retrospective studies have suggested that younger patient age, cause of hydrocephalus, and more frequent revisions are correlated with shunt infections. A recent retrospective case control study of 820 consecutive VP shunt placements identified four independent risk factors for infection. Each year of decreasing age was associated with a 4% increase in the risk of infection. The other risk factors included insertion of a shunt into a premature neonate, use of a neuroendoscope, and shunt insertion after a previous shunt infection [66].

Table 6
Pathogens

Organism	Enger [72] n=9	Odio [58] n=59	Ronan [57] n=41	Kontny [56] n=28	Mancao [55] n=29[a]	McGirt [66] n=92	Total n=258
S epidermidis	7 (78)	27 (46)	7 (17)	16 (57)	14 (48)	49 (53)	120 (47)
S aureus	1 (11)	17 (29)	12 (30)	1 (4)	7 (24)	24 (26)	62 (24)
Gram negatives	—	15 (25)	10 (24)	2 (7)	3 (10)	8 (9)	38 (15)
Viridans streptococcus	—	6 (10)	—	—	—		6 (2)
Enterococcus	—	3 (5)	2 (5)	—	—	4 (4)	9 (3)
Mixed	—	—	—	5 (18)	3 (10)	—	8 (3)
Other[a]	2 (22)	—	—	4 (14)	2 (7)	4 (4)	12 (5)

Values listed as number (percent).

Dashes indicate that no organisms in a category were isolated.

[a] Other culture results include *Candida* spp (n = 2) [72]; no growth (n = 4) [56]; *Corynebacter* (n = 1) and group B *Streptococcus* (n = 1) [55]; and *Proprionibacterium* (n = 4) [66].

Treatment

To date only one prospective randomized study has been conducted regarding the treatment of shunt infections [67]. It is generally accepted that optimal management of a shunt infection includes removal of the shunt and placement of a temporary ventricular reservoir until resolution of infection. In the retrospective studies that addressed shunt removal, this strategy clearly was associated with better outcome. An analysis of treatment options for shunt infections that included 17 studies published over the past 30 years revealed that the combination of shunt removal and antibiotics successfully treated 88% of 244 infections, whereas antibiotic therapy alone was successful in only 33% of 230 infections [68].

Empiric antibiotic therapy should include broad-spectrum antibiotics that cover the major pathogens associated with shunt-related infections. Because staphylococcal species are the most commonly found pathogens, vancomycin is recommended for gram-positive coverage, especially given the high prevalence of *S epidermidis* and the increasing prevalence of methicillin-resistant *S aureus.* The array of pathogenic gram-negative organisms is significantly larger. The report of *P aeruginosa* in several series and case reports, in combination with its propensity to adhere to foreign material, warrants including pseudomonal coverage in empiric therapy. Ceftazidime and fluoroquinolones have excellent pseudomonal coverage and penetrate the CSF well. Therapy can be tailored further based on the identification and susceptibility of the causative organism. If appropriate systemic therapy fails to eradicate infection, vancomycin and the aminoglycosides can be given intrathecally. Rifampin, which has better CSF penetration than vancomycin, is often added for gram-positive shunt infections that fail to clear on vancomycin monotherapy. Strong evidence that this strategy is successful is not available, however [69].

Prevention

Despite aseptic technique in the operating room, surgical contamination of some extent is inevitable. With that in mind, several studies, which have been largely inconclusive, have examined the benefit of antibiotic prophylaxis for shunt placement surgeries [65,70]. More recently, VP shunts impregnated with clindamycin and rifampin have produced successful results in animals models. Two small clinical trials in humans are promising, and this technique warrants further investigation [64,71].

Summary

Practicing hospitalists will be called on increasingly to manage infections associated with CVCs, whether in an intensive care setting, the emergency department, or an inpatient unit. Knowledge of the various types of catheters is key, because the presentations, risk factors, pathogens, and management vary significantly by type [72].

VP shunt infections represent another challenge for practitioners. Children may present with signs and symptoms that highly suggest shunt infection, or they may present with fever with an indwelling device. Determining the site of infection is essential, because removal of the shunt often is required for definitive treatment. Careful evaluation is needed to avoid inappropriate procedures and provide appropriate therapy of an identified source.

Skin flora, such as CoNS and *Proprionibacterium acnes* (for ventricular shunts), cause most infections. Management of device-related infections includes device removal for some Ca-BSIs and all VP shunt-related infections. The isolation of certain organisms (eg, *S aureus, Candida* spp) in children with central catheters should prompt consideration of disseminated infection. Future research may determine the impact of increasing catheter use in non–intensive care hospital settings and in home care. New technologies, such as antimicrobial-impregnated CVCs and ventricular shunts, show promise in reducing the infection rates of these devices.

References

[1] Mermel LA, Farr BM, Sherertz RJ, et al. Guidelines for the management of intravascular catheter-related infections. Clin Infect Dis 2001;32(9):1249–72.
[2] Neville HL, Lally KP. Pediatric surgical would infections. Semin Pediatr Infect Dis 2001;12: 124–9.
[3] Richards MJ, Edwards JR, Culver DH, et al. Nosocomial infections in pediatric intensive care units in the United States: National Nosocomial Infections Surveillance System. Pediatrics 1999;103(4):e39.
[4] Elward AM, Hollenbeak CS, Warren DK, et al. Attributable cost of nosocomial primary bloodstream infection in pediatric intensive care unit patients. Pediatrics 2005;115(4):868–72.
[5] Wisplinghoff H, Seifert H, Tallent SM, et al. Nosocomial bloodstream infections in pediatric patients in United States hospitals: epidemiology, clinical features and susceptibilities. Pediatr Infect Dis J 2003;22(8):686–91.
[6] National Nosocomial Infections Surveillance (NNIS) System Report. Data summary from January 1992 through June 2004, issued October 2004. Am J Infect Control 2004;32(8):470–85.
[7] Shah SS, Manning ML, Leahy E, et al. Central venous catheter-associated bloodstream infections in pediatric oncology home care. Infect Control Hosp Epidemiol 2002;23(2):99–101.
[8] O'Grady NP, Alexander M, Dellinger EP, et al. Guidelines for the prevention of intravascular catheter-related infections. Pediatrics 2002;110(5):e51.
[9] Hu KK, Lipsky BA, Veenstra DL, et al. Using maximal sterile barriers to prevent central venous catheter-related infection: a systematic evidence-based review. Am J Infect Control 2004;32(3):142–6.
[10] Darouiche RO, Raad II, Heard SO, et al. A comparison of two antimicrobial-impregnated central venous catheters. N Engl J Med 1999;340(1):1–8.
[11] Shah SS, Downes KJ, McGowan KL, et al. Time to blood culture positivity in children with central venous catheters [abstract]. Pediatr Res, in press.
[12] Gorelick MH, Owen WC, Seibel NL, et al. Lack of association between neutropenia and the incidence of bacteremia associated with indwelling central venous catheters in febrile pediatric cancer patients. Pediatr Infect Dis J 1991;10(7):506–10.

[13] Raad II, Luna M, Khalil SA, et al. The relationship between the thrombotic and infectious complications of central venous catheters. JAMA 1994;271(13):1014–6.

[14] Brun-Buisson C, Abrouk F, Legrand P, et al. Diagnosis of central venous catheter-related sepsis: critical level of quantitative tip cultures. Arch Intern Med 1987;147(5):873–7.

[15] Maki DG, Weise CE, Sarafin HW. A semiquantitative culture method for identifying intravenous-catheter-related infection. N Engl J Med 1977;296(23):1305–9.

[16] Raad I, Hanna HA, Alakech B, et al. Differential time to positivity: a useful method for diagnosing catheter-related bloodstream infections. Ann Intern Med 2004;140(1):18–25.

[17] Blot F, Nitenberg G, Chachaty E, et al. Diagnosis of catheter-related bacteraemia: a prospective comparison of the time to positivity of hub-blood versus peripheral-blood cultures. Lancet 1999;354(9184):1071–7.

[18] Blot F, Schmidt E, Nitenberg G, et al. Earlier positivity of central-venous versus peripheral-blood cultures is highly predictive of catheter-related sepsis. J Clin Microbiol 1998;36(1):105–9.

[19] Seifert H, Cornely O, Seggewiss K, et al. Bloodstream infection in neutropenic cancer patients related to short-term nontunnelled catheters determined by quantitative blood cultures, differential time to positivity, and molecular epidemiological typing with pulsed-field gel electrophoresis. J Clin Microbiol 2003;41(1):118–23.

[20] Li J, Plorde JJ, Carlson LG. Effects of volume and periodicity on blood cultures. J Clin Microbiol 1994;32(11):2829–31.

[21] Chandrasekar PH, Brown WJ. Clinical issues of blood cultures. Arch Intern Med 1994;154(8): 841–9.

[22] Schelonka RL, Chai MK, Yoder BA, et al. Volume of blood required to detect common neonatal pathogens. J Pediatr 1996;129(2):275–8.

[23] Isaacman DJ, Karasic RB, Reynolds EA, et al. Effect of number of blood cultures and volume of blood on detection of bacteremia in children. J Pediatr 1996;128(2):190–5.

[24] Mermel LA, Maki DG. Detection of bacteremia in adults: consequences of culturing an inadequate volume of blood. Ann Intern Med 1993;119(4):270–2.

[25] Weinstein MP, Murphy JR, Reller LB, et al. The clinical significance of positive blood cultures: a comprehensive analysis of 500 episodes of bacteremia and fungemia in adults. II. Clinical observations, with special reference to factors influencing prognosis. Rev Infect Dis 1983; 5(1):54–70.

[26] Reimer LG, Wilson ML, Weinstein MP. Update on detection of bacteremia and fungemia. Clin Microbiol Rev 1997;10(3):444–65.

[27] Maraqa NF, Gomez MM, Rathore MH. Outpatient parenteral antimicrobial therapy in osteoarticular infections in children. J Pediatr Orthop 2002;22(4):506–10.

[28] Edmond MB, Wallace SE, McClish DK, et al. Nosocomial bloodstream infections in United States hospitals: a three-year analysis. Clin Infect Dis 1999;29(2):239–44.

[29] Smith TL, Pullen GT, Crouse V, et al. Bloodstream infections in pediatric oncology outpatients: a new healthcare systems challenge. Infect Control Hosp Epidemiol 2002;23(5):239–43.

[30] Tokars JI. Predictive value of blood cultures positive for coagulase-negative staphylococci: implications for patient care and health care quality assurance. Clin Infect Dis 2004; 39(3):333–41.

[31] Sohn AH, Garrett DO, Sinkowitz-Cochran RL, et al. Prevalence of nosocomial infections in neonatal intensive care unit patients: results from the first national point-prevalence survey. J Pediatr 2001;139(6):821–7.

[32] Sinkowitz RL, Keyserling H, Walker TJ, et al. Epidemiology of vancomycin usage at a children's hospital, 1993 through 1995. Pediatr Infect Dis J 1997;16(5):485–9.

[33] Garrett DO, Jochimsen E, Murfitt K, et al. The emergence of decreased susceptibility to vancomycin in Staphylococcus epidermidis. Infect Control Hosp Epidemiol 1999;20(3):167–70.

[34] Smith TL, Pearson ML, Wilcox KR, et al. Emergence of vancomycin resistance in Staphylococcus aureus: glycopeptide-intermediate Staphylococcus aureus working group. N Engl J Med 1999;340(7):493–501.

[35] Weiner E. Catheter sepsis: the central venous line Achilles' heel. Semin Pediatr Surg 1995;4: 207–14.

[36] King DR, Komer M, Hoffman J, et al. Broviac catheter sepsis: the natural history of an iatrogenic infection. J Pediatr Surg 1985;20(6):728–33.

[37] Hartman GE, Shochat SJ. Management of septic complications associated with Silastic catheters in childhood malignancy. Pediatr Infect Dis J 1987;6(11):1042–7.

[38] Flynn PM, Shenep JL, Stokes DC, et al. In situ management of confirmed central venous catheter-related bacteremia. Pediatr Infect Dis J 1987;6(8):729–34.

[39] American Academy of Pediatrics. Staphylococcal infections. 26th edition. Elk Grove Village (IL): American Academy of Pediatrics; 2003.

[40] Benjamin Jr DK, Miller W, Garges H, et al. Bacteremia, central catheters, and neonates: when to pull the line. Pediatrics 2001;107(6):1272–6.

[41] Raad I, Davis S, Khan A, et al. Impact of central venous catheter removal on the recurrence of catheter-related coagulase-negative staphylococcal bacteremia. Infect Control Hosp Epidemiol 1992;13(4):215–21.

[42] Raad II, Bodey GP. Infectious complications of indwelling vascular catheters. Clin Infect Dis 1992;15(2):197–208.

[43] Rosen AB, Fowler Jr VG, Corey GR, et al. Cost-effectiveness of transesophageal echocardiography to determine the duration of therapy for intravascular catheter-associated Staphylococcus aureus bacteremia. Ann Intern Med 1999;130(10):810–20.

[44] Fowler Jr VG, Li J, Corey GR, et al. Role of echocardiography in evaluation of patients with Staphylococcus aureus bacteremia: experience in 103 patients. J Am Coll Cardiol 1997;30(4): 1072–8.

[45] Valente AM, Jain R, Scheurer M, et al. Frequency of infective endocarditis among infants and children with Staphylococcus aureus bacteremia. Pediatrics 2005;115(1):e15–9.

[46] Raad II, Sabbagh MF. Optimal duration of therapy for catheter-related Staphylococcus aureus bacteremia: a study of 55 cases and review. Clin Infect Dis 1992;14(1):75–82.

[47] Hanna H, Afif C, Alakech B, et al. Central venous catheter-related bacteremia due to gram-negative bacilli: significance of catheter removal in preventing relapse. Infect Control Hosp Epidemiol 2004;25(8):646–9.

[48] Blumberg HM, Jarvis WR, Soucie JM, et al. Risk factors for candidal bloodstream infections in surgical intensive care unit patients: the NEMIS prospective multicenter study. The National Epidemiology of Mycosis Survey. Clin Infect Dis 2001;33(2):177–86.

[49] Lecciones JA, Lee JW, Navarro EE, et al. Vascular catheter-associated fungemia in patients with cancer: analysis of 155 episodes. Clin Infect Dis 1992;14(4):875–83.

[50] Eppes SC, Troutman JL, Gutman LT. Outcome of treatment of candidemia in children whose central catheters were removed or retained. Pediatr Infect Dis J 1989;8(2):99–104.

[51] Nucci M, Anaissie E. Should vascular catheters be removed from all patients with candidemia? An evidence-based review. Clin Infect Dis 2002;34(5):591–9.

[52] Zaoutis TE, Greves HM, Lautenbach E, et al. Risk factors for disseminated candidiasis in children with candidemia. Pediatr Infect Dis J 2004;23(7):635–41.

[53] Pappas PG, Rex JH, Sobel JD, et al. Guidelines for treatment of candidiasis. Clin Infect Dis 2004;38(2):161–89.

[54] Yogev R. Cerebrospinal fluid shunt infections: a personal view. Pediatr Infect Dis 1985;4(2): 113–8.

[55] Mancao M, Miller C, Cochrane B, et al. Cerebrospinal fluid shunt infections in infants and children in Mobile, Alabama. Acta Paediatr 1998;87(6):667–70.

[56] Kontny U, Hofling B, Gutjahr P, et al. CSF shunt infections in children. Infection 1993; 21(2):89–92.

[57] Ronan A, Hogg GG, Klug GL. Cerebrospinal fluid shunt infections in children. Pediatr Infect Dis J 1995;14(9):782–6.

[58] Odio C, McCracken Jr GH, Nelson JD. CSF shunt infections in pediatrics: a seven-year experience. Am J Dis Child 1984;138(12):1103–8.

[59] Anderson CM, Sorrells DL, Kerby JD. Intra-abdominal pseudocysts as a complication of ventriculoperitoneal shunts: a case report and review of the literature. Curr Surg 2003;60(3): 338–40.

[60] McClinton D, Carraccio C, Englander R. Predictors of ventriculoperitoneal shunt pathology. Pediatr Infect Dis J 2001;20(6):593–7.

[61] Brook I. Meningitis and shunt infection caused by anaerobic bacteria in children. Pediatr Neurol 2002;26(2):99–105.

[62] Chiou CC, Wong TT, Lin HH, et al. Fungal infection of ventriculoperitoneal shunts in children. Clin Infect Dis 1994;19(6):1049–53.

[63] Baird C, O'Connor D, Pittman T. Late shunt infections. Pediatr Neurosurg 1999;31(5):269–73.

[64] Aryan HE, Meltzer HS, Park MS, et al. Initial experience with antibiotic-impregnated silicone catheters for shunting of cerebrospinal fluid in children. Childs Nerv Syst 2005;21(1):56–61.

[65] Morris A, Low DE. Nosocomial bacterial meningitis, including central nervous system shunt infections. Infect Dis Clin North Am 1999;13(3):735–50.

[66] McGirt MJ, Zaas A, Fuchs HE, et al. Risk factors for pediatric ventriculoperitoneal shunt infection and predictors of infectious pathogens. Clin Infect Dis 2003;36(7):858–62.

[67] James HE, Walsh JW, Wilson HD, et al. Prospective randomized study of therapy in cerebrospinal fluid shunt infection. Neurosurgery 1980;7(5):459–63.

[68] Schreffler RT, Schreffler AJ, Wittler RR. Treatment of cerebrospinal fluid shunt infections: a decision analysis. Pediatr Infect Dis J 2002;21(7):632–6.

[69] Brackbill ML, Brophy GM. Adjunctive rifampin therapy for central nervous system staphylococcal infections. Ann Pharmacother 2001;35(6):765–9.

[70] Pople IK, Bayston R, Hayward RD. Infection of cerebrospinal fluid shunts in infants: a study of etiological factors. J Neurosurg 1992;77(1):29–36.

[71] Govender ST, Nathoo N, van Dellen JR. Evaluation of an antibiotic-impregnated shunt system for the treatment of hydrocephalus. J Neurosurg 2003;99(5):831–9.

[72] Enger PO, Svendsen F, Wester K. CSF shunt infections in children: experiences from a population-based study. Acta Neurochir (Wien) 2003;145(4):243–8 [discussion 248].

PEDIATRIC CLINICS

OF NORTH AMERICA

ELSEVIER
SAUNDERS

Pediatr Clin N Am 52 (2005) 1209–1219

Index

Note: Page numbers of article titles are in **boldface** type.

Order your subscription today. Simply complete and detach this card and drop it in the mail to receive the best clinical information in your field.

Please Print:

Name _____

Address_____

City_____ State _____ ZIP _____

Method of Payment

❏ Check (payable to **Elsevier**; add the applicable sales tax for your area)

❏ VISA ❏ MasterCard ❏ AmEx ❏ Bill me

Card number _____ Exp. date _____

Signature _____

Staple this to your purchase order to expedite delivery

❏ **Adolescent Medicine Clinics**		
❏ Individual	$95	
❏ Institutions	$133	
❏ *In-training	$48	
❏ **Anesthesiology**		
❏ Individual	$175	
❏ Institutions	$270	
❏ *In-training	$88	
❏ **Cardiology**		
❏ Individual	$170	
❏ Institutions	$266	
❏ *In-training	$85	
❏ **Chest Medicine**		
❏ Individual	$185	
❏ Institutions	$285	
❏ **Child and Adolescent Psychiatry**		
❏ Individual	$175	
❏ Institutions	$265	
❏ *In-training	$88	
❏ **Critical Care**		
❏ Individual	$165	
❏ Institutions	$266	
❏ *In-training	$83	
❏ **Dental**		
❏ Individual	$150	
❏ Institutions	$242	
❏ **Emergency Medicine**		
❏ Individual	$170	
❏ Institutions	$263	
❏ *In-training	$85	
❏ Send CME info		
❏ **Facial Plastic Surgery**		
❏ Individual	$199	
❏ Institutions	$300	
❏ **Foot and Ankle**		
Individual	$160	
Institutions	$232	
❏ **Gastroenterology**		
❏ Individual	$190	
❏ Institutions	$276	

❏ **Gastrointestinal Endoscopy**		
❏ Individual	$190	
❏ Institutions	$276	
❏ **Hand**		
❏ Individual	$205	
❏ Institutions	$319	
❏ **Heart Failure (NEW in 2005!)**		
❏ Individual	$99	
❏ Institutions	$149	
❏ *In-training	$49	
❏ **Hematology/ Oncology**		
❏ Individual	$210	
❏ Institutions	$315	
❏ **Immunology & Allergy**		
❏ Individual	$165	
❏ Institutions	$266	
❏ **Infectious Disease**		
❏ Individual	$165	
❏ Institutions	$272	
❏ **Clinics in Liver Disease**		
❏ Individual	$165	
❏ Institutions	$234	
❏ **Medical**		
❏ Individual	$140	
❏ Institutions	$244	
❏ *In-training	$70	
❏ Send CME info		
❏ **MRI**		
❏ Individual	$190	
❏ Institutions	$290	
❏ *In-training	$95	
❏ Send CME info		
❏ **Neuroimaging**		
❏ Individual	$190	
❏ Institutions	$290	
❏ *In-training	$95	
❏ Send CME inf0		
❏ **Neurologic**		
❏ Individual	$175	
❏ Institutions	$275	

❏ **Obstetrics & Gynecology**		
❏ Individual	$175	
❏ Institutions	$288	
❏ **Occupational and Environmental Medicine**		
❏ Individual	$120	
❏ Institutions	$166	
❏ *In-training	$60	
❏ **Ophthalmology**		
❏ Individual	$190	
❏ Institutions	$325	
❏ **Oral & Maxillofacial Surgery**		
❏ Individual	$180	
❏ Institutions	$280	
❏ *In-training	$90	
❏ **Orthopedic**		
❏ Individual	$180	
❏ Institutions	$295	
❏ *In-training	$90	
❏ **Otolaryngologic**		
❏ Individual	$199	
❏ Institutions	$350	
❏ **Pediatric**		
❏ Individual	$135	
❏ Institutions	$246	
❏ *In-training	$68	
❏ Send CME info		
❏ **Perinatology**		
❏ Individual	$155	
❏ Institutions	$237	
❏ *In-training	$78	
❏ Send CME inf0		
❏ **Plastic Surgery**		
❏ Individual	$245	
❏ Institutions	$370	
❏ **Podiatric Medicine & Surgery**		
❏ Individual	$170	
❏ Institutions	$266	
❏ **Primary Care**		
❏ Individual	$135	
❏ Institutions	$223	

❏ **Psychiatric**		
❏ Individual	$170	
❏ Institutions	$288	
❏ **Radiologic**		
❏ Individual	$220	
❏ Institutions	$331	
❏ *In-training	$110	
❏ Send CME info		
❏ **Sports Medicine**		
❏ Individual	$180	
❏ Institutions	$277	
❏ **Surgical**		
❏ Individual	$190	
❏ Institutions	$299	
❏ *In-training	$95	
❏ **Thoracic Surgery (formerly Chest Surgery)**		
❏ Individual	$175	
❏ Institutions	$255	
❏ *In-training	$88	
❏ **Urologic**		
❏ Individual	$195	
❏ Institutions	$307	
❏ *In-training	$98	
❏ Send CME info		

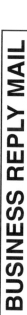

BUSINESS REPLY MAIL

FIRST-CLASS MAIL   PERMIT NO 7135   ORLANDO FL

POSTAGE WILL BE PAID BY ADDRESSEE

PERIODICALS ORDER FULFILLMENT DEPT
ELSEVIER
6277 SEA HARBOR DR
ORLANDO FL 32821-9816